Advance Praise for
Fibromyalgia: Up Close & Personal
by
Mark J. Pellegrino, MD

"Dr. Pellegrino's *Fibromyalgia: Up Close & Personal* is a must have for both patients and healthcare professionals. It is written in a clear, easy to follow manner with humor and is an excellent book to have on hand to answer ALL your questions! This is a must read for ALL healthcare professionals, attorneys, family, friends, neighbors, co-workers of fibromyalgia patients and patients alike."

Sue Alexander
FM Support Group Leader
Sacramento, CA

"Many a fibromyalgia patient has wished that her/his physician could see what it is *really* like to live with FM for just one day. Others have wished their doctor simply had more time to openly discuss many of the complicated or difficult topics related to FM. With his specialized medical training, his extensive clinical experience, and his own personal challenges with FM, Dr. Pellegrino is able to bring a unique blend of information, insight, and hope to readers with *Fibromyalgia: Up Close & Personal*.

This book is not only reader-friendly, but also rich in content covering diagnosis, treatment and research on FM as well as the successful handling of the specific challenges of FM in daily life. Of special interest are his comprehensive and up-to-date discussion of medications and his expanded material on post-traumatic fibromyalgia, a field in which he has become a national expert. Perhaps most of all, as an FM 'survivor' himself, Dr. Pellegrino has much to offer as an inspiration and example to patients and medical professionals alike."

Tamara K. Liller
President & Director of Publications
National Fibromyalgia Partnership, Inc.
Linden, VA

"This book should prove to be enlightening to all fibromyalgia patients. I would encourage my patients to refer to this for information about this potentially disabling but manageable condition. I found the information to be most helpful to both patients and physicians for understanding and management of fibromyalgia."

Angela M. Stupi, MD
Rheumatology
Wexford, PA

"I think Dr. Pellegrino's style of writing is great. I really like the way he has laid out his treatment protocol so we know what to look for in our own treatment. The section on Medications and Injections for FM is one of the best I have ever seen on this topic!"

Lynn Wagar
FM Support Group Leader
St. Cloud, MN

"I have been practicing Physiatry and treating fibromyalgia patients for 17 years. Since I have read Dr. Pellegrino's first book on fibromyalgia, I have recommended his books to my patients as the 'Bible' to have at their bedside to consult again and again. As a physician I always learn something new with his book updates. I am certain that *Fibromyalgia: Up Close & Personal* will contribute further to the well being of thousands and thousands of people trying to improve the quality of their lives while coping with fibromyalgia."

Silvia Knoploch, MD
Physical Medicine
Norwalk, CT

"I am one of the few people with FM who is incapacitated due to the unrelenting, unspeakable pain of this dratted disease. I particularly like Dr. Pellegrino's style of writing exactly as he talks. I thought he had reached his zenith with *The Fibromyalgia Supporter*, but not so. *Fibromyalgia: Up Close & Personal* is his very best. No matter what I read in any of his earlier books, I get 'high' on Pellegrino!"

Ann LeBlanc
FM patient
Tallahassee, FL

"Very well written, clear and concise. The information is very useful not only for patients but also for physicians interested in obtaining good information about fibromyalgia. I recommend the book without reservations."

Pedro L. Escobar, MD
Physical Medicine
Tucson, AZ

"Excellent source of information for the physician, the patient and for those with an interest in fibromyalgia."

James R. Ryba, MD
Rheumatology
Fountain Valley, CA

Fibromyalgia
Up Close & Personal

Mark J. Pellegrino, M.D.

The material in *Fibromyalgia: Up Close and Personal* is presented for informational purposes only. It is not meant to be a substitute for proper medical care by your doctor. You need to consult with your doctor for diagnosis and treatment. This material is not intended to substitute for the advice of a qualified attorney or other professional. You should consult a qualified professional for advice about your specific situation.

PRINTED IN THE UNITED STATES OF AMERICA

ISBN 1-890018-50-3 FIBROMYALGIA: UP CLOSE AND PERSONAL

By Mark J. Pellegrino, M.D.
Anadem Publishing, Inc.
Columbus, Ohio 43214
614•262•2539
1•800•633•0055
World Wide Web: www.anadem.com

Library of Congress Cataloging-in-Publication Data

Pellegrino, Mark J.
 Fibromyalgia : up close & personal/ with Mark J. Pellegrino.
   p. cm.
 Includes bibliographical references and index.
 ISBN 1-890018-50-3 (pbk.)
 1. Fibromyalgia. I. Title.

 RC927.3.P36633 2004
 616.7'42—dc22
                              2004017094

DEDICATION

I dedicate this book to Mary Ann, my wife of 22 years, my best friend, and my soul mate, and to my children, Maria, Dominic, and Rocco, who have my heart always.

TABLE OF CONTENTS

Introduction

I have fibromyalgia. I am also a fibromyalgia survivor. When I was 28 years-old, I was officially diagnosed with this disorder. I was in the midst of my Physical Medicine and Rehabilitation residency program when I started having severe pain all over, especially in my neck and shoulders. One of my residency instructors examined me and discovered my painful tender points, and I was diagnosed with fibromyalgia.

Since my diagnosis, I have tried to learn as much as I could about fibromyalgia by researching, reading, attending conferences, treating patients, and ultimately, by personal experiences. I have been able to look back and realize that I had various symptoms as a child and probably was at a risk of getting fibromyalgia some day. As a patient and a physician, I have come to appreciate how complex this condition really is, and that every individual is affected differently. Some people with fibromyalgia are hardly bothered by this condition, whereas others are incapacitated because of the pain.

As a medical doctor specializing in Physical Medicine and Rehabilitation, I have treated thousands of patients over the years. I have seen many different types of problems, including fibromyalgia, and I have come to appreciate how painful conditions interfere with a patient's ability to perform everyday activities and enjoy life. As fibromyalgia became the most common condition I saw, I became committed to helping these patients reach their fullest abilities and try to have the best quality of life possible, despite having fibromyalgia.

Over time, my personal and professional experiences in fibromyalgia evolved. I realized that no one treatment cures fibromyalgia, but different treatment approaches can help the pain and improve quality of life. Since I began private practice in 1988, I have diagnosed and treated over 15,000 people with this disorder. My approach has been to help all patients deal with their symptoms, first, by helping them understand fibromyalgia, and second, to encourage them to use successful strategies to become a fibromyalgia survivor.

I have learned to become a fibromyalgia survivor, not through reading medical journals or attending symposiums, but through experience with the patients I have come to know and treat over the years. Today I continue an active clinical practice and am working together WITH fibromyalgia patients to solve OUR problems.

As part of my therapy, I enjoy writing. It helped me accomplish one of my main goals: educating people about fibromyalgia. I have published numerous books on fibromyalgia over the years, including one of the first ever, *Fibromyalgia: Managing the Pain* in 1993. The *Fibromyalgia Survivor* published in 1995, contained detailed strategies for coping with this painful disorder, while maintaining a positive outlook. *Inside Fibromyalgia*, published in 2001, was an expanded updated version that combined my philosophy, personal and professional experiences, and management strategy.

The title of this book, *Fibromyalgia: Up Close and Personal,* was chosen because it accurately reflects my daily personal and professional experiences with this painful condition. I see it up close in my patients, and I deal with it on a personal basis every day. I understand fibromyalgia. I have it, plus I see it all the time in my practice. I tried to write about fibromyalgia in a way that helps you understand it, but also to let you know I understand it too.

In this book, I've combined the accumulated professional and personal experiences to help you gain insight and useful knowledge. This latest updated publication incorporates an additional three years of clinical experience and research information since my last book. I have expanded the section on post-traumatic fibromyalgia, and have tried to organize the book into practical and informative sections. There are various diagrams to help you understand and "digest" the information easier.

Throughout this book, I have included articles and passages that may be considered "diversionary writings." I take the title *Fibromyalgia: Up Close and Personal* to heart, and I have written about several special patients up close and a number of personal experiences from over the years. Not all patients I see have fibromyalgia, and I have many personal experiences not related to fibromyalgia. Sometimes a good outcome, a humorous story, or a lighter look at dealing with pain can be therapeutic, regardless of whether it deals specifically with fibromyalgia. I hope you find these diversional writings uplifting should you choose to read them.

My simple philosophy in treating fibromyalgia is to find whatever works. This includes a responsible and successful home program and a good mental outlook. We are all constantly reminded that fibromyalgia is a part of us, and it is an ongoing obligation and personal struggle because of this condition. This book will show you some ideas and strategies that have worked for me and my patients. I hope this book helps you in a few more battles against fibromyalgia along the way and improves the quality of your life.

By arming ourselves with knowledge, experience, and some timely guidance, we all have the chance to overcome the effects of fibromyalgia and ultimately conquer it. I hope you too can become a fibromyalgia survivor. Better yet, I hope you can ultimately become a fibromyalgia victor!

Mark J. Pellegrino, M.D., F.M.S. (Fibromyalgia Survivor) and F.M.V. (Fibromyalgia Victor)

SECTION I—DIAGNOSING FIBROMYALGIA

This section reviews the basics of fibromyalgia, from what it is to how it is diagnosed. The first step toward becoming a fibromyalgia victor is…having fibromyalgia! For the experienced person who was diagnosed long ago, this section will be a review. For the newly diagnosed person, I think this section will help provide you with a summary of how you got your diagnosis and set a basic framework for where to go from here. I've introduced a lighter look at fibromyalgia in this section, which I hope you will enjoy.

Imagine This...

You've been healthy all of your life. You've had some aches and pains from time to time just like everyone else, but the pains always went away. If you overexert yourself from playing a game of volleyball, you notice your legs will hurt. If you carry a heavy bag of salt into the basement, you might hurt your back a little. Or you may have had a lot of stress followed by a headache, or done too much on the job and ached. This never stopped you, though. You just took some aspirin, maybe rubbed some muscle creams on the sore areas or rested a little bit, and you felt better.

One day, you woke up and noticed severe pain in your neck and shoulders. At first you thought, "I must have slept the wrong way." Or maybe you did something the night before that caused some pain. But when you tried your usual remedies, such as taking a few aspirin and resting, the pain didn't go away. In fact, the pain got worse and moved around. It spread until you hurt all over.

Your doctor found nothing wrong. Numerous tests were run, and they all came back normal. Medicine didn't help. Nothing helped the pain. And it got worse. No one could tell you what was wrong.

You don't understand it. "How can this be happening to me?" you wonder. "What is wrong with me?" Your whole body feels like it is on fire. Your nerves seem to be amplifying every pain signal a hundredfold, and you can't ignore the pain. It prevents you from doing simple things that you used to take for granted, things like reaching up, bending over, sleeping, or concentrating. You are having great difficulty doing anything. You can no longer get through your day without pain, you can't work without pain, you can't even function without pain, and no one seems to understand your pain because you look okay. Your life is spinning out of control. It feels like there is no end in sight for your pain.

That's what fibromyalgia does.

Chances are if you are reading this, you aren't imagining this at all; fibromyalgia is a reality for you, and you are not alone...

...and there is hope.

Fibromyalgia: Up Close & Personal

Fibromyalgia Overview

What It Is

Fibromyalgia is a common condition that causes widespread pain, fatigue, poor sleep, and stiffness, as well as other symptoms. It is a chronic condition recognized as a distinct medical entity with characteristic findings, mainly painful tender points. The name fibromyalgia comes from the Latin words "fibro," meaning fibrous tissue such as tendons, ligaments, and bursa; "my," meaning muscle; and "algia," meaning pain. Fibromyalgia used to go by other names, including fibrositis, rheumatism, tension myalgia, and myofibrositis. In the past, some physicians used the term "psychogenic rheumatism" to describe what they thought were patients' symptoms that were "all in their patients' heads."

Because muscle pain is more commonly reported in fibromyalgia, we used to think the problem arose from the muscles. Ongoing research has revealed that the underlying problem lies within the nerves, not the muscles. A process called central sensitization occurs in the brain and spinal cord which results in amplified pain, the hallmark symptom of fibromyalgia. Even though muscles hurt, the hypersensitive nerves in fibromyalgia are directing the muscles to hurt.

The pain of fibromyalgia usually consists of generalized aching, a sense of "I hurt all over." Certain parts of the body are particularly painful, and the pain may move around and be accompanied by severe muscle spasms. The pain can fluctuate from day to day and often flares up. It can be aggravated by various physical, environmental, and emotional factors, and the pain can become so intense that it interferes with one's ability to perform daily activities or work. Some people with fibromyalgia may have only mild discomfort, and others may be completely disabled by it. Some seem to be like pain magnets and attract all sorts of pain!

In addition to pain, fibromyalgia also causes numerous other symptoms and associated conditions. Fatigue is a major problem that can fluctuate in severity and cause functional limitations, just like the pain does. Stiffness, numbness, headaches, poor sleep, decreased memory and concentration, chest pain, irritable bowel syndrome, and temporomandibular joint (TMJ) dysfunction are other symptoms and conditions commonly present with fibromyalgia, and each can cause separate problems and limitations as part of the overall fibromyalgia.

Fibromyalgia is a treatable condition. Many treatments are available including education, medicine, therapy, injections, and supplements to help reduce the pain and fatigue and improve the quality of life. Even if the condition cannot be completely cured, it can be healed.

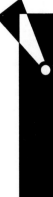

Fatigue is a major problem that can fluctuate in severity and cause functional limitations, just like the pain does. Stiffness, numbness, head-aches, poor sleep, decreased memory and concentration, chest pain, irritable bowel syndrome, and temporomandibular joint (TMJ) dysfunction are other symptoms.

Fibromyalgia is a recognized disease and has its own accepted diagnostic code: **729.1**. The term "fibromyalgia" or "fibromyalgia syndrome" is a medically correct name for this condition, although sometimes other names are still used. Regardless of the name, we are talking about the same condition.

Despite its rightful recognition and acceptance throughout the medical, legal, Workers' Compensation, and Social Security systems, fibromyalgia is not without controversy. A few doctors say fibromyalgia does not exist and is an imagined disorder. To this issue I would say everyone has a right to an opinion, even if it's wrong. This book will address all aspects of fibromyalgia in detail. It will not give an "equal" view from the disbelievers for the simple reason that this is my book. Let the disbelievers write their own books!

What It Is Not

Fibromyalgia can cause symptoms that resemble arthritis or neurological disorders, but it is different from these disorders.

- Unlike arthritis, fibromyalgia does not cause joint swelling or deformities, even though it may cause pain in the tissues or a feeling of swelling around the joints.

- Fibromyalgia does not cause paralysis or progressive neurological problems like multiple sclerosis or Lou Gehrig's disease.

- It is not a ruptured disc or a pinched nerve, even though your symptoms may resemble those caused by a pinched nerve.

- It is not a tumor.

It does not turn into one of these conditions, although people with fibromyalgia can certainly get other conditions over time that are unrelated to fibromyalgia. Other conditions can worsen fibromyalgia pain or co-exist with fibromyalgia. Even though fibromyalgia is not life-threatening or crippling, it is very much a painful condition that can cause severe problems. We may look okay on the outside, but we are definitely hurting on the inside.

Who Gets It?

Anyone can get fibromyalgia. Millions and millions of people have it worldwide, with about 2%–5% of the overall population estimated to have fibromyalgia. Women are diagnosed more frequently than men, about seven to ten times more. Symptoms usually appear between the ages of 25 and 45. I see a lot of men with this disorder in my practice, although I certainly see many more women. Children can also have fibromyalgia. Because fibromyalgia has hereditary components, I frequently see children of a parent who has been diagnosed with fibromyalgia.

Symptoms may be present for years, even though the diagnosis may not be made until a later age. Once you are officially diagnosed with the disorder, you continue to have it as you get older; thus the prevalence of fibromyalgia increases in the population as the age increases. According to Dr. Robert Bennett, a fibromyalgia researcher, about 3½% of 20-year olds will meet the American College of Rheumatology (ACR) definition of fibromyalgia. Among 70-year olds, 12% have fibromyalgia.

Not all people with chronic widespread pain have fibromyalgia. Dr. Daniel Clauw and Dr. Leslie Crofford found only about 20% of individuals in the population with chronic widespread pain meet the 11 of the 18 tender point criteria (see Chapter 5). One possible explanation is that some of these people have a more regional form of fibromyalgia, or have myofascial pain syndrome which can cause generalized pain even with fewer than 11 of 18 tender points present. Over the years I've seen numerous patients with regional pain, widespread aching and fewer than 11 of 18 tender points, many of whom went on to develop full-blown fibromyalgia over time. If we include those with regional fibromyalgia, myofascial pain or widespread pain that have fewer than 11 of 18 tender points, the overall population with fibromyalgia may be closer to 5–10% instead of 2%.

Once you are officially diagnosed with the disorder, you continue to have it as you get older; thus the prevalence of fibromyalgia increases in the population as the age increases.

Fibromyalgia has been around for a long time even though its "official" name is only about 15 years old. The medical literature before the late 1900's contained some descriptions of persistent pains in patients without evidence of infection or surgical problem. The description sounds like fibromyalgia. Florence Nightingale is believed to have suffered from this disorder. In 1904, Dr. Sir William Gowers, a British neurologist (1845–1915) first described the condition of "fibrositis" as a cause of chronic low back pain. Fibrositis became the "first" name for what we know as "fibromyalgia" today.

The original name was based on the reported microscopic inflamed area seen in a fascia (fibrous tissue) that intertwines with the muscle. The name "fibrositis" implies that the cause of the chronic pain is fibrous tissue inflammation. We now know this is not the case. With the advent of more sophisticated microscopes and carefully designed research studies, medical investigators have shown that there is no actual inflammation in the fascia of these patients, even though these people have chronic muscle pains. At first, many doctors concluded that "fibrositis" did not even exist because the original microscopic inflammation changes reported were found to be wrong. Instead of investigating further to explain the cause of the chronic pain, many doctors concluded that these patients didn't have real pain, but only imagined symptoms. Without a consistent reported abnormality to validate the condition, fibromyalgia sat by the mainstream medical wayside for a number of years.

Doctors with special interest in pain disorders continued to diagnose and treat these patients with painful muscle problems and normal tests. These doctors used different names for these conditions, including fibrositis, fibromyositis, and myofascial pain syndrome. In the 1960s and 1970s, Dr. Janet Travell popularized the terms "myofascial pain syndrome" and "trigger points" for those with painful muscle spasms and referred pain. In 1981, Dr. Muhammad Yunus described criteria for diagnosing patients with fibrositis.

Articles and descriptions about fibrositis were appearing in specialty medical journals for Physical Medicine and Rehabilitation and Rheumatology, and the name "fibromyalgia" was emerging as the name of choice. In 1987, Dr. Goldenberg published an important overview article on fibromyalgia in the most widely read scientific journal, the *Journal of the American Medical Association (JAMA)*. This article and the accompanying editorial by Dr. Bennett validated the existence of fibromyalgia as a legitimate medical condition recognized by the American Medical Association. It also marked the crossover of fibromyalgia from specialty journals to widely read journals by all doctors.

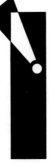

Fibromyalgia has been around for a long time even though its "official" name is only about 15 years old.

Since the late 1980's, an explosion of research and publication on fibromyalgia has occurred. In 2000, over 200 reports on fibromyalgia appeared in the medical literature. The medical landscape on chronic pain is no longer sparsely dotted with articles on fibrositis/fibromyalgia, it is colored by them. It is recognized by various medical organizations, including the American Medical Association, the World Health Organization, the Bureau of Worker's Compensation System, Medicare, Social Security, the insurance industry and the court systems. As I mentioned earlier, controversies continue to the present day, but those who understand and treat fibromyalgia will agree that it is a legitimate medical condition with unique characteristics requiring individualized treatment.

I don't expect that the controversies surrounding fibromyalgia will disappear as long as there are people who don't understand or believe in fibromyalgia. Not only does it exist, it is a chronic and permanent condition for which there is no cure at this time. A lot can be done for this condition, however, and the challenge is not only to fully understand fibromyalgia, but to minimize its effect on the individual and the community until a cure is found.

If You Want To Know More

1. Bennett RM. *Fibromyalgia, the commonest cause of widespread pain.* Compr Ther 1995; 21: 269–75.

2. Bennett RM. *Emerging concepts in the neurobiology of chronic pain: evidence for abnormal sensory processing in fibromyalgia.* Mayo Clin Proc 1999; 74: 385–98.

3. Clauw DJ, Crofford RJ. *Chronic widespread pain and fibromyalgia: what we know, and what we need to know.* Best Pract Res Clin Rheumatol 2003; 17: 685–701.

4. Goldenberg DL. *Fibromyalgia syndrome: an emerging but controversial condition.* JAMA 1987; 257: 2782–7.

5. *ICD–9 CM Professional for physicians.* Vols. 1 & 2, 6th ed. Saint Anthony's Publishing, 2003.

6. Mulholland RC. *Historical perspective: Sir William Gowers.* Spine 1996; 21: 1106–10.

7. Pellegrino MJ. *Inside fibromyalgia.* Columbus, OH: Anadem Publishing, 2001.

8. Rao SR. *The neuropharmacology of centrally-acting analgesic medications in fibromyalgia.* Rheum Dis Clin N Am 2002; 28(2): 235–59.

9. Travell JG, Simons D. *Myofascial pain and dysfunction: the trigger point manual.* Vol 1. Lippincott, Williams & Wilkins, 1983.

A Lighter Look At Fibromyalgia

Fibromyalgia is not a funny condition. It causes severe pain and disabilities, and it affects every aspect of our lives. Sometimes, however, we need to take a break from our pain and try to laugh. Some of the funniest people I know have fibromyalgia. I try to use humor and enjoy humor in my everyday life whether or not I'm dealing with fibromyalgia. In this book, I attempt humor in many forms, and I hope you find at least one attempt funny! I wanted to introduce this chapter near the book's beginning so you could understand my humor attempts throughout the book, especially if you don't find them funny!

Laughing is therapeutic, especially when we can laugh at ourselves. Norman Cousins wrote a classic article in the *New England Journal of Medicine* that became the first chapter of his book, *Anatomy of an Illness*. In it he describes how laughter helped him overcome a painful connective tissue disease. Physiologically, laughing helps us by:

- Increasing release of endorphins, our natural painkillers

- Improving blood flow and relaxing muscles

- Stimulating the brain centers that tell us to feel good

- Temporarily blocking pain signals

- Improving body's homeostasis, including our immune function.

If we can learn to laugh at ourselves, we may find it easier to cope with fibromyalgia. I've always tried to keep my sense of humor in spite of my pain, and I've appreciated over the years that people with fibromyalgia, as a group, have a great sense of humor. You know all of the bad things about the condition and how it affects your everyday life. Whenever we think we are feeling a little bit better, something will happen to remind us we still have pain. There is so much we can't control: the weather; what others think or do; and what life's next surprise will be.

Maybe, though, we can learn to approach our fibromyalgia with a lighter attitude. I say that if we are stuck with this miserable daily pain, we should try to laugh at it. It is like dark humor. In some aspects it is sad, but we can make humor of the situation to better cope with it. Plus, we are more fun to be around if we are funny or at least trying to be positive.

There are various ways we can poke fun at our fibromyalgia; you know, take a light look and lighten up.

Think Of Advantages Of Having Fibromyalgia

Perhaps not all of fibromyalgia has to be bad. Think of some good things that happen from having fibromyalgia. It provides convenient excuses for our mistakes: "I forgot the meeting? Oh, sorry, must be my fibromyalgia, it affects my memory." "Darn, I broke the glass. That fibromyalgia makes me drop things."

It saves you money. No need to purchase alarm clocks, self-installed appliances, or vacuum cleaners. Since you can't do anything else, it enables you to spend more time watching TV and adding to your knowledge. You can learn all about what movie stars like to eat and what cars they drive, natural habitats for iguanas and other lizards, and other interesting information. It allows you to eliminate unenjoyable activities such as mowing the lawn, visiting certain relatives, and cleaning out the garage.

The best reason of all for making jokes about our fibromyalgia is that only people with fibromyalgia will understand. We have our own club. We're special indeed!

Look At Things In A Different Light

Think about situations you get into with fibromyalgia and add your own unique flavor to emphasize a point and make it humorous. One way to do this is to come up with some funny definitions of common situations that happen with fibromyalgia.

A few years back I created fibronyms, or words that take on a unique meaning when pertaining to fibromyalgia. Throughout this book, I've inserted some fibronyms for your light reading and hopefully heavy amusement.

Examples Of Fibronyms:

Mack truck: A popular vehicle that frequently runs over fibromyalgia patients while they are asleep.

Groan-up: Adult fibromyalgia patient.

Pain pal: A fibromyalgia colleague who understands what we are going through.

Ambidextrous: The ability to be equally clumsy with both hands.

Make Up A Funny List

We are already experts at organizing lists because we are so absentminded and forgetful. Write down a list of things that you would like to see or how you would like something to be. These are things you can't change, but they can be described in a different way. A funny list can help. Here is an example of a top ten list. Others are provided throughout the book.

Top Ten Fibromyalgia Self-Help Books That Never Became Best Sellers

1. How to Cure Fibromyalgia

2. Learn to Speak Assertively to Your Muscles

3. How to Blame Others For Your Fibromyalgia

4. Be Positive in Spite of Miserable, Depressing Pain in Every Despicable Muscle of Your Body

5. Yes, Every Problem You've Ever Had is From Fibromyalgia!

6. Teach Your Spouse, Family, Friends, and Doctor to Completely Understand Fibromyalgia

7. Smother Your Pain With Love

8. Planning a Vacation? Don't Forget to Bring Along Your Fibromyalgia

9. Use Your Pain to Win the Lottery!

10. How to Function on Only 2 Hours of Stage IV Sleep

Use Humorous Reinforcement

We know what increases our pain and causes flare-ups, and we need to continuously remind ourselves of things to do and not to do. To lighten your view, think of funny ways to cause increased pain and flare-ups.

To demonstrate this I've come up with FLAWS, which stands for Fibromyalgia **F**amous **LA**st **W**ord**S**. FLAWS are what we say or hear just before a flare-up. Look for FLAWS within this book!

Examples of FLAWS:

- "This shouldn't take too long."

- "No thanks, I can lift this myself."

- "Mom, throw us the frisbee!"

Mentally Send Funny Messages

People are always trying to think of clever and humorous greeting cards and answering machine messages. Imagine funny messages that you would send someone with fibromyalgia about some aspect of it.

Examples of personalized fibromyalgia greeting cards:

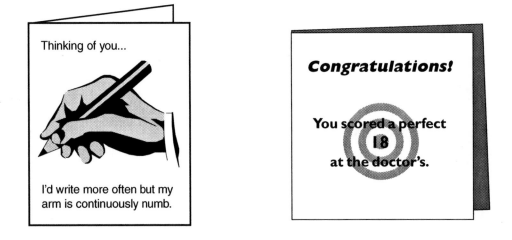

An example of a personalized answering machine message related to fibromyalgia:

"Hello, you've reached the Smith residence. I'm unavailable because of my fibromyalgia. I'm either at the doctor's, getting massotherapy, taking a hot shower, or spending time in the bathroom. Leave a message, and if I remember to check the machine, I'll call you back."

Look for other examples in the book.

Pain Power

We have the worst pain with fibromyalgia, more than anyone else without fibromyalgia. Imagine your pain can give you more control and power. Because of your pain, you are able to create unique and humorous situations. Pretend that you have a lot of control over your fibromyalgia rather than no control. If anyone else tells you about how bad her pain is, you can do better!

I came up with "how bad is my pain …" to give us some power! Patients will always say to me, "my pain is so bad that …" Common examples include, "My pain is so bad that it feels like a hot poker is sticking me." Or, "My pain is so bad I feel like a Mack truck ran over me."

So here is how I imagine what you may really want to tell me to give your pain more power:

"How bad is my pain?"

"My pain is so bad that … A hot poker tickles me."

"My pain is so bad that … Mack trucks swerve to avoid running over me."

"My pain is so bad that … In the Complete Encyclopedia of Pain, I am Volumes 7–12."

"My pain is so bad that … Hungry mosquitoes avoid me."

"My pain is so bad that … Others take narcotics when they see me."

"My pain is so bad that … The sound of a dental drill is actually soothing to me."

Personal Perspective

by Mark J. Pellegrino

Oxymorons

I am fascinated with a unique word called oxymoron. It takes root from a word meaning "fool" and has come to mean a word or a combination of words with apparent contradictory meanings. Oxymorons abound in everyday language; familiar examples include **jumbo shrimp**, **cruel kindness** and **bittersweet**. Children's fairy tales introduced us to **sweet lemons** and **sour grapes**. Hollywood has given us the **Living Dead**, the **Cowardly Lion**, and the **Hero Villain**, as well as movies such as **True Lies**, **Eyes Wide Shut** and **Ladies' Man**. History has provided us with the **Virgin Birth**, the **Civil War**, and **Democratic Leadership**. One of my favorites is: "**This Page Intentionally Left Blank**." One doesn't have to be a **graduate student** to figure these out, but I may be **thinking out loud**.

Medicine has also contributed to the oxymoron list. Numerous medical oxymorons exist: **smokeless cigarettes** and **living wills** are two examples, but these may be **incorrect facts**. I saw a good one inside a diet booklet: **silent pain**. I'm sure the person who wrote that one did not have fibromyalgia!

I have not been able to figure out **status post sudden death**. Is that better than **unsuccessful resuscitation** or an **uneventful death**?

What is the prognosis when a **benign malignancy** is removed? Is it **guardedly optimistic**? It depends on the surgeon's best **educated guess**.

What should I recommend when someone complains of **pain centered in the left back** with a **numb feeling** in the legs? I should probably assess for a **down-going Babinski's**. If there is **unsteady balance**, **absent reflexes**, or **slow rapid alternating movements**, I would worry about a neurological condition that could eventually lead to **incomplete paraplegia**.

Can people really have brainstem **CVAs**, **occluded blood flow**, **bilateral hemisphere lesions**, or **irregular rhythms**? I had another example, but it was **found missing**. I imagine that any of these conditions could cause **disrupted homeostasis**.

For the physiologically astute: can one have a **lengthening contraction** causing **deltoid adduction**? Of course, that is a **proven theory**!

What about those with fibromyalgia? Does this **invisible condition** have its unique oxymorons, or is it pure **science fiction** full of **false hopes**? I think it's a **safe bet** to say fibromyalgia is loaded with oxymorons.

For example, I saw an **anxious patient** the other day, **Mary Devores**, who said I was her **first choice for a second opinion** regarding fibromyalgia. Mary was a **young 65** and said she's been in **bad health** for many years and complains of pain all over with **weak muscles**. She also has **restless sleep** and said a sleep study showed poor **sleep activity**. She was told she may have **non-inflammatory arthritis** based on X-rays that showed **early chronic changes**. Plus, two of her **adult children** showed similar symptoms. She said the symptoms made her think in **slow motion** and her mind often **draws a blank**, and this caused **functional limitations** in her job as a social worker. She said she felt **all alone**.

I examined her and found **painful tender points**. I diagnosed fibromyalgia and prescribed a **daily pain patch twice a day** and told her to use **Icy Hot** lotion. She didn't require surgery so I wrote an **aggressive conservative**

continued on next page...

Personal Perspective

continued from previous page...

therapy program that included a **stationary bike** and **relaxation exercises**. I told her she may **hurt good** to get better, and it was no **easy task** to overcome fibromyalgia. She had to find her own **unique routine** and learn the difference between **good pain** and bad pain. We discussed **wholesome** dietary strategies, and I told her it's okay to indulge in **diet ice cream** with **white chocolate** chunks from time to time (This sounds **sinfully good**!). She followed the advice **almost exactly** and made nice progress.

As you have noticed, I highlighted the oxymorons for your convenience. I hope you found these oxymorons to be **intellectually stimulating**. I am a **sensitive guy**, but I won't be offended if you didn't like it. You may have differing opinions on some, but we can **agree to disagree**. It's whether you see the glass as **half empty or half full**; it's probably the **same difference**, though. Personally, I thought this was a **well-written and humorous article**.

Mark J. Pellegrino, M.D.

(Currently on **working vacation**, eating a **breadless sandwich**, trying to fix a **clogged drain** caused by unused oxymorons)

Humor has its proper place. It is not to be used inappropriately or to offend anyone. Humor is a choice. You can choose whether or not to read something, and you decide whether or not you find it funny. It is your choice and your responsibility. Humor is not something that should ever be thrust in your face, because it can offend or shock you. Fibromyalgia humor is truly only understood by people with fibromyalgia; everyone else will just look at you with a confused expression.

I have been in situations where fibromyalgia humor was thrust upon unwitting people who did not have it. This has occurred on several occasions in a court room setting. I would be providing medical testimony about a particular fibromyalgia patient that I am treating, and the opposing attorney would begin to question me about humor that I had written. Imagine the jury members' surprise, shock, and disbelief when an attorney introduces a fibromyalgia humor book in a setting as serious as a court room. I never imagined that my attempts to help patients use humor would ever be used in such a shocking and negative way in a courtroom.

I realize now that some attorneys will use whatever they can to influence the jury. So, remember that humor, especially humor about a serious medical condition, needs to be used appropriately and responsibly so as not to offend anyone.

Fibromyalgia makes us more understanding, compassionate, appreciative and perceptive. When we are laughing, there is a period of time when we aren't noticing any pain. And every time we laugh, we send a message to our muscles and nerves that we are not going to let them win. Don't be afraid to use humor to help you manage your fibromyalgia. And if you enjoy some of the humor attempts in this book, go ahead and laugh out loud. It makes me feel better!

▶ If You Want To Know More

1. Cousins N. *Anatomy of an illness as perceived by the patient*. Bantam Books, 1981.

2. Pellegrino MJ. *Laugh at your muscles*. Columbus, OH: Anadem Publishing, 1995.

3. Pellegrino MJ, Dawkins B. *Laugh at your muscles II*. Columbus, OH: Anadem Publishing, 1997.

Symptoms Of Fibromyalgia

Fibromyalgia Patient:

"Is it possible for everything wrong with me to be from fibromyalgia?"

Doctor:

"Of course not. I'm sure that of the hundreds of symptoms you just described, one or two are not from fibromyalgia!"

Patients with fibromyalgia are concerned about all the symptoms they have, but they are equally concerned about being perceived as a hypochondriac. They can't help what they feel; however, when they share all their different symptoms with me during the first visit, inevitably they may ask "Am I nuts?"

Well, we all tend to go a little nuts when we get fibromyalgia (me included), but the condition is very much a whole body, multi-system problem, which means it causes numerous symptoms from head to toe. This chapter is meant to review the most common symptoms and problems associated with fibromyalgia. Many patients have all the symptoms and more! Some "only" have the pain. All are bothered by the symptoms, which are real and part of the fibromyalgia.

Pain

The main complaint with fibromyalgia is pain. Several key phrases describe severe pain: "I hurt all over," "My pain moves around," and "I feel like I've been run over by Mack truck." Whenever I hear these phrases, I think of fibromyalgia.

The pain may be described as a constant ache, nagging, or throbbing. The muscles are not the only painful areas. Other soft tissues, such as ligaments, tendons, and bursa can be painful. Typical pain locations include the head and neck, shoulders (especially between the shoulder blades), low back and hip muscles. Certain areas may cause sharp, stabbing pains. Patients can point to exact areas and note they are very painful to touch.

The pain may appear to wander to different sites; the low back may be sore today, and tomorrow, the neck hurts. These wandering symptoms may lead you to think you are going crazy! The pain isn't really wandering. Think of being wired with Christmas lights capable of different blinking patterns. At any given time, each bulb has potential to light up and stay lit for a while, or stay off for a while. Wherever there is a bulb, the potential to "light up" is already there. Our body consists of many potentially painful areas all the time capable of "lighting up." We know these areas hurt because when we press on them they tell us. Sometimes these areas spontaneously hurt (light up), and if different areas hurt at different times, we feel as if the pain is actually moving from one area to another.

At first, I was convinced that there could be no possible physical condition that would cause pain to wander, and therefore I must be imagining things. Once I learned that fibromyalgia can indeed cause wandering pains, I knew I was not as crazy as I thought. I now wonder whether other people should be paying us to marvel at our Fibromyalgia Holiday Light Display!

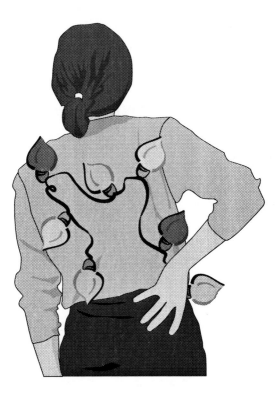

About half of the time, patients report a gradual progression of pain. The pain begins in one location such as the shoulder, but over time other areas become affected until pain is no longer localized but rather generalized throughout the body. Sometimes the onset is so gradual that patients can't even remember the beginning of their pain. Other times, the pain begins after a specific trauma and patients can recall the exact moment when they first had pain. Over half of the patients attribute their symptoms to some type of trauma or severe stress.

Usually a person describes multiple "types" of pain when fibromyalgia is present. Generalized "ache all over" type pain may be accompanied by severe stabbing pains in certain regions, and other areas may have burning or radiating pains. There is usually chronic pain, but often flare-ups occur and certain areas or the whole body become severely painful. Invariably, the pain interferes with everyday activities, including work, hobbies, and recreation. Interpersonal relationship problems occur frequently. Almost everyone with fibromyalgia reports disruption of their functional abilities because of pain.

Modulating Factors

Certain factors modulate fibromyalgia pain, either worsening or improving it. Physical activities can cause flare-ups in the pain. Performing strenuous activities such as moving furniture or gardening can increase pain even after you've stopped the activity. Too much activity is an obvious cause of increased pain, but too little activity can be just as bad.

I learned first-hand how decreased activities could worsen my fibromyalgia. During my residency, I became involved in so many projects that I was unable to continue my exercise program on a regular basis. Gradually, I noticed increased pain in my low back. My back seemed to go into spasms very easily, even with minimal activity such as bending over to pick-up a tissue. I realized that my body had come to expect a certain physical activity level, and by not keeping up with my program, I became more vulnerable to flare-ups. Once I resumed my regular exercise program, my symptoms improved within a short period of time, and I felt more "stable" in my back. I learned not to neglect my exercises, because I (and my back) would pay the price.

Certain positions that require sustained isometric muscle contractions, such as holding our arms out in front of us for a long time, are not tolerated well by people with fibromyalgia. Our muscles do not like sustained contractions, and they tell us by saying "OUCH!" People who have jobs that require reaching (typing, assembly line work, or driving are examples) will often have increased pain, especially in the neck, shoulders, and back.

Weather changes affect our symptoms. Cold, damp weather and cold drafts or air conditioning drafts are major enemies for us. Likewise, cold water will cause muscle pain to flare-up, and we don't do well in pools where the water temperature is below 90° F. We tend to do better in warm, dry weather and climates. Many of my patients try to escape to Arizona for "therapeutic" vacations. (I live in Northeast Ohio, which seems like one of the worst places in the world for fibromyalgia!) Hot, humid weather can aggravate the pain whereas hot, dry weather is preferred.

Emotional stress certainly plays a role in fibromyalgia flare-ups. Stress is part of life, but during times of increased stress, we usually experience increased fibromyalgia pain. Most people will experience more pain when they have a flu virus, and sometimes even after getting a flu vaccine. A lot of women notice a flare-up of their symptoms before their period starts and increased premenstrual syndrome (PMS) symptoms. Likewise, the pain symptoms can increase during early menopause.

Sometimes there is no obvious reason why pain flares up. This is common in fibromyalgia, and it can be very frustrating because you may be doing all of the "right" things.

Fatigue

Next to pain, fatigue is the major complaint in people with fibromyalgia. Fatigue is actually a combination of physical and mental factors. Fibromyalgia muscles already have low energy stores and tire easily. Any activity, whether usual or "out of the ordinary," can cause fatigue. Going shopping at the mall, playing a game of basketball, and walking up several flights of steps are activities that can cause sudden increased fatigue in the muscles.

A steel worker described his leg fatigue at the end of the work day as turning him into a Slow-Mo camera. He felt like his legs were working in super slow-motion, with each move requiring detailed concentration.

Fatigue can be unpredictable and strike the muscles suddenly. Another one of my patients described her fatigue as a feeling of driving along and idling at a stop-light, when suddenly the car runs out of gas and stalls (she is not an auto mechanic by the way!)

Extreme fatigue has a mental component as well as a physical one. Neurasthenia is a medical term that describes the extreme lack of energy and feeling of mental exhaustion. This mental fatigue makes it hard to concentrate or focus on a task. We feel like we are in a fog.

Concentration and Memory Problems (Fibrofog)

Fibromyalgia can cause considerable difficulties with our thinking, and this can vary from day to day. These difficulties include forgetfulness, absentmindedness, confusion, short-term memory difficulties, extreme mental fatigue, and something else…but I can't remember what. We refer to these symptoms as "fibrofog." Further review of fatigue and fibrofog are found in Section IV.

We are the people who have to stop and think about which side is right and which side is left. We also are the worst group of people to ever ask for directions, especially since we get lost all of the time!

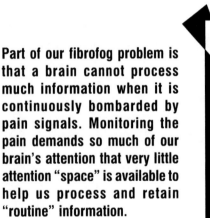

Part of our fibrofog problem is that a brain cannot process much information when it is continuously bombarded by pain signals. Monitoring the pain demands so much of our brain's attention that very little attention "space" is available to help us process and retain "routine" information.

Many people are extremely concerned that this indicates a deterioration of their brain function or dementia, but that is not the case. We demonstrate normal learning and memory although we process information more slowly because of our fibromyalgia. Part of our fibrofog problem is that a brain cannot process much information when it is continuously bombarded by pain signals. Monitoring the pain demands so much of our brain's attention that very little attention "space" is available to help us process and retain "routine" information.

Our fibrofog is one of our most frustrating problems. We can read the same thing over and over and still not understand a word we read. We can see a close relative and suddenly forget her name. We drive past freeway entrances and exits and constantly discover new routes home—inadvertently! Countless times I cannot remember a specific word or person's name, or anything else important! I'm frequently absent of mind (NO, that's not a typo!). On the other hand, fibrofog is something you can have the most fun with, if you really try. What else can be more exciting than trying to find your misplaced car keys when they're right in your pocket, or wondering how the cereal got in the refrigerator and the milk in the cupboard?

Poor Sleep

Poor sleep is a hallmark of most patients with fibromyalgia. Patients report that the quality of their sleep is poor, and when they awake in the morning they do not feel well rested (non-restorative sleep). You may not have trouble falling asleep, but often your sleep is characterized by frequent awakening especially in the early morning hours, and lack of a deep, sound sleep. Dr. Harvey Moldofsky performed studies which demonstrated disruptions of the deep sleep stage in many with fibromyalgia.

I do not have difficulty falling asleep but I usually wake up around 4:00 AM. I feel ready to conquer the world at that time, but I realize that it is too darn early to get up. So I lay there in bed. Every fifteen minutes I find myself glancing at the clock and never falling back into a deep sleep. When it is finally time to get up, I feel completely exhausted and must use every self-motivation technique as well as great effort to drag myself out of bed.

Many people have trouble falling asleep and wake often. Others suffer from a condition called sleep apnea characterized by irregular breathing and periods of breathing cessation (apnea) during sleep. Whatever the cause(s), a lack of deep sleep certainly contributes to fatigue during the day. Our batteries are not getting recharged adequately during the night.

Headaches

We get a lot of tension, migraine, sinus and mixed headaches with fibromyalgia. Tension headaches are also called muscle contraction headaches, and they usually begin at the base of the neck and extend upward to the back of the head and frequently into the temples. Many people describe a band-like squeezing headache. Migraine headaches are vascular headaches in which some event triggers the blood vessels to constrict and then dilate. This causes a severe headache that may be located inside the head or behind the eyes and may be accompanied by nausea, vomiting, eye pain, and facial numbness. Sinus headaches are common because we often have a lot of allergies with fibromyalgia.

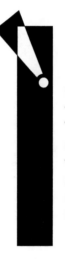

Many people with fibromyalgia have headaches with both tension and migraine features. They describe daily tension headache with aching pain, and then on a fairly regular basis, perhaps once a week or twice a month, a severe migraine headache occurs.

Many people with fibromyalgia have headaches with both tension and migraine features. They describe daily tension headache with aching pain, and then on a fairly regular basis, perhaps once a week or twice a month, a severe migraine headache occurs. Various factors can trigger a migraine headache including certain foods, exposure to certain odors, stresses, weather changes, and menstrual cycles.

Frequent severe headaches are particularly tough for patients. Head pain is much more disruptive than pain in other locations, so it will interfere more with work abilities, daily activities, and interactions with others.

Chest Pain

Non-cardiac chest pain can be of particular concern because patients fear that this may represent heart disease. Usually there is no problem with the heart. Rather, the pain comes from muscles in the chest wall and rib areas, that is, the pectorals and intercostal muscles. The ligaments and tendons around the chest area (sternum or breast plate) can become painful. This is called costochondritis and it can mimic heart pain. Large-busted women and women who have fibrocystic breast disease (painful cysts in the breasts) often have more chest pain with their fibromyalgia. Fear and anxiety triggered by chest pain can make the pain worse.

When I first started seeing people with fibromyalgia, I noticed many had atypical chest pain as their "first" symptom. They may have had a heart work-up at first, which was negative. Ultimately they received a diagnosis of fibromyalgia with associated musculoskeletal chest pain. I published these results in 1989 and have since come to appreciate how common chest pain is in fibromyalgia, whether it is the initial symptom or develops after the fibromyalgia has already been diagnosed.

If you have unexplained chest pain, always get it checked out. If it's found to be related to your fibromyalgia, you can relax a little knowing it's not a heart problem and focus on managing the fibro-related pain.

Mitral Valve Prolapse

Mitral valve prolapse (MVP), often present in fibromyalgia, can contribute to chest wall pain. MVP is a condition when one of the heart valves, the mitral valve, bulges excessively during the heartbeat. It can be diagnosed by listening with a stethoscope for a characteristic click-murmur. The diagnosis is confirmed with a sound wave test (echocardiogram). Although it sounds scary, most doctors feel that MVP is usually a benign condition.

I conducted a study at the Ohio State University which showed that the majority of people with fibromyalgia also had MVP. The mitral valve is mostly connective tissue, not a muscle. This study supports the belief that fibromyalgia involves tissues other than muscles.

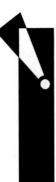

Chest pain in fibromyalgia is usually benign, but people with fibromyalgia can have other problems, too, including heart problems. Remember, if you experience new chest pain, consult a physician at once.

MVP usually does not cause problems in fibromyalgia patients, but sometimes it can be more severe and cause cardiac problems that require specific medications. Antibiotics may be prescribed before certain surgeries or procedures such as dental work. Atypical chest pain and shortness of breath can occur. Chest pain in fibromyalgia is usually benign, but people with fibromyalgia can have other problems, too, including heart problems. Remember, if you experience new chest pain, consult a physician at once.

Morning Stiffness & Joint Pains

Stiffness and joint pain are usually present in fibromyalgia. These symptoms are mostly related to pain at the muscle and tendon insertions into the joint area, and not actual joint pathology or inflammation. Morning stiffness is a common complaint, so not only are we sleeping poorly, but when we wake up in the morning we are so stiff that we can hardly move. This stiffness can also occur after prolonged periods of sitting or standing in one position. Usually once we get up and start moving around, we tend to loosen up.

Temporomandibular Joint (TMJ) Dysfunction

Over a third of patients with fibromyalgia have pain in the jaw and temple areas related to TMJ dysfunction. TMJ dysfunction can cause a variety of symptoms such as headaches, ringing in the ears, face numbness, and dizziness. Other jaw and "face" symptoms frequently reported include facial twitching, flushing, and a fullness or swelling sensation.

Swallowing Difficulties

Swallowing may be difficult at times, as if a tight band is constricting our throats. This may trouble us if we are having a hard time swallowing a piece of food. These symptoms may fluctuate and

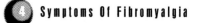

seem to worsen if we are more tense and nervous. We have a lot of muscles in the throat for fibromyalgia to bother.

Throat pain and fullness may occur. Many feel hoarse or have problems vocalizing. Still others have a condition called esophageal reflux where acid and stomach contents can "backflow" up to the throat and cause irritation and pain. All these problems are seen more often in people with fibromyalgia.

Neurological Symptoms

Various neurological symptoms are present in fibromyalgia. These include numbness or tingling especially in the arms and legs and particularly in the hands or feet. These symptoms can mimic a pinched nerve or carpal tunnel syndrome. Other sensory symptoms include feelings of burning, itching and swelling. Finger swelling is common and rings may become tight on the finger. Any abnormal sensation is known as a paresthesia.

Weakness is a common complaint as well. This weakness is not due to neurologic damage from a pinched nerve, for example, but rather a weakness related to muscle pain and fatigue and overall loss of strength and stamina. If muscles hurt, they prevent us from using them properly, hence we feel weak.

People complain of sensitivity to temperatures and often get hot flashes and cold hands and feet. Night sweats are common. Some people even develop a condition known as Raynaud's phenomenon, which is characterized by intermittent attacks of red, white or blue discoloration of the fingers or toes. Cold temperature or stress usually brings on these neurovascular changes.

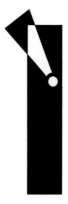

Some people even develop a condition known as Raynaud's phenomenon, which is characterized by intermittent attacks of red, white or blue discoloration of the fingers or toes.

Other neurological symptoms include dizziness, light-headedness, and vertigo or spinning sensation. We often become very sensitive to louder noises or may notice ringing in our ears (tinnitus). We may have balance problems or lack of coordination. We have to be careful that we don't get up too fast because we are more prone to a drop in blood pressure known as neurally-mediated hypotension. This can cause us to get light-headed and feel like we are going to faint. Fainting is definitely not recommended for those who have fibromyalgia!

Frequently, patients complain of mainly right-sided (or left-sided) pain. If the person is right handed, usually the right side will hurt more, but that's not always the case. Sometimes the non-dominant side will be more painful. The one-sided involvement may be related to neurological mechanisms which cause one side of the brain to be more sensitive to pain.

Visual Symptoms

Certainly we do not expect our eyes to be spared from fibromyalgia, do we? Up to a third of those with this condition have dry eyes, which may make it impossible to wear contacts. We notice that our eyes are particularly sensitive to smoke or that environments with very dry air cause vision difficulty. Eye muscles can get painful or go into spasms with fibromyalgia, so we have difficulty with moving our eyes, focusing, reading and tracking.

Eye muscle spasms combined with dry eyes can cause eye pain and headaches. Many patients have to change their glasses prescriptions frequently because of fibromyalgia-related vision fluctuations and changes in visual acuity. Fibromyalgia does not cause retinal detachments or glaucoma.

A particular visual difficulty experience is what I call "visual overload." This occurs when we try to process a lot of visual information at once. It becomes confusing and overwhelming to us. A common example of this occurs when you are reading a paragraph in a book, and you have read the paragraph 3 times and still have no clue what you just read. It's like fibrofog in the eyes, a combination of cognitive and visual problems.

I have these particular visual difficulties in stores. For example, if I need to find a can of olives and I try to scan all of the colorful cans stacked on a shelf about ten feet high and the length of a football field, I become dizzy and overwhelmed with this visual overload. I am unable to focus and scan and try to spot that can of olives. So, instead of my eyes giving me organized information like "cans of green beans, cans of corn, cans of carrots, cans of olives," they give me jumbled bits of information like this: "bright-yellow label, cans of corn, don't they come in frozen boxes, too?; little girl smiling, green and orange design on a can, that one isn't centered, what's behind this box?; don't forget you have to get ice-cream too, my back is getting sore, did I know that guy? WHAT AM I LOOKING FOR AGAIN?"

Leg Pains

Many people develop leg pains and cramps, especially in the calves, or an intense feeling of restlessness in the legs. This sensation occurs particularly when you lie down at night and is often not relieved until you move the leg or literally get up and walk around. This is called restless leg syndrome. Nocturnal myoclonus is another leg problem that consists of involuntary jerking of the legs during sleep. The nighttime leg symptoms are usually worse if you have been more active and on your feet during the day. These conditions are felt to be related to a neurologic mechanism where there is difficulty "turning off the switch" when you are trying to relax. Your throbbing leg pains are blocked out during the day by all the other sensory bombardments (from the eyes, ears, muscles, etc.). At night, all these other sensory inputs disappear as we lay down, turn off lights, and tune out noise. The leg pains and other sensations are no longer blocked out—and we feel them.

Allergies/Chemical Sensitivities

Many patients with fibromyalgia have allergies or sensitivities. These may be due to environmental substances such as dust or pollen, or they may be medications or foods. We are hypersensitive to odors, noises, weather changes, bright lights, various chemicals, food additives, and more. We get a lot of nasal congestion, sinus headaches, nausea, itching, and rashes. We probably have a dysfunctional allergy and immune system responsible for these problems.

Our allergies/sensitivities often make us very sensitive to prescription medicines, so we have more side effects or don't tolerate medicines. We get more colds, sinus infections and yeast infections because of our dysfunctional immune system.

I am particularly sensitive to smells. Cigarette smoke, perfumes and colognes, and incense will often make me nauseated and cause my eyes to water. Particular enemies are the plug-in scents and those most annoying perfume and cologne inserts in magazines.

Personal Snapshot

by Mark J. Pellegrino, M.D.

The Invasion Of Sample Scents (first published in *Fibromyalgia Frontiers*)

I've always had a keen sense of smell. I assumed it was hereditary, although no one else in my family could ever sniff out a Reese's peanut butter cup in the back of a sock drawer. Perhaps some of my Italian ancestors liked bloodhounds (I mean REALLY liked them) and instead of inheriting all the old factories, I got the olfactories. If anyone had spoiled milk or bad meat queries, questions regarding body odors, or needed confirmation if someone had smoked something, I (my nose) was consulted. I was the Ann Landers of Olfaction.

As I trained to become a doctor, I learned that some diseases produced a characteristic odor that nasally-astute doctors could recognize. A foul odor on breath could mean fetor oris, common in dental or tonsillar infections. Fruity acetone breath smells are common in diabetic ketoacidosis or starvation acidosis. A curious musty odor can signal severe liver disease. Alcohol on the breath indicates the person has been imbibing, whereas garlic on the breath means keep at least 10 feet away from where the person was speaking!

It wasn't until I was diagnosed with fibromyalgia at the end of my Physical Medicine and Rehabilitation residency that I learned of a reason for my extranasal perception. Most individuals with fibromyalgia have a dysfunctional autonomic nervous system which can cause hypersensitivity to smells. Odor-producing molecules come into contact with the nasal membranes and generate a nerve signal that travels from the olfactory nerve to the smell center of the brain. The autonomic nerves convey sensitivity and intensity characteristics to the smells, so fibromyalgia people with hypersensitive autonomic nerves will notice odors more. In layman's terms, fibromyalgia is why I get sick if I wear cologne.

My hypersensitive sense of smell has not interfered with my medical practice. From time to time, I would have an acute pheromone attack in the office which temporarily interfered with my clinical abilities (it is very difficult to see my patients if the eyes are flowing like the Mississippi River, or to talk to them if the larynx is narrowed like the Isthmus of Panama). I can remember my most nasally (geographically) challenging patients: the two-pack a day smoking housewife who oozed Chanel Number 5 from every body cell, the beer drinking construction worker who lunched at a Mexican buffet, the owner of horse stables who didn't have time to change before her appointment, and the sweet elderly lady I saw in January who owns a wood-burning stove that she uses to heat her house in the winter.

No matter what happened in my office, odorously speaking, I knew I could always count on home being a safe haven for smells, a place where I could relax without worry of uncontrolled or unexpected nasal attacks. If some magazine advertiser wanted me to scratch and sniff, I never scratched. I decided what I would smell. That is until one day when my home was invaded by the sample scents.

I'll never forget the first time it happened. I was leafing through a magazine when suddenly, my eyes began to water, my throat felt scratchy, my nose began to itch, then became stuffy, followed by a wave of nausea. I noticed a harsh aromatic scent and immediately realized that foreign odor molecules were attacking me. I leapt into action, reconnoitering the terrain for any enemies. I checked the trash can, the garbage disposal, and the refrigerator—negative. I looked for those darn plug-in scents and found none. Then I retraced my steps back to the magazine and spotted the intruder—a sample perfume scent insert in the magazine. This pheromone-packed insert was potent enough to cause me an allergic-type reaction. No one else in my family noticed these smells. Only I suffered from the unwanted pheromone invasion of my personal space.

I removed the insert that day and have done so innumerable times since. I learned inserts usually arrived in pairs, so I routinely sought out these two in each magazine that entered my house, wrapping them up in newspaper, disposing of them, then washing my hands. Afterwards, I would read the magazine if I was still interested and wasn't too tired.

continued on next page...

A close relationship exists between smell and sexual function in many species of animals, and all the perfume and cologne ads are ample evidence that humans are a targeted species. Undoubtedly, something other than nausea was the intended reaction of these scented pieces of paper, so I'm sure the scent manufacturers didn't have me in mind when they concocted their marketing campaigns.

So what's next, scented medical journals? Perhaps the Annals of Pathology should have formaldehyde-scented inserts? How about opening up an issue of Pulmonary Medicine and getting a whiff of cigarette smoke? Or chocolate aroma wafting from the spring issue of Nutritional News. Any suggestions for the Journal of Proctology?

If I could nominate a smell to represent fibromyalgia pain, I would vote for the smell of burnt popcorn. It's irritating and a nuisance, but not damaging to the nostrils. Sometimes you can imagine tasty popcorn odors in the midst, but an acute whiff of burn smells makes you realize you're only pretending the popcorn doesn't have a problem. So you try to accept the smell, but it's so hard to get used to, and if you try to remove the popcorn from the room, the smell still lingers and seems to go with you wherever you go.

Humans can distinguish up to 4000 different odors, including Lysol's Disinfecting Spring Waterfall scent. If fibromyalgia is amplifying them all, well… that stinks! Call me old fashioned, but I prefer the simpler times and smells. I guess I prefer old-fashioned olfaction, and so does my fibromyalgia.

Irritable Bowel Syndrome Or Spastic Colon

About half of the patients describe frequent bouts of constipation and/or diarrhea accompanied by abdominal pain, bloating and upset stomach. Irritable bowel syndrome may have been a problem in the past, or it may be an ongoing problem as part of the overall fibromyalgia. Many patients with severe gastrointestinal symptoms require specific medicines and treatments "separate" from the fibromyalgia treatments.

Irritable Bladder/Interstitial Cystitis

The sister of irritable bowel syndrome causes symptoms of a bladder infection with frequent painful urination, but a urine test does not reveal any evidence of infection. Some people have been found to have benign microscopic blood in the urine. Severe bladder problems may require a urologic evaluation.

Pelvic Pain

Both sexes may report pelvic pain, but it is more common in women. The low back, sacroiliac, and pelvic muscles may be particularly painful. Women may develop endometriosis (painful uterine tissue growing in various locations of the pelvic cavity) or vulvodynia (painful, itching vulva and vaginal region). Irritable bowel syndrome can refer pain to the pelvic area.

Women with fibromyalgia often complain of extremely painful periods, or premenstrual syndrome. A few of their husbands complain to me about this as well! (about their wives' PMS, that is)

Plantar Fasciitis

Many people with fibromyalgia complain of pain in their feet. Heel pain, arch pain, toe pain, and entire foot pain are commonly reported. A condition known as plantar fasciitis is seen commonly in fibromyalgia. This is characterized by arch and heel pain especially, usually worse in the morning when one steps out of bed and first puts weight on the feet. Knife-stabbing pains in the bottom of

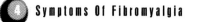

the feet are described. Once the person is up and walking around for a few minutes, the pain tends to subside.

Foot pain is more common in individuals who stand and walk all day, especially on hard surfaces, or who have to wear uncomfortable shoes. People with fibromyalgia seem more prone to getting tendinitis and the feet have many tendons that are candidates to be painful.

Skin Problems

The skin is the largest organ of our body, so it certainly won't be left out when we have fibromyalgia. Many people feel as if their skin is inflamed and describe burning or a sunburn feeling. Even light touch hurts the skin. Other skin problems include rashes, itching, dryness and easy bruising. People with fibromyalgia are more prone to allergies and yeast infections which can further contribute to skin rashes and itching.

Weight Gain

This common problem develops for a number of reasons in fibromyalgia. First, the increased pain interferes with our ability to be as active as we used to be, so we can't burn off calories as well. Plus, our metabolism and carbohydrate tolerance changes and we're more prone to weight gain. Also, many medicines used to treat fibromyalgia can cause weight gain as a side effect. Weight gain and dietary strategies are discussed in more detail later in this book.

Muscle Spasms

Inherent to our fibromyalgia is a tendency for our muscles to tighten up. The muscles are lacking in energy molecules, and these energy molecules are necessary to actively "relax" the muscles. A lack of energy in the muscle means less ability to relax and more tendency to tighten up or go into a spasm. Often we experience fibromyalgia flare-ups because of sudden spasms in the muscles.

Depression

Depression is commonly seen in conditions that cause chronic pain such as fibromyalgia. Up to half of patients become clinically depressed over the course of their fibromyalgia. Symptoms of low self-esteem, frequent crying spells, feeling of helplessness, and a bleak outlook are common. Some people have been diagnosed with depression before they were diagnosed with fibromyalgia.

Anxiety Disorder And Panic Attacks

Many people experience episodes of extreme anxiety and near panic. They may feel their heart racing, palpitations, chest tightness and find it difficult to get their breath. There may be a feeling of impending doom. We appear to be extremely sensitive to adrenaline, the main hormone that causes anxiety and panic attacks.

We frequently have "silent" anxiety attacks. I say silent because to the outside world nothing is apparent. When we first encounter a stressful situation, we look calm, cool and collected. But on the inside we feel like a runaway train is rushing through our blood vessels.

Fibromyalgia "Personality"

I think people with fibromyalgia have a certain type of personality. People with fibromyalgia tend to be compulsive, highly organized, perfectionists, time-oriented, and anxious. We like to do things ourselves because we know it will get done exactly the way we want. We cannot trust others to "get the job done right," so we end up doing almost everything ourselves. It really bothers us when others do not respect the details and time as we do.

Because we are so compulsive, we are not satisfied with just getting a job done; we want it to be the best job ever done. Consequently, no matter what we do, whether at work or home, we are always putting pressure on ourselves to do the best that we can. Even if we would change our job to testing recliner chairs, we would still be stressed out because we would want to be the best recliner chair testers ever!

Summary Of Symptoms

This long chapter has pointed out various symptoms and associated conditions seen with fibromyalgia. Believe it or not, there are still more symptoms and associated conditions. I've only mentioned the most common ones. I didn't describe all possible symptoms because I wanted to have room in this book to write about other things!

As you will soon know (hopefully!) when reading about the abnormalities in the central nervous system later in this book, nearly all the fibromyalgia symptoms can be traced to one culprit: dysfunctional hypersensitized nerves. The autonomic nerves are especially affected as these nerves are wired to everything: pain, spinal cord, hormones, immune system, blood vessels, mood, heart rate, sleep quality, resistance to allergens, urge to go to the bathroom, hormone responses, and even personality. A problem with these nerves can lead to widespread and yet distinct nerve "symptoms."

Looking to design a perfect guinea pig to study dysfunctional autonomic nerves? Look in the mirror!

It's not our fault that we have all these symptoms. The fact that we have so many does not make us all hypochondriacs, it makes us people with fibromyalgia.

▶ If You Want To Know More

1. Bennett RM. *Fibromyalgia: the commonest cause of widespread pain.* Comp Ther 1995; 21: 269–75.

2. deGier M, Peters ML, Vlaeyen JW. *Fear of pain, physical performance, and attentional processes in patients with fibromyalgia.* Pain 2003; 104: 121-30.

3. Hudson JI, Pope HG. *The relationship between fibromyalgia and major depressive disorder.* Rheum Dis Clin North Am 1996; 22: 285-303.

4. Moldofsky H, Scarisbrick BS, England R, et al. *Musculoskeletal symptoms and non-REM sleep disturbance in patients with "Fibrositis Syndrome" and healthy subjects.* Psychosomatic Medicine 1975; 37(4): 341.

5. Pellegrino MJ, Van Fossen D, Gordon CA, et al. *Prevalence of mitral valve prolapse in primary fibromyalgia: a pilot investigation.* Arch Phys Med Rehabil 1989; 70: 541–3.

6. Pellegrino MJ. *Atypical chest pain as an initial presentation of primary fibromyalgia.* Arch Phys Med Rehabil 1990; 71: 526–8.

7. Pellegrino MJ. *Inside fibromyalgia.* Columbus OH: Anadem Publishing, 2001.

Clinical Evaluation Of Fibromyalgia

Concerned Patient:

"Doctor, I hurt all over."

Confused Doctor:

"Who's Al Over?"

The medical evaluation of the fibromyalgia patient includes a history and a physical exam. The medical history is an account of events in a patient's life that have relevance to the particular problem that brings the patient to see the doctor. It is a discussion between you and the doctor about why you are seeing the doctor. Your chief complaint when you see the doctor is usually PAIN! Lots of it!!

The medical history is not simply an unprompted narrative by the patient. If given the chance, many people with fibromyalgia could talk for hours about what's wrong with them! Rather, the medical history is more of a specialized form of information gathering. Knowing which questions to ask is one of the most important tools in making the diagnosis of fibromyalgia. For this reason, your physician should be properly trained to work with fibromyalgia patients. As I ask questions, I record and evaluate the symptoms, but this is not the only data I need. The patients' feedback about their condition is also critical to this fact-finding mission. Think of your medical history as your "fibromyalgia resume." Its purpose is to highlight the most relevant facts, background information, and symptoms in the same way a resume does for a job interview.

There are consistent features in the medical history of someone with fibromyalgia. When I take the history of a patient who is complaining of pain, I note key features. Below are types of questions that I might ask and typical answers given by people with fibromyalgia.

1. Where is the pain?

Typical answers: "I hurt all over." "I ache all over, but I have severe headaches and neck pain." "My back hurts me especially, but so do my head, shoulders, arms, hips, legs, hands, and feet."

Most people with fibromyalgia will complain of generalized pain but may have regions that are relatively more painful. People can literally hurt everywhere on their body.

2. When did the pain start?

Typical answers: "I've had pain since I was young; I remember having growing pains as a kid;" "Years ago my back started to hurt, but then it seemed to spread to other areas over time;" "It started after I got mono in college;" "It began in 1985 when I had a lot of stressful things happen to me;" "My pains began at 1:48 PM on April 15, 1993 when I was sitting at a red light and was rear-ended by another car."

Sometimes the pain onset is so gradual that patients cannot remember the beginning of the pain. Other times, the pain began after a trauma and the exact moment is remembered.

3. What caused your pain?

Typical answers: "A motor vehicle accident;" "A work injury;" "A stressful event;" "I don't know, nothing that I can relate to."

Over half of patients attribute their symptoms to trauma or severe stress. The rest cannot identify any specific cause.

4. What aggravates your pain?

Typical answers: "Any weather change, especially cold, damp weather;" "Air-conditioning drafts will aggravate my pain;" "If I bend or lift or overdo any activity;" "Stress."

5. What helps your pain?

Typical answers: "Heat feels good;" "If I lay down and rest this usually helps;" "I get my husband (or wife) to massage my muscles;" "If I move around and try to stay active."

Modulation factors were described in the last chapter. Helpful clues are obtained when people describe what makes the pain worse or better.

6. Describe the pain.

Typical answers: "I feel like I've been run over by a Mack truck;" "It is a dull ache but often there are sharp pains;" "It is a constant pain that radiates up and down my arms and legs."

Usually a person describes multiple "types" of pain when fibromyalgia is present.

7. How has the pain interfered with your life?

Typical answers: "I can barely work, and when I get home I am so exhausted I can hardly do anything;" "I used to exercise 3 days a week, and now it is too painful to try to move;" "My husband (wife) complains that I never want to do anything with him (her) anymore."

Nearly everyone with fibromyalgia will report some disruption of their abilities due to pain. Included are activities of daily living, work, hobbies, recreational activities, interpersonal relationships.

8. What has been done for this pain?

Typical answers: "I've tried everything, and nothing seems to work;" "I've seen my family doctor and he has prescribed medicines;" "I've tried to do stretches and take walks."

Various treatments, including medicines and therapies, usually have been tried before I first see a patient. Many patients may have found a fairly successful home program, but their fibromyalgia still flares up from time to time.

9. Do you have symptoms other than pain?

Typical answers: "Yes doctor, in fact I wrote things down so I wouldn't forget them. Where is my list? Here it is. I have fatigue, difficulty sleeping, irritable bowel syndrome, depression, anxiety, headaches, TMJ problems …"

Many symptoms and conditions associated with fibromyalgia contribute to the patient's pain or may interfere with the treatment and recovery. These associated conditions may require separate treatment approaches altogether in addition to the overall fibromyalgia treatments.

When giving their histories, patients may say one thing but they really mean something else. Sometimes I have to read deeper into what people are telling me. Let me share some examples of what you may say, and what you really mean!

What You Say . . .	What You Mean . . .
It's a terrible toothache.	My teeth are the only part of me that doesn't hurt.
I used to walk 3 miles a day.	It hurts me to drive 3 miles.
I used to have a photographic memory.	Doctor, my brain is out of film.
I used to go on vacations.	The only things that travel now are my pains.
Do you see many people with fibromyalgia?	I sure hope I don't know more about this condition than you do!

Patients may minimize their pain in a doctor's office. They may be embarrassed to admit it, or worry that the doctor may think it isn't real. Your pain is REAL, so tell us about it.

A detailed history of the pain and other symptoms of fibromyalgia enables the doctor to think about fibromyalgia as a possible diagnosis. The history is only part of the clinical exam, however, and not sufficient alone to diagnose fibromyalgia. The physical exam must be done and must be consistent with fibromyalgia.

Physical Exam

The purpose of the physical examination is to detect any abnormalities or patterns of abnormal changes that help the physician determine the diagnosis. An abnormality detected by a physician during the physical exam is called an objective finding. It is one that is verifiable and reproducible by the examining physician. It would also be found by another knowledgeable physician who examines the same patient.

Many patients will complain that previous doctors have examined them and found nothing wrong. They may have been told that their exam was normal, and this causes confusion and frustration because the patients are hurting, but the doctor is telling them that they are normal. The physical examination in the fibromyalgia patient is NOT normal. Fibromyalgia patients have characteristic abnormalities, particularly tender points.

Tender Points

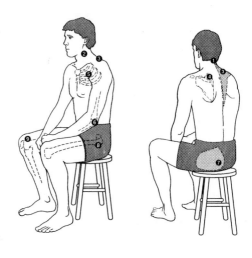

The main findings on physical examination are the tender points. Tender points are areas in the soft tissue (the muscles, tendons, and/or ligaments) that are very sensitive and painful when pressed. These tender points are found in distinct locations of the body. They do not move around and can be found in multiple locations of the body.

The presence of tender points is the main criterion used to identify fibromyalgia. According to a landmark study by the American College of Rheumatology published in 1990, fibromyalgia is diagnosed when an individual has a history of widespread pain present for at least 3 months, and at least 11 of 18 positive tender points in characteristic locations (see figures). The pain is considered widespread when all of the following are present: Pain is in both sides of the body, pain is above and below the waist, and pain is along the spine.

These are "signature" areas that distinguish individuals with fibromyalgia from those with chronic muscle pain from other causes. The 18 tender points are located in nine areas of the body, both sides, in pairs.

These signature areas include:

1. The occiput. This is in back of the head where the suboccipital muscles connect to the skull.

2. Low cervical muscle. This is along the neck muscle in front of the fifth, sixth, and seventh cervical vertebrae.

3. Trapezius muscle. This broad muscle extends from the neck to the shoulder. The tender point is in the mid point of the upper part of the muscle.

4. Supraspinatus muscle. This muscle is located at the top of the shoulder blade, and the tender point is located near the spine.

5. The second rib. This costochondral area is right below the collarbone.

6. Lateral epicondyle. This is located at the top of the forearm and is also called the "tennis elbow" area.

7. Outer gluteus maximus. This is the buttock muscle and should be painful in the upper outer portion.

8. Greater trochanter. This is part of the femur or thigh bone which has a knobby protrusion right below the hip joint, covered by a bursa (fluid-filled sac).

9. Medial knee. This painful area is right above the inside of the knee.

Positive Tender Point

A positive tender point is one that is painful upon palpation with enough pressure to cause my thumbnail to blanch (about 4 kilograms of force). Palpation is the art of using the sense of touch to feel for abnormalities. The tips of the fingers and thumb are the medical examiner's most sensitive "instruments" for examining the soft tissue for the presence of painful tender points. I prefer to use my thumb for palpating. The patient may indicate pain by saying "ouch" or grimacing, or by trying to withdraw and avoid the pressure. The area must hurt or be painful to be positive; it can't just be "tender."

While we are on the subject of tender points, I want to call to attention one of my pet peeves: the name "tender point." By definition, a tender point is positive when it is painful. If it is just tender, it is not a positive tender point. Why don't we call them painful points? I explain to my patients that sometimes things aren't logical! I call these areas painful tender points.

Painful tender points can be found in essentially any muscle, but usually are present in larger muscles such as the neck, shoulder, back and hips. Examining for painful tender points is a process of "mapping out" the soft tissues to determine where the painful areas are, both in the designated signature areas, and in areas that are painful, but not part of the designated 18 tender points. Mapping helps in the diagnosis of fibromyalgia and helps determine the response to treatments.

Fibronym:

Painstaking: The diligent care and effort taken when palpating and mapping out the painful tender points.

People with fibromyalgia are painful all over with palpation compared to someone without fibromyalgia. Indeed, studies have indicated that people with fibromyalgia are sensitive to painful stimuli throughout the body, not just in the American College of Rheumatology defined locations (Granges and Littlejohn, 1993). The tender points are more painful than "control" areas, or areas expected to be less sensitive or painful. Examples of control areas are the inside of the forearms, the front of the legs below the knees, and the back of the hands.

Many patients do not realize they have so much muscle pain until their muscles are palpated on exam. Painful tender points may not be spontaneously painful. "Latent" tender points are common, and they usually aren't so latent immediately after the exam! The spontaneously "active" tender points are what the patients notice and what ultimately brings them to the doctor.

The "11 of 18" criterion has been agreed upon for academic and research purposes to enable a consistent fibromyalgia diagnosis using a "gold standard." In the clinical setting, however, fewer tender points may be present and still indicate fibromyalgia (Wolfe, 1994). Indeed, many patients with fibromyalgia have fewer than 11 painful tender points in characteristic locations, but have other typical symptoms. If I find 10 of 18 painful tender points on someone with a typical history of fibromyalgia, I don't say, "You have nothing wrong with you!" I make the diagnosis of fibromyalgia if it best fits the overall exam.

I give newly diagnosed patients with fibromyalgia a tender point "scorecard." This bookmark scorecard contains a tender point diagram which I label accordingly for the patient and indicate a tender point score. This scorecard doesn't rank up there with the driver's license and Social Security card identifications, but may compete with the "Free car wash with a fill-up" coupon!

Tender point counts can differ from exam to exam on the same patient. It would not be unusual for someone to have 14 of 18 positive on the first exam, and on the follow-up exam a month later, 12 of 18 are positive. The pattern and numbers of tender points are important in the diagnosis, but the exact locations and total numbers are less important when following a patient over time. I map out the painful areas and document them. The patients may improve but still have the same number of positive tender points (or even more!). More tender points may have become "latent" with treatment instead of remaining "active," hence the overall improvement despite the same tender point count. The number of tender points does not correlate with the severity of the overall pain. People with 11 of 18 positive tender points can have worse pain that those who have all 18 points positive.

While we cannot compare tender points among different patients, we can look at the tender points in a given patient and correlate them to the severity of his/her pain. For example, someone whose tender point score decreased from 14 to 11 of 18 after treatment will usually report less pain overall. Individual tender point scores are more meaningful than scores for the entire population, especially when correlating responses to treatment.

Tender Point Exam Paradox

I often encounter a situation during examination of a patient for tender points which I call the tender point exam paradox. In this situation, the patient complains of pain all over and when I perform a detailed tender point exam, I find that the person reports pain everywhere palpated; that is, the whole body is a painful tender point.

I am unable to separate out distinct tender points in designated areas because soft tissues are equally painful everywhere. Technically I have not really isolated any specific tender points as defined by the American College of Rheumatology criteria since the entire body is painful.

The paradox is that even though the person may have fibromyalgia (with severe widespread pain, sensitive skin, and intolerance of any palpation), he/she is not able to meet the tender point criteria at the time of my exam. When this happens I'll explain to the patient how fibromyalgia can lead to widespread body sensitivity or cause chronic pain syndrome which accounts for the whole body pain upon exam. If chronic pain syndrome is present, I may recommend a different type of treatment program (see Chapter 27).

Regional Fibromyalgia

Many people have regional pain and clustering of painful tender points, that is, fewer than 11 of 18 designated ACR tender points. I believe that regional fibromyalgia is part of the fibromyalgia spectrum, and is essentially synonymous with a condition called myofascial pain syndrome. My own view is that the 11 of 18 tender points in the ACR criteria is an excellent diagnostic tool to be used as a guideline for generalized fibromyalgia, but there are many patients (including those with regional fibromyalgia) who have fewer than 11 painful tender points on a given examination date.

Trigger Points

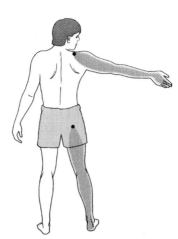

If pressing on a particularly painful tender area causes pain, numbness, or tingling to radiate or spread to another area, this spot is called a trigger point. A trigger point is another typical finding in patients with fibromyalgia and was first described by Dr. Janet Travell. If I were to press on an area in your mid-trapezius muscle and you felt numbness radiating down your entire right arm into the hand, that area in the trapezius muscle would be called a trigger point. It could also be a painful tender point as well.

These trigger points can cause confusion since they may mimic a pinched nerve. Rather, the trigger areas in the muscles are causing radiating symptoms to distant locations (see figure).

Trigger points arise from shared neurological links between seemingly unrelated body parts. These seemingly unrelated parts actually shared a common tissue during the body's early fetal development. After these tissues divided and formed specialized parts, a common sensory neurological link remained and could "communicate" (refer pain) in certain situations. For example, if a man is having a heart attack, he may experience numbness in the left arm. There is no problem with the left arm, per se. Rather, the heart muscle is being damaged, and because it has sensory connections to the left arm, it sends referred symptoms down the left arm. The injured heart muscle acts as a trigger point in this situation.

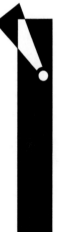

The human body has hundreds of potential trigger points. They can develop wherever fibromyalgia pain develops and are very common after trauma to muscles. Trigger points can cause numbness, headaches, dizziness, ringing in the ears, jaw pain, sciatica, and many other symptoms. If trigger points are spontaneously irritated, they may cause constant symptoms. If pressing on these trigger points during the exam causes them to be "activated," the physician may be able to reproduce some of the patient's subjective complaints such as referred pain and numbness. This valuable information can help distinguish between symptoms caused by a trigger point and those caused by a pinched nerve.

> **The human body has hundreds of potential trigger points. They can develop wherever fibromyalgia pain develops and are very common after trauma to muscles. Trigger points can cause numbness, headaches, dizziness, ringing in the ears, jaw pain, sciatica, and many other symptoms.**

Ropey muscles

What exactly do these tender points feel like? Fibromyalgia muscles have a peculiar consistency that feels like ropey bands or nodules. This band-like or ropey consistency is an important abnormal finding in fibromyalgia. Sometimes these taut ropey bands involve a larger area and form a fibromyalgia nodule, a firm lump that can be palpated within the muscle. This tightness, ropiness, or nodular consistency represents localized muscle spasms that can be detected with palpation by an experienced physician. These ropey muscle findings can vary in size depending on how much of the muscle is in a spasm. Usually the painful tender points will have palpable localized spasms.

Normal muscle has a texture of firm gelatin. Imagine that you take this firm gelatin and put in some grapes and strands of carrots and a couple chunks of pineapple, and when you palpate the gelatin fruit salad, you can imagine the lumpy, bumpy consistency (grapes and chunks) and ropey consistency (carrot strands). This is what the fibromyalgia muscles feel like.

Other Exam Findings

Other physical exam abnormalities can be present in fibromyalgia. These include:

1. **Dermatographism** (Latin for "skin writing"). Scratching with a finger along the skin will cause a red mark or rash to form in patients with dermatographism. This phenomenon is most pronounced in the skin overlying painful muscles. This is thought to be due to dysfunctional autonomic nerves that "overreact" to the pressure and cause a low grade skin irritation.

2. **Decreased skin sensation**. Light touch and pin prick sensations may be decreased in fibromyalgia patients. Affected body parts include hands, feet, arms, legs, and face. Only one side of the body may be affected. Patients still feel these sensations, but they are not "normal." This is felt to be caused by an autonomic nervous system dysfunction.

3. **Goosebumps.** This frequent finding is another result of a dysfunctional autonomic nervous system. These are usually noticed in the legs during the palpation of painful tender points, but can be seen in the arms also. These goose bumps are medically known as piloerections (this has nothing to do with Sex and Intimacy, Chapter 39).

4. **Decreased range of motion**. Still another physical exam abnormality is decreased joint range of motion due to painful, tense muscles. Full joint flexibility depends on the muscles' ability to relax and allow the joint to move. Tight painful muscles prevent the joints from moving freely through their range.

The physical examination of a person with fibromyalgia should NOT reveal the following abnormalities:

1. "True" weakness (from nerve damage)
2. Loss of reflexes
3. Joint swelling, heat, or inflammation
4. Atrophy or wasting of muscles
5. Abnormal muscle tone

If any of these physical findings are present, a condition in addition to, or other than, fibromyalgia must be present. I've mentioned various physical exam abnormalities in a person with fibromyalgia. The most important and meaningful findings are the painful tender points in characteristic locations. It is this abnormal pattern of painful tender points that enables doctors to objectively identify fibromyalgia.

In case you are wondering, I've found that some tender point locations are more commonly "positive" than others. Based on my experience, I award the top 2 tender point pairs to the trapezial and cervical areas. The least common 2 tender point pairs are the medial knee and costochondral areas. Many people achieve a perfect tender point score, 18 of 18 (remember we are perfectionists). I tell people that the tender point test is one test they don't want to ace! But most do, anyway! What is the most common tender point score? I would have to say, 14 of 18, which happens to be my score.

If You Want To Know More

1. Granges G, Littlejohn G. *Pressure pain threshold in pain-free subjects, in patients with chronic regional pain syndromes, and in patients with fibromyalgia syndrome.* Arthritis Rheum 1993; 36: 642–6.

2. Pellegrino MJ. *Inside fibromyalgia.* Columbus OH: Anadem Publishing, 2001.

3. Terval JG, Simons D. *Myofascial pain and dysfunction: the trigger point manual.* Vol. I, Lippincott, Williams & Wilkins, 1983.

4. Wolfe F, Smythe HA, Yunus MB, et al. *The American College of Rheumatology 1990 Criteria for the Classification of Fibromyalgia. Report of the Multicenter Criteria Committee.* Arthritis Rheum 1990; 33: 160–72.

5. Wolfe F. *When to diagnose fibromyalgia.* Rheum Dis Clin N Am 1994; 20: 485–501.

Diagnostic Testing In Fibromyalgia

You would expect a condition that is so painful and causes so many symptoms and associated conditions to have numerous abnormal lab tests and X-rays, right? Well, the answer is: not really. We know that a lot of measurable abnormalities are present in fibromyalgia, but no single lab test or X-ray is considered diagnostic. In fact, routine labs and other tests are usually normal. There are specialized tests in which fibromyalgia patients may test positive, but these tests are not considered routine, nor are they positive in all patients with fibromyalgia.

In the last chapter, I described objective tender point abnormalities in a typical pattern that were characteristic findings in fibromyalgia, the 11 of 18 painful tender points. These tender points are found through physical examination, not laboratory tests or X-rays. If characteristic tender points are present on exam in a patient with widespread muscle pain for more than 3 months duration, fibromyalgia is fairly straightforward. Few conditions cause chronic widespread muscle pain as fibromyalgia does. But numerous conditions cause overlapping symptoms and can mimic fibromyalgia. Examples of these conditions include polymyalgia rheumatica, rheumatoid arthritis, lupus, hypothyroidism, myopathy, osteoarthritis, multiple sclerosis, mononucleosis, blood disorders, and more. Other times, fibromyalgia coexists with one of these other conditions, either being "caused" by this other condition or coincidentally present along with this other condition. Many conditions mimicking fibromyalgia can be ruled out by a careful history and physical examination. Certain specialized laboratory and other types of testing may be helpful also.

Although many lab tests are normal in fibromyalgia, this does not mean nothing is wrong. A normal test result simply means the particular test did not detect any abnormality. If an X-ray, a test to look at bones, is normal, it does not mean that fibromyalgia is not present. Rather, it means the X-ray of the bones was normal. Likewise, an abnormal test does not necessarily mean a particular condition is present. Your doctor has to correlate this test abnormality with your clinical examination. For example, if a magnetic resonance image (MRI) of the brain shows abnormal white spots suggesting multiple sclerosis, but the person has a completely normal neurologic examination and no symptoms whatsoever, the doctor would not diagnose multiple sclerosis without more evidence.

Any diagnostic test in medicine has its limitations. Each test measures something specific; it may detect something, quantify something, or observe something. Depending on what test is being done and what is being measured, the physician might be able to make certain diagnoses or rule them out. Physicians, however, cannot rule out a diagnosis based on a particular test if the test is not "measuring" that particular diagnosis. In other words, a blood sugar lab test won't show a broken bone.

A common example of a false positive in fibromyalgia is a positive ANA (antinuclear antigen), which is a screen for lupus. Many people with fibromyalgia have a positive or elevated ANA result, yet they do not have the clinical disease of lupus.

Another concept to understand with medical testing is that not everyone with a particular disease will test "abnormal" for it and, conversely, some normal people without the disease will test "positive" for it. When an individual has a disease but tests normal, we call this test a false negative, which means it should have tested positive. When a test is positive, but the person really doesn't have the disease that is being tested, we call this test a false positive, which means it should have tested negative.

A common example of a false positive in fibromyalgia is a positive ANA (antinuclear antigen), which is a screen for lupus. Many people with fibromyalgia have a positive or elevated ANA result, yet they do not have the clinical disease of lupus. In these people, the high ANA is a false positive. Most of you will tell me you have had a billion tests done before your diagnosis of fibromyalgia was made. Many times you go to another doctor and proceed to have yet another billion tests done. The results are always the same: normal! You just happen to have fibromyalgia, and various lab studies, electrical studies, X-rays and other radiographic imaging are normal because these tests look for other conditions which you don't have.

I've written a brief review of some common categories of testing that may be done to evaluate the cause of your pain or to rule out specific conditions other than fibromyalgia. Some tests are very expensive, others are invasive. In fibromyalgia, various tests can show abnormalities. Certain laboratory studies, specialized radiographic studies, and some electrical studies can be abnormal but are not necessary to diagnose fibromyalgia. These specialized tests are not routinely done for fibromyalgia, because they are more often used in research centers. The following is a summary of some of these tests. You and your doctor need to decide what testing may be needed, if any. Don't assume that any test abnormalities are due to fibromyalgia or some serious problem. Your doctor will guide you through the test results.

Laboratory Tests

In patients with persistent pain, laboratory studies are often done to look for any abnormalities in the body's electrolytes, muscle enzymes, bone enzymes, or other areas that might provide clues to the source of pain. Useful laboratory screening tests include erythrocyte sedimentation rate, serum creatinine kinase, complete blood count, thyroid function tests, and perhaps tests for rheumatoid factor and antinuclear antibody (Goldenberg 1987). If a patient has true muscle inflammation (not from fibromyalgia), the sedimentation rate might be elevated. If the patient has anemia, the hemoglobin and hematocrit on the complete blood count might be low. There are hundreds of lab tests that measure the body's major functions, but your physician will select the ones that will give the most useful information for your particular problem.

I usually order screening lab tests in patients who have not had any recent blood work if I suspect fibromyalgia. Remember, some people can also have another condition present that is causing fibromyalgia, and the clinical exam is revealing "only" the fibromyalgia.

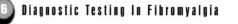

Routine Screening Lab Tests:

> **Complete blood count with differential and platelets**. This checks for anemia, abnormal white blood counts, or platelet abnormalities that could signal a blood disorder, a bone marrow problem, iron deficiency, and more.

> **Sedimentation rate**. This is considered a nonspecific marker for inflammation. If it is high, additional testing might be necessary to look for conditions such as rheumatoid arthritis, lupus, or myositis.

> **Thyroid function studies**. These measures for abnormal thyroid problems, such as hypothyroidism or hyperthyroidism, and can also determine if the person has "relatively" low levels of thyroid although still within the normal range.

Certain laboratory studies have been found to be abnormal in fibromyalgia. These tests are not considered "routine" labs, but specialized labs. Here is a summary of these labs.

Serotonin

Serotonin is a neurotransmitter and a hormone. It is important in the brain's ability to control pain, maintain an upbeat mood or outlook, be motivated, and concentrate on a task. It has been described as the "brightness switch" of the brain, and a low serotonin level is equivalent to turning down the brightness switch on your brain's TV.

Serotonin is usually low in patients with fibromyalgia. One place that serotonin is stored is in the platelets of the blood, and Dr. I. Jon Russell discovered that serotonin storage in the platelets of fibromyalgia patients is low compared to normal people. Low serotonin is also closely related to clinical depression, so it is not surprising that many people with fibromyalgia will also have clinical depression at some time during the course of their syndrome.

Substance P

This is a small protein neurotransmitter that is found mainly in the spinal column. It has several purposes; one is the transmission of pain signals (think P for pain). Substance P can also help block pain signals. It is not unusual for neurotransmitters (small proteins) to perform different, seemingly opposite functions. One portion of the substance P molecule produces pain while another blocks the pain sensation and controls its severity.

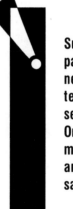

Substance P can also help block pain signals. It is not unusual for neurotransmitters (small proteins) to perform different, seemingly opposite functions. One portion of the substance P molecule produces pain while another blocks the pain sensation and controls its severity.

Dr. Russell has also discovered that substance P is significantly high in the spinal cord fluid of patients with fibromyalgia, and because fibromyalgia causes so much pain this likely means that the "bad" function of substance P is overriding the good.

Nerve growth factor (NGF)

NGF is another small protein that causes the growth and repair of nerves. Researchers found that NGF in spinal fluid of fibromyalgia patients is significantly elevated compared to normal people (*J Rheumatol*, 1999). Excesses of NGF are probably contributing to pain, perhaps causing hypersensitization of the nerves.

The regeneration (growth/repair) of nerves is actually a painful process. For example, patients who have had nerve trauma or spinal cord injury will often experience severe burning, tingling type pain that corresponds to the attempted regeneration of the nerves. NGF may be producing this type of pain in people with fibromyalgia even though there has been no obvious nerve injury.

Neuropeptide Y

This small protein is a breakdown product of the hormone norepinephrine, a primary brain hormone. Levels of neuropeptide Y are found to be low in patients with fibromyalgia, particularly when a stress, such as the tilt-table test described later in this chapter, is applied to the autonomic nervous system. This finding suggests that the autonomic nervous system is dysfunctional, particularly when it is stressed. Among other things, this dysfunction causes low blood pressure, fast heart rate, and anxiety.

Growth hormone

The "master" hormone in the body is growth hormone, secreted by the pituitary gland. Growth hormone's many functions include buildup of proteins, breakdown of fatty tissues, and enhanced metabolism. In the blood stream, growth hormone breaks down to various particles. One of them is IGF 1 (insulin-like growth factor 1). Dr. Bennett has been researching growth hormone in patients with fibromyalgia and has found that the IGF 1 levels (and hence growth hormone levels) are low in many patients. Low growth hormone may contribute to various fibromyalgia symptoms including fatigue, feeling cold, and lack of motivation.

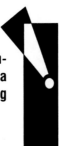

Low growth hormone may contribute to various fibromyalgia symptoms including fatigue, feeling cold, and lack of motivation.

Thyroid antibodies

Thyroid studies, as previously mentioned, are usually normal in patients with fibromyalgia. A number of people with underactive thyroid or relatively low functioning thyroid may have thyroid labs that are normal (false negative lab results). Looking at the microsomal thyroid antibodies may provide an additional clue as to whether there is a condition known as autoimmune thyroiditis. Dr. Arflott Bruusgaard performed a study that found 16% of people with fibromyalgia have positive thyroid antibodies. Does this mean that these people have a thyroid problem in addition to fibromyalgia? Remember, fibromyalgia has many subsets, and one may cause thyroid problems that need specific treatment.

Cortisol

This hormone is our natural steroid hormone secreted in response to stress. Different researchers have found that the adrenal glands in people with fibromyalgia produce less cortisol than normal. Having fibromyalgia and its associated elevated stress may ultimately wear down our stress response mechanisms to the point where our adrenal glands have a hard time producing enough cortisol. Too little cortisol means an inability to handle the body's stresses well, causing us to be at risk for infection, fatigue, and anxiety.

Magnesium

Magnesium is a mineral that plays a major role in key body functions. A primary role of magnesium is to help the muscles manufacture energy molecules known as ATP. Dr. Thomas Romano performed a study that found low magnesium levels in the muscles of patients with fibromyalgia. Measurement of the total body magnesium level is usually within the normal range, but selectively deficient in muscles, probably reducing the muscles' energy metabolism abilities and increasing their pain and spasm. When muscles relax, they require energy (ATP). Muscle relaxation is an active, not passive, process. Anything that decreases ATP in the muscles will decrease the muscles' ability to relax, and thus, increase muscle spasms. Measuring red blood cell levels of magnesium as opposed to serum magnesium gives a better reading of intracellular magnesium level (inside the cells, including muscles). Serum magnesium levels measure extra cellular magnesium (in the blood and serum).

Antipolymer antibody (APA)

Antipolymer antibodies are complex proteins that were first discovered in the blood of some women who had silicone breast implants (Dr. Tenenbaum's research). The APA is thought to be a marker for an immunological response and has been found to be high in a subset of patients with fibromyalgia. A study by Dr. Russell Wilson, *et al.*, found that 61% of people with severe fibromyalgia had positive APA reactivity, and 30% of those with mild fibromyalgia had increased APA. The APA reactivity may someday have a role as a laboratory marker in the diagnosis and assessment of certain types of fibromyalgia.

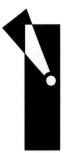

A recent study…found that 61% of people with severe fibromyalgia had positive APA reactivity, and 30% of those with mild fibromyalgia had increased APA.

Vitamin B$_{12}$ level

If fatigue, numbness, and tingling are problems, I frequently order this test to make sure it is not low, as Vitamin B$_{12}$ deficiency can cause these symptoms. I find many people with fibromyalgia have a "low normal" B$_{12}$ level; that is, it is still within the normal range but at the lower end.

Radiographic Imaging Tests

X-rays

X-rays are pictures that tell us whether the bones have normal density, whether there is a fracture, whether the bones are in proper position, or whether any bony diseases are present. X-rays do not "see" muscles or discs. There may be abnormal positioning of the bones on the X-ray that gives us clues that something has occurred in the soft tissues such as the muscles, ligaments, or discs. An example is a cervical spine X-ray taken shortly after a whiplash injury that shows "straightening." A normal cervical spine has a curvature called a lordosis. If a whiplash has occurred and spasms have resulted, the cervical spine may tighten up. X-rays may show a straightening or a reversal of the normal cervical lordosis.

Often X-rays will show "incidental" abnormalities such as some arthritis changes, disc deterioration, or calcifications. However, X-rays of anyone over the age of 29 will show bony changes from wear and tear, especially in weight bearing bones (spine, knees, and hips). We must not misinterpret these X-ray changes, particularly normal aging changes, as the "cause" of the pain. Normal aging changes are usually not painful.

Sometimes the X-rays reveal conditions such as osteoarthritis, osteoporosis, scoliosis, or calcified tendons, that indicate something else is present in addition to, or instead of, fibromyalgia.

Computerized tomography (CAT scan)

A CAT scanner uses thousands of small X-ray beams to take picture "slices" of the part being tested. A computer generates an image that combines all these slices to form a "whole" picture of that body part. This picture can show brain white and gray matter, blood, ruptured discs, fractured bones, and more. A CAT scan can be taken of the head to look for a brain hemorrhage, for example, after a concussion. It can evaluate the spine for any ruptured or herniated disc. In fibromyalgia, the CAT scan is almost always normal. If it is abnormal, something else is present.

Bone scan

This specialized imaging study uses labeled calcium particles injected into the patient's blood stream. These particles are taken up by the bone. If the bone is inflamed in a particular area, more of these particles will accumulate there and show up as a "hot spot." Although we feel as if our muscles have a bunch of "hot spots," our bone scans are usually normal.

Myelogram

A myelogram is performed when a dye is injected into the spinal column in the low back. The dye fills up the spinal fluid spaces that surround the spinal cord and nerve roots, and when an X-ray picture is taken, the dye shows up on the film and gives an anatomical view of the spinal cord and nerve roots. Any abnormality within the spaces, particularly a protruding or herniated disc, can be detected. A myelogram can also detect severe narrowing of the spinal column called spinal stenosis.

The myelogram is no fun at all, and in patients with fibromyalgia, it is usually normal. Some fibromyalgia patients have been found to have narrowing of their cervical spinal column, called cervical spinal stenosis.

Cervical CAT scan and myelogram

A subgroup of people with fibromyalgia was found to have a higher incidence of cervical spinal stenosis (narrowing of the cervical spinal canal) and Arnold-Chiari malformation (birth defect where the lower part of the brain protrudes into the cervical spinal canal). Many of these conditions don't cause any noticeable symptoms. This stenosis can cause compression of the cervical spinal cord and perhaps contribute to the neck and shoulder pain of fibromyalgia. Some patients have noted improvement in their fibromyalgia symptoms following surgery to relieve spinal stenosis problems. Cervical cord compression in fibromyalgia needs to be studied further.

SPECT scan

This is a specialized imaging of the brain. SPECT stands for Single Photon Emission Computerized Tomography and examines brain function by measuring brain blood flow. Drs. James Mountz and Laurence Bradley have identified abnormalities in patients with fibromyalgia. Specific parts of the brain that process pain, the thalamus and caudate nucleus, have shown decreased blood flow on the SPECT scan. If these parts of the brain do not function well, the result may be more pain. This research may lead to a better understanding of the brain's role in inhibiting pain.

Positron emission tomography (PET)

A PET scan can be another sensitive test for pinpointing brain abnormalities by measuring the rate of glucose metabolism. Glucose metabolism correlates with the activity of a cell. Active cells use glucose as food, and active cells are functioning cells.

An injection of a tracer glucose is given to the patient, and after thirty minutes or more, the PET scan is taken to study the glucose metabolism in different regions of the brain. Dr. J.C. Hsieh coordinated a study of PET scanning in patients with fibromyalgia and found increased glucose activity in specific parts of the brain, namely the anterior cingulate cortex.

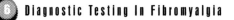

Magnetic resonance imaging (MRI)

This specialized imaging is accomplished by placing the patient in a powerful magnetic field, then beaming radio waves into the field, which causes tissue particles to orient themselves in a specific pattern in the magnetic field. The images generated by the MRI machines are remarkably sharp and give detailed pictures of the anatomy of the spine, soft tissues, and organs, depending on what part is being scanned.

This testing is a valuable tool in the diagnosis of tumors, disc herniations, and ligament tears. In fibromyalgia the routine MRIs are usually completely normal. However, a study using a super fast form of MRI, called functional MRI (or fMRI) confirmed what we always knew—we have real pain. Two researchers, Dr. Richard Gracely and Dr. Daniel Clauw, published a study in the May 2002 issue of *Arthritis and Rheumatism*.

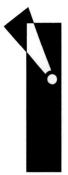

In fibromyalgia the routine MRIs are usually completely normal. However, a study using a super fast form of MRI, called functional MRI (or fMRI) confirmed what we always knew— we have real pain.

In the study, 60 fibromyalgia patients and 60 without the disease underwent fMRI to see if any measurable differences were found in response to painful signals from applied pressure to the subject's thumbnail.

The fibromyalgia patients reported pain with mild pressure, while the control subjects reported little pain with the same pressure. The fibromyalgia patients had more areas of their brain "light up" on the fMRI when they felt pain compared to the control subjects. Furthermore, some areas of the fibromyalgia brains stayed "quiet" while the same areas in the controls became active.

This "illuminating" study suggests that fibromyalgia patients have enhanced responses to pain in some brain regions and diminished or inhibitive responses in other regions. This study offers the first objective method for collaborating the pain reported by those with fibromyalgia, and supports the notion of neurobiological amplification of pain signals. This study also suggests that brain inhibition of pain may be turned off in fibromyalgia, as evidenced by the "quiet" areas in fibromyalgia patients. Without normal pain inhibition, pain signals can amplify unchecked and not be blocked.

Electrical Studies

Whereas laboratory studies measure the presence and quantity of a particular unit and X-rays show the bone anatomy, electrical studies measure the function of certain body organs. Persons with chronic or persistent pain may undergo various electrical studies to look for any measurable functional abnormality.

Electroencephalogram (EEG)

In the waking individual with fibromyalgia, who has various electrodes attached to the scalp and hooked to a machine that measures electrical currents and activities of the brain's nerves, this testing will be normal. Even with a severe, splitting headache, the EEG should be normal, since headaches usually do not cause changes in our brain waves. The EEG can detect seizures or damage to the brain, neither of which is part of fibromyalgia.

Dr. Stuart Donaldson in Canada did a research study looking at EEGs in patients with fibromyalgia after a trauma. He found an increase in the low frequency brain waves (the theta waves) in these patients. This increase in theta activity means the brain is functioning in a "slow" mode and may

In fibromyalgia, many people will demonstrate a characteristic sleep abnormality where the deep part of sleep, stage IV sleep, is abnormal.

explain some of our fibrofog. This testing may help clarify how the pain causes the brain's electrical patterns to change.

Another EEG test, the sleep study, measures brain activity during various sleep cycles. In fibromyalgia, many people will demonstrate a characteristic sleep abnormality where the deep part of sleep, stage IV sleep, is abnormal. Dr. Harvey Moldofsky has done the important pioneer research studies on these types of abnormalities in fibromyalgia.

Electromyelogram (EMG)

This specialized test measures the function of nerves and muscles. Since people with fibromyalgia often have numbness and weakness, this test is commonly performed to look for any nerve irritation. Small electrical shocks resembling static shocks are given to stimulate the nerves and record the function. A needle electrode is inserted into different muscles to measure if they are working properly. Electrodiagnostic testing can help identify certain problems such as a radiculopathy, carpal tunnel syndrome, neuropathy, or myopathy.

Unless a person with fibromyalgia has one of these conditions, the electrodiagnostic testing will be normal. Many people with fibromyalgia can also get carpal tunnel syndrome, which is very common. However, fibromyalgia does NOT cause carpal tunnel syndrome, nor does it cause any typical electrodiagnostic abnormality.

Electrocardiogram (EKG or ECG)

This test measures the electrical function of the heart and may be ordered in individuals with chest pain. Chest pain is common in fibromyalgia, but EKGs are usually normal because the chest pain is not due to cardiac muscle or heart involvement. Rather, the chest and rib muscles and the soft tissues around the ribs are the usual source of the pain.

Tilt-table testing

This testing is one way to investigate the autonomic nerve function in people with fibromyalgia. The autonomic nerves control blood pressure and heart rhythm, and tilt-table testing involves monitoring blood pressure, pulse, and the EKG.

An individual having a tilt-table test lies down flat on a table and is monitored. The table is then slowly tilted up and the blood pressure, pulse, and EKG are continuously monitored for any changes. In people with fibromyalgia, about 25% have a significant drop in blood pressure and an increase in pulse rate. These abnormalities are felt to represent dysfunctional sympathetic nervous system activity causing inability to respond to stress. In the case of the tilt-table, the stress is gravity acting upon the body.

Tilt-table testing is abnormal in many with chronic fatigue syndrome as well. Dr. J.E. Naschitz published a recent study in which he performed a head-up tilt-table test of forty persons with chronic fatigue syndrome. He found a distinct hemodynamic instability score (a measure of blood pressure and heart rate change in tilt test) and the results of these with chronic fatigue syndrome may differ from those with fibromyalgia taking the same test. There seems to be a distinctive dysautonomia (or dysfunctional autonomic nerves) in chronic fatigue syndrome that is different from other conditions causing fatigue, even fibromyalgia, according to Dr. Naschitz. Chronic fatigue syndrome may be separate from fibromyalgia or a measurably different subset within fibromyalgia.

Summary Of Testing

Many tests have shown some abnormalities in people with fibromyalgia. I have not mentioned every test. Ongoing studies are showing additional abnormalities and giving us some clues as to the pathology of fibromyalgia. Functional MRIs may provide an exciting tool to further clarify the abnormal neurobiology in fibromyalgia. Some additional research is discussed in Section II: Understanding Fibromyalgia. With ongoing research, we may some day see a specific test that is accepted as a good marker for fibromyalgia and is readily available and not cost prohibitive. Such a test does not exist at this time.

If You Want To Know More

1. Giovengo SL, Russell IJ, Larson AA. *Increased concentrations of nerve growth factor in cerebrospinal fluid of patients with fibromyalgia.* J Rheumatol 1999; 26: 1564–9.

2. Gracely RH, Petzke F, Wolf JM, et al. *Functional magnetic resonance imaging evidence of augmented pain processing in fibromyalgia.* Arthritis Rheum 2002; 46 (5): 1333–43.

3. Hsieh JC, Belfrage M, Stone-Elander S, et al. *Central representation of chronic ongoing neuropathic pain studied by positron emission tomography.* Pain 1995; 63(2): 225–36.

4. Milhorat TH, Chou MW, Trinidad EM, et al. *Chiari I malformation redefined: clinical and radiographic findings for 364 symptomatic patients.* Neurosurg 1999; 44(5): 1005–17.

5. Moldofsky H. *Sleep and fibrositis syndrome.* Rheum Dis Clin N Am 1989; 15: 91–103.

6. Mountz JM, Bradley LA, Alarcon GS. *Abnormal functional activity of the central nervous system in fibromyalgia syndrome.* Am J Med Sci 1998; 315: 385–96.

7. Naschitz JE, Rosner I, Rozenbaum M, et al. *The head-up tilt test with hemodynamic instability score in diagnosing chronic fatigue syndrome.* Q J Med 2003; 96: 133–42.

8. Petzke F, Clauw DJ. *Sympathetic nervous system function in fibromyalgia.* Curr Rheumatol Rep 2000; 2(2):116–23.

9. Romano TJ. *Serum magnesium levels may not indicate low tissue magnesium levels.* Arch Int Med 1997; 157: 460.

10. Rosner MJ. *Decompression of craniovertebral stenosis leads to improvement in FMS and CFIDS symptoms.* New Dimensions in Fibromyalgia Symposium, Portland, Oregon, September 1997, http://www.nfra.net/Stenos3.htm

11. Russell IJ, Orr MD, Littman B, et al. *Elevated cerebrospinal levels of substance P in patients with the fibromyalgia syndrome.* Arthritis Rheum 1994; 37: 1593–601.

12. Tenenbaum, SA, Rice, JC, Espinoza, LR, et al. *Antipolymer antibodies, silicone breast implants, and fibromyalgia.* Lancet 1997; 349: 1172–3.

13. Wilson RB, Gluck OS, Tesser JR, et al. *Antipolymer antibody reactivity in a subset of patients with fibromyalgia correlates with severity.* J Rheumatol 1999; 26: 402–7.

14. Wolfe F, Russell IJ, Vipraio G, et al. *Serotonin levels, pain threshold, and fibromyalgia symptoms in the general population.* J Rheumatol 1997; 24: 555-9.

Who Diagnoses Fibromyalgia?

Official Diagnosis

Fibronym:

Expert: Someone who doesn't know any more than you do about fibromyalgia, but uses slides.

Fibromyalgia is an "official" diagnosis which must be made by a doctor. Examples of qualified doctors include M.D.'s (Medical Doctors), D.O.'s (Osteopathic Doctors), D.C.'s (Chiropractors), or N.D.'s (Naturopathic Doctors). According to the Medical/Legal Guidelines of the Medical Practice Acts, only qualified or licensed doctors can render a medical diagnosis.

Due to their education, training, and experience, certain medical specialists, particularly rheumatologists and physiatrists (a specialist in Physical Medicine and Rehabilitation), have particular expertise in diagnosing and treating musculoskeletal problems such as fibromyalgia. A rheumatologist is a specialist in rheumatic conditions, which include a variety of disorders (such as arthritis, lupus, and gout) characterized by inflammation, degeneration, or derangement of connective tissue structures in the body, especially joints, muscles, bursa, tendons, and fibrous tissues. A physiatrist (pronounced fiz-e-AH-trist) is a specialist who deals with the diagnosis, treatment, and prevention of conditions causing pain, weakness, and functional impairment like injuries, stroke, and paraplegia. Both of these specialty programs require additional years of residency training, usually 4 years, after medical school is completed.

Much of today's research and literature refers to a rheumatologist as the main specialist treating fibromyalgia. I certainly recognize and appreciate the work the rheumatologists have done on fibromyalgia over the years, but as a physiatrist myself, I will be naturally biased and say that my field is uniquely trained and suited in the diagnosis and treatment of fibromyalgia (see Chapter 13).

One does not have to be a specialist in Rheumatology or Physical Medicine and Rehabilitation to diagnose and treat fibromyalgia. There are many knowledgeable physicians who are interested in working with fibromyalgia patients. In fact, I work with many primary care physicians, (*i.e.*, family practitioners and internists) who may have diagnosed fibromyalgia themselves or suspect it and have referred patients to me for further evaluation and recommendations. I think it is important for every patient to have a primary care doctor who is willing to work with her or him in treating this condition.

I also see many patients who refer themselves to me. They may have read about symptoms of fibromyalgia and feel it fits them and want confirmation or additional evaluation by a specialist. It is not surprising for patients to tell me on their first visit that they were talking to a sister, an aunt, a bank teller, a hairdresser, or a co-worker's nephew's fiancée who said they sound like they have fibromyalgia and should get checked out!

Many people have said they read my handout or book or something on fibromyalgia, and it was like reading about their life. They are convinced that they have fibromyalgia even before their evaluation because they read about it and it fits them, and they are usually right. I consider the "read-and-fit" test to be a diagnostic test!

There are many non-physician medical professionals who are knowledgeable and experienced in fibromyalgia, including physical therapists, massotherapists, and nutritionists. Many patients who have been diagnosed with fibromyalgia were first directed to their physician by one of these medical professionals who suspected fibromyalgia. A person "enters the books" when he or she goes to a doctor and receives the official diagnosis of fibromyalgia.

One does not have to be a specialist in Rheumatology or Physical Medicine and Rehabilitation to diagnose and treat fibromyalgia. There are many knowledgeable physicians who are interested in working with fibromyalgia patients.

You need an "official" diagnosis, as your pain could be caused by a number of conditions other than fibromyalgia. Diagnosing yourself isn't wise; make sure you see a qualified doctor. Your doctor can determine what tests may be needed to rule out other conditions. I've seen many people who thought they had fibromyalgia but turned out to have something else. You can't pick up a pamphlet and make an official diagnosis on yourself.

Undiagnosed Fibromyalgia

Many people have fibromyalgia but have not been diagnosed yet. It is like the proverbial saying, "if a tree falls in a forest and no one is around to hear it, does it make a sound?" In fibromyalgia talk, it is saying "if someone has symptoms of fibromyalgia and tender points, but no doctor has actually examined the person and made the diagnosis, does this person have fibromyalgia?"

The answer is yes. That person has undiagnosed fibromyalgia (this sounds like an oxymoron). Doctors wait for people to come to us with symptoms before making a diagnosis. That is the nature of our work. It would be pretty silly if we went door-to-door asking people if they had any medical problems that they would like treated today. Only the people who seek out medical attention for their symptoms can be diagnosed with fibromyalgia.

However, if we go out into the community, for example, when we perform research projects or studies, we will find fibromyalgia in people who have never gone to the doctor. Or we may find people who have been diagnosed with another problem, but they really have fibromyalgia. Fibromyalgia is probably more like an iceberg, with the tip representing the ones who go to doctors for diagnosis and treatment.

729.1

The medical organization has a code for every medical condition. This allows a standard means of classifying, indexing, and communicating conditions among health providers including the insurance industry. The current industry standard for classifying medical conditions is the ICD-9 system which stands for the International Classification of Diseases, ninth revision. The World Health Organization developed the official version. Any recognized condition from Acne to Zoster has a number. If you're in the book, you are a condition! The number 729.1 of the ICD-9 classification is fibromyalgia. It's officially in the book!

As I mentioned earlier, fibromyalgia is recognized worldwide, not just by the insurance industry. The American Medical Association, the World Health Organization, the Bureau of Workers' Compensation, Medicare and Social Security, the court system, the Centers For Disease Control, as well as millions of patients and their health care providers worldwide have all formally accepted fibromyalgia as a valid painful medical condition with specific diagnostic criteria. Not every doctor diagnoses and treats fibromyalgia however, so you need to find a doctor who can help you.

Finding A Doctor

How does one find a doctor who understands fibromyalgia and is willing to treat it? Your doctor should be understanding, knowledgeable, and willing to learn. He or she should be eager to work with you and be open-minded, and also be willing to work with other medical professionals.

Patients have told me how they go about finding these doctors.

1. **Trial and error**. Unfortunately, many patients have had to see a number of doctors before finding one who would work with them. This effort is certainly time consuming, costly, and inefficient, but those who have gone this route are certainly wiser in the end, even if they still hurt!

2. **Word of mouth**. If a friend or family member can put in a good word, your odds of finding a good doctor increase.

3. **References**. Various physician reference agencies are available in your community either through medical organizations or state and local medical societies. These organizations would have names of specialists in Rheumatology or Physical Medicine and Rehabilitation.

4. **Fibromyalgia newsletters and databases on the Internet** have the names of physicians who are interested in treating fibromyalgia, and have been "verified" by patients who have seen these doctors. This technique is a more formalized "word-of-mouth" approach.

5. **Self-research**. Call and ask doctors if they see patients with fibromyalgia, if they are comfortable with treating patients with fibromyalgia, and if they accept patients with

fibromyalgia and prescribe treatments. You will not likely talk to the doctor himself or herself for this phone interview, but the staff should be very knowledgeable and helpful in getting answers to your questions.

6. **Referral from your primary care doctor**. Perhaps the ideal situation is to have your primary care doctor, whom you trust, make a referral to someone who knows and understands fibromyalgia. If your primary care doctor is agreeable, he/she would appreciate the additional input. This technique ensures that your primary care doctor will continue to be an informed team player in your attempts to optimize fibromyalgia treatments. Sometimes traveling longer distances may be necessary to see a specialist, and it may not be practical for you to follow-up with a specialist on a frequent basis due to the long distance. Following up with your primary care doctor who works closely with your specialist would be an ideal and practical situation.

7. **Networking with other patients**. You can meet them at a local support group, a lecture, a course on fibromyalgia, a health food store, and just about anywhere else! People who have fibromyalgia are everywhere and they love to talk.

Not Everybody Diagnoses Fibromyalgia

There are many doctors, including rheumatologists and physiatrists, who want nothing to do with fibromyalgia. Working with chronic pain patients can be demanding and challenging. Some physicians do not feel comfortable or talented in this area. Their strengths may lie in treating acute problems or in research. It is better that they recognize that aspect of their personality and let it be known they choose not to see these patients.

But, for whatever reason, some physicians choose to go beyond that. Instead of quietly refusing to see patients with fibromyalgia, they feel it necessary to voice negative opinions regarding fibromyalgia. Examples of these opinions/statements include:

1. Fibromyalgia simply does not exist.

2. Fibromyalgia is a wastebasket diagnosis used when you don't know what else is wrong.

3. Fibromyalgia is basically a name for depressed ladies with pain.

4. Fibromyalgia is overblown and out of control.

Remember, these statements are made by physicians who have no experience in treating fibromyalgia (because they won't see anybody with it!). Yet they choose to make statements about fibromyalgia under the guise of medical credibility! However, everyone has a right to his or her opinion. You have a right to find a doctor who believes you and wants to help you.

Ultimately, the doctors who are willing to work with you to treat your fibromyalgia have at least one thing in common: they respect your condition, and they respect you. By getting a proper diagnosis of a legitimate condition from a trained physician, you are being validated, and you are being treated with respect.

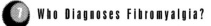

Top Ten Responses When a Doctor Says Fibromyalgia Doesn't Exist

1. I'm sorry, I CAN'T HEAR YOU!

2. Let me tell you 729.1 reasons why it does.

3. Hey, your shoelaces are untied.

4. Are you talking to me? Are you talking to ME?

5. I must insist it does exist.

6. Did someone say something; I can't see anyone?

7. And your opinion doesn't exist either.

8. Sure it does; it lives in the real world where real doctors see it everyday.

9. And I believe you from the bottom of my 18th tender point.

10. I guess the rest of the world is wrong then; thanks for enlightening me.

Putting It All Together

Fibromyalgia can be difficult to diagnose by a doctor not familiar with this condition. Many of the symptoms of fibromyalgia mimic those of other disorders such as hypothyroidism, inflammatory diseases, multiple sclerosis, and arthritis. Plus, those with fibromyalgia can have other conditions in addition to the fibromyalgia. Diagnostic confusion can result.

The person with fibromyalgia will describe a typical history, one filled with chronic widespread pain. The pain may have been localized at first, and may have been triggered by an injury or illness. The pain never disappeared over time, but rather worsened and became widespread. In addition to pain, numerous other symptoms such as poor sleep, fatigue, headache, and fibrofog may be present.

As discussed in Chapter 5, the key finding on physical exam is the painful tender point. A trained doctor can palpate the abnormal areas and find these tender points. When at least 11 of 18 painful tender points are present, one is said to meet the American College of Rheumatology-defined criteria for fibromyalgia.

People can have fibromyalgia with fewer than 18 positive tender points if they have typical symptoms, and the examining doctor feels the overall clinical picture is consistent with fibromyalgia. Regardless of what preceded the patient's visit to the doctor, if the symptoms and clinical exam fit, the diagnosis of fibromyalgia can be made.

As I've emphasized, fibromyalgia is not a diagnosis that is made by performing some specialized test. Nor is it a diagnosis that cannot be made if there is no specialized test to detect it. Diagnostic tests such as laboratory studies, X-rays, or electrical studies are not necessary to make a diagnosis of fibromyalgia. There are various test abnormalities present in fibromyalgia, but there is no single lab test that indicates fibromyalgia 100% of the time. The key diagnostic test remains the physical exam finding of the painful tender points.

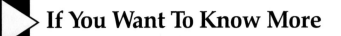

If You Want To Know More

1. *ICD-9 CM professional for physicians.* Vols. 1 & 2. 6ᵗʰ ed. St. Anthony's Publishing, 2003.

2. Pellegrino MJ. *Inside fibromyalgia.* Columbus, OH: Anadem Publishing, 2001.

SECTION II—UNDERSTANDING FIBROMYALGIA

This section focuses on what I know about the pathology of fibromyalgia based on my interpretation of what's been researched and my own experiences. First I describe "normal" pain, then move on to abnormal pain. Chronic pain is "abnormal" pain and it includes fibromyalgia. Emotional aspects contribute to all types of pain and I've discussed these aspects as well. Confused? I hope it will be more clear when you finish this section. If it is, you've accomplished an important part of becoming a Fibromyalgia Victor: you've understood it (or at least some of it)! I know this section is complicated, but hopefully it helps.

Our knowledge of this complicated condition continues to change and evolve as more and more research is done and clinical experience is accumulated. Understanding fibromyalgia is really half the battle . . . so go forth and win knowledge!

Normal Pain

Pain is a bad word. All we have to do is watch any TV commercial or look in a magazine and we will see multiple advertisements constantly telling us that pain is bad and we need to do something about it. Every year we spend billions of dollars on medicines and devices for our pain. If you factor in medical costs, lost wages, and Workers' Compensation, we are spending probably 100 billion dollars a year in treating pain.

Pain may be a warning that something is wrong, and it may evoke fear that something is terribly wrong with our bodies, such as a heart attack or cancer. But pain is essentially a part of living. In fact, the average person experiences pain every day, and the average American over 45 has at least 2 painful conditions (Dr. Ernest W. Johnson). Dr. Johnson, my mentor at Ohio State University, also says: "Pain is a part of living. It is an expected and necessary part of our interface with the environment. Pain is a privilege, a reminder of being alive."

This is for "normal" pain, though. Pain in fibromyalgia is different from the everyday aches and pains. As we will learn in the next chapter, it is amplified pain that can't be ignored. It is *not* a privilege! In this chapter, we'll try to understand regular "normal" pain.

I find it fascinating to look back in history and see how pain was viewed. In prehistoric times, pain was believed to be caused by demons entering the body through wounds and swimming around, and the treatment was to open new wounds to allow fluids with the demons to escape. During the Renaissance, the heart was perceived as the pain center. It wasn't until the 1800's that the nervous system was understood to be the cause of the pain. We now know that pain is a complicated process of the nervous system, and in fibromyalgia, pain gets even more complicated.

Normal Pain

Pain is a normal built-in process to give us information about our body and the world it is in. Acute pain warns us that something is wrong and tells us that we had better do something about it—fast. Not feeling pain would be dangerous to our health. We wouldn't be able to tell if we were having a heart attack, a broken bone, appendicitis, or a ruptured brain aneurysm.

Nerves

The normal transmission of pain begins at specialized nerve endings of skin, muscles, bones, and other tissues. These specialized nerves are pain sensitive cells called nociceptors. Nociceptors are programmed to respond to specific noxious or painful stimulations that could be potentially harmful to the body. When you drop a pan on your foot, you activate the foot nociceptors and initiate a chain reaction.

The nociceptors release chemicals called neurotransmitters, which create tiny electrical currents that travel up the nerves into the spinal cord via a nerve relay system. Once the signal reaches the spinal cord, specialized nerve tracts called spinal neurons relay the signals upward to the brain.

Spinal Cord

The spinal neurons are highly specialized and dynamic in their responses. Spinal neurons can respond to nociceptive stimuli and transmit this information upward, but they can also block signals, sensitize them, or desensitize them. Spinal neurons act like a dynamic filter when pain signals traveling from the tissues reach the spinal cord.

The dynamic spinal cord pain filter can do several things with these arriving peripheral pain signals. It can allow the signals to pass as they are, like an open filter. It may let signals pass at first, but then it tends to slow them down and after a while may stop them altogether like a concentrating filter. Once a certain "concentration" of the signal is passed through, fewer similar signals are allowed to penetrate

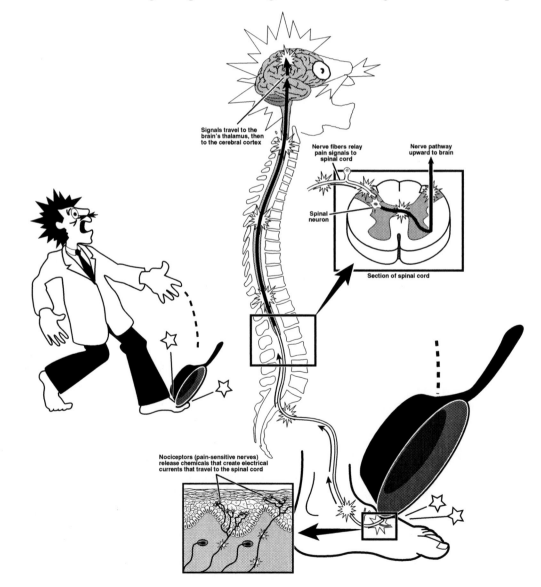

the filter. This is known as attenuation, or weakening of successive neurological signals over time. An example of this occurs when you wrap a fairly tight rubber band around your wrist. At first the band feels tight, perhaps slightly annoying. After a minute or so, you don't even realize the rubber band is there.

Another option is for the spinal filters to amplify the incoming signals. This is done by specialized receptors called NMDA receptors. If the signals are augmented, the filter acts as a hyperconcentrating filter. An example of normal amplified signals might occur when someone is tickling you, but does not occur when you try to tickle yourself!

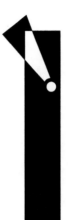

The spinal neurons are highly specialized and dynamic in their responses. Spinal neurons can respond to nociceptive stimuli and transmit this information upward, but they can also block signals, sensitize them, or desensitize them.

The spinal dynamic filter can also block out some signals like a filter that can let water pass but traps the debris. The "debris" could be unwanted pain signals that are not allowed to pass through the spinal neurons. A specialized system called diffuse noxious inhibitory control (DNIC) exists in the spinal neurons to block out a variety of input so the brain isn't overloaded. If the DNIC system works well, it filters out signals before they become amplified by the NMDA receptors.

The spinal cord neurons and the pain filtering system do a combination of all these mechanisms in a dynamic fashion. After the signals are processed at the spinal cord level, the modified signals are relayed up to the brain.

Brain

It isn't until the signals reach the brain that a phenomenon called nociperception occurs, which is when the brain detects pain, and therefore, you first perceive the original signal (the pan falling on your foot) to be painful. This whole process happens in milliseconds. Normally, the pain signal travels at a speed of 112 m.p.h., so you will feel pain immediately when you drop a pan on your foot. The pain signals are closely connected to your motor nerves, too, which enables an immediate physical reaction to pain. For example, if you put your hand on a hot stove, you reflexively move your hand off of the stove. If you drop a pan on your foot, the motor neurons reflexively tell your mouth to open and say something like "Darn, I wish I hadn't dropped the pan on my foot." Or perhaps a different choice of words would be added!

The brain perceives pain and it interprets the incoming pain signals from the spinal cord centers. Specifically, the information relayed to the brain deals with: What type of pain is it? Pain can be perceived as a burning, numbness, tingling, ache, stabbing, tearing, itching, swelling, crawling or a combination. Where is the pain? How intense is the pain? Is the body still being injured? Why did you drop a pan on your foot? Did you think your foot was a stove?

The brain, like the spinal neurons, can modify the signals. The brain is more highly specialized than the spinal cord, more like a gourmet chef instead of a filter. The brain adds "flavor" to all the incoming ingredients (signals) and prepares the final entrée (modified pain signals) for our culinary sampling (nociperception). The modified brain signals tell us what kind of pain it is, how it affects us, how we feel about it, and what we are able to do about it: the "flavors" of pain.

A "light" recipe from *The Fibromyalgia Chef:*

Fruit Medley Salad

Pureed mental fog

½ c. canned sliced sleep (can use poor quality)

2 dried eyes (whole)

1½ c. firmly packed painful muscles (chunky style)

1 c. of night sweat

1 t. stomach acid

1 very ripe bloated stomach (leave pit in)

1 dash of lightheadedness

In blender, combine all ingredients and process until unbearably offensive. Pour mixture into doctor's office, let simmer, and then bring to boil. Remove from doctor's office, let cool slightly, and transfer mixture to another doctor's office, bring to boil again. Repeat these steps until mixture finds acceptable doctor's office, where it can naturally gel and be served immediately.

The process of getting the pain signals from the nociceptors to the brain is fairly constant and universal in all normal humans. That is not to say that the neurological system is constant, unchanging, and always produces the exact same response in everyone. We know that the nervous system in the spinal cord is dynamic and has a lot of variations from individual to individual. It would be like saying that all humans are equipped with a radio broadcasting system representing the nerve endings and spinal cord. This radio system has multiple channels representing different neurological pathways to the brain. Whenever signals are broadcast, our brains receive these signals at once, but each of us gets signals through different channels. Our radios are always turned on and we each always have an "open" channel for our pain to be relayed, but we are not all using the same channel at any given time.

I've managed to compare our brains to a gourmet chef and a radio in one page! Can you think of anywhere else you could get this unique image of a wrinkly, rotund chef wearing a radio and headphones, humming to the song *We Will Rock You* while preparing a gourmet meal over the stove? Only in my book on fibromyalgia!

Unique Pain

Even though the signals get to our brain in a fairly constant way, we aren't saying that all individuals perceive pain the same way. In fact, part of what makes us unique is that we each perceive pain differently, uniquely. Using the radio station and chef analogy, that would mean that we all receive the pain radio signals to our brain fairly equally, but some of us interpret the pain with a more "country" flavor while others give it a more "rock-n-roll" taste, and still others interpret their pain to have a more "oldies" taste. I imagine the radio station for fibromyalgia would be something like "no rhythm with the blues."

The unique individual component of pain is interpreted at 2 centers of the brain known as the limbic system and the cerebral cortex. The limbic system is a structure that includes the thalamus and hippocampus, amygdala, locus ceruleus, and cingulate gyrus. It is a complex unit that gives an "emotional component" to pain. Fear, anxiety, and depression can modulate one's perception of how bad pain is, and one's pain threshold can be elevated or lowered based on emotional responses generated by the limbic system.

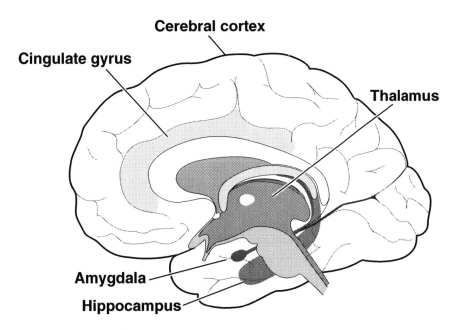

The cerebral cortex is the intelligence center of the brain where pain information is ultimately interpreted, processed, responded to, and stored. It is the most advanced part of our brain that makes us human. The cortex ultimately completes our sensory and motor pain experience with the emotional aspect contributed from the limbic system. In our cortex, we experience, learn, behave, and memorize in unique ways as a result of pain experiences. Individual brain responses to pain are shaped by factors such as genetics, learned responses, and previous experiences.

Childhood experiences with pain will influence how pain is perceived later in life. What is the first thing we do when a child cuts his knee? We say, "Oh no, you've got a boo-boo, let me put a bandage on it." And then, every grown-up who sees the bandage says to the child "Oh you poor thing, you've got a boo-boo, let me kiss it. How does it feel?" The child learns at a very young age that pain hurts, but one can be rewarded with attention and other good things! Cultural differences also contribute to a child's pain learning experience. Pain experiences can have both "negative" components (it hurts!) and "positive" ones (get attention, get candy).

It doesn't take long for people to recognize a pattern that if they hurt and look like they hurt, other people will immediately notice the pain. In fact, people can learn that acting like they have pain (pain behaviors) even if no pain is present will still cause other people to react as if pain were present. A person can learn to signal pain behaviors to others to indicate pain. A facial grimace, a groan, or grabbing one's back may be signals to call others' attention to pain. These are examples of pain behaviors that can be learned, and sometimes they are used to avoid undesired chores such as taking out the garbage or visiting in-laws!

Another example of how pain can be perceived and learned differently is the expectation of what happens from the pain. For example, most mothers will tell me that giving birth is the worst pain they have ever experienced, yet many mothers have been pregnant many times. Why is that? Quite simply, despite the severe pain during delivery, the outcome of their pain was good, that is, a new life was born. This is a highly positive reward from experiencing severe pain. On the other hand, an individual with chronic muscle pain with no end in sight may experience the pain as the worst imaginable. Nothing good is expected from this never-ending pain. In our culture we have learned that pain is bad, and we have learned "responses" to pain. The pain isn't less real because of our perceptions and learned responses. As we will see, the pain is physiologically worse in fibromyalgia because of a number of neurobiological changes that occur.

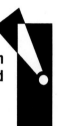

Childhood experiences with pain will influence how pain is perceived later in life.

The International Association for the Study of Pain (IASP) defines pain as an unpleasant sensory or emotional experience associated with actual or potential tissue damage (Merskey and Bogduk, 1994). This definition states that pain can be present whether or not there is tissue damage. Even anticipation of pain may activate pain memories and cause painful unpleasantness without actual nociceptive nerve signals (Dr. Bradley, 2000).

Pain is always subjective and unpleasant, by definition. Pain is difficult to measure, standardize, or reproduce because its perception is influenced by multiple factors such as personal beliefs, education, culture differences, learned experiences, and genetics. But we know pain exists even if we can't always measure it. In fibromyalgia, our seventh sense has to work overtime!

Differences In Pain Between Men And Women

There are sex differences in the perception of pain. According to recent research women are more sensitive to pain than men, but are better able to cope with it, recover more quickly, and are less likely to let pain control their lives. Men tend to cope poorly with pain and suffer in silence. It is probably a macho thing, literally, because research suggests that the presence of the hormone testosterone (at higher levels in men) increases pain tolerance. Women (with their high estrogen and low testosterone) have a lower pain threshold, but their sensitivity to pain probably increases their awareness of potential health problems and they seek health care sooner than men.

Another factor that may cause sex differences in pain is that women have a bigger corpus callosum. The corpus callosum is the part of the brain that connects the right and left halves of the brain. A bigger corpus callosum means that women connect both sides of the brain better. Thus, the female brain halves can work together simultaneously better than those of men, who are suffering with small corpus callosums and use only one side of the brain at a time. These differences allow women to incorporate more information simultaneously when solving a pain problem and use their keener sense of pain as a call to action to overcome pain.

Men and women differ in how they process pain signals at the spinal cord level, that is, they have different dynamic pain filters. Dr. Roland Staud (*Pain*, 2003) found that the inhibitory filters (the DNIC system) in normal women did not work as well as in normal men. This suggests that normal women are more prone to developing amplified, chronic pain then men because of less ability to inhibit persistent pain signals. This, in part, can account for the higher prevalence of fibromyalgia among women.

Drs. Fillingim and Edwards (*Pain*, 2003) studied the DNIC system in "younger" healthy people with an average age of 22, and "older" healthy people with an average age of 63, and found that the DNIC system worked better in the younger group than in the older group, with men and women affected the same.

Pain thresholds were also found to decrease with age in both men and women. Pain thresholds are a measure of how much a pain signal hurts, which is a way to measure the pain filtering system, the DNIC system. This study supports the finding that the DNIC system undergoes an age-related deterioration in both men and women, hence lower pain thresholds with increasing age. The next chapter will look at "abnormal" pain in fibromyalgia.

If You Want To Know More

1. Adams RD, Victor M. *Principles of Neurology.* 7th Ed. McGraw-Hill, 2001.

2. Alberts KR, Bradley LA, Alarcon GS. *Anticipation of acute pain and high arousal feedback in women with fibromyalgia, high pain anxiety, and high negative affectivity evokes increased pain and anterior cingulate cortex activity without nociception.* Arthritis Rheum 2000; 43(9-suppl): 637.

3. Edwards RR, Fillingim RB, Ness TJ. *Age-related differences in endogenous pain modulation: a comparison of diffuse noxious inhibitory controls in healthy older and younger adults.* Pain 2003 Jan; 101(1-2): 155–65.

4. Flor H. *Cortical reorganisation and chronic pain: implications for rehabilitation.* J Rehabil Med 2003; 41 Suppl: 66–72.

5. Kest B, Wilson SG, Mogil JS. *Sex differences in supraspinal morphine analgesia are dependent on genotype.* J Pharmacol Exp Ther 1999; 289: 1370–5.

6. Melzack R, Wall DP. *The challenge of pain.* Basic Books, 1983.

7. Mersky H, Bogduk N. *Classification of chronic pain: descriptions of chronic pain syndromes and definition of pain.* 2nd ed. IASP Press, 1994.

8. Rao SG. *The neuropharmacology of centrally-acting analgesic medications in fibromyalgia.* Rheum Dis Clin N Am. 2002; 28(2): 235-59.

9. Staud R, Robinson ME, Vierck CJ, et al. *Diffuse noxious inhibitory controls (DNIC) attenuate temporal summation of second pain in normal males but not in normal females or fibromyalgia patients.* Pain 2003; 101: 167–74.

10. Vance LM. *The role of culture in the pain experience.* Pain Clinic 2003; 4: 10–23.

A Disease Of Amplified Pain

In the last chapter, I described "normal" pain. A normally functioning pain pathway will continuously monitor the body and its environment. Different types of pain can be identified, but the 2 main types are acute and chronic.

Acute Pain

Acute pain can be a brief warning signal such as touching a hot stove with no damage done to the tissue. Or there could be tissue damage as occurs with any number of conditions including muscle strains, ligament sprains, bone fracture, ruptured disc, skin burn, or a pinched nerve. In acute pain, healing is the body's expected outcome, and hopefully the pain will be able to go away completely. The healing may take anywhere from a few days for a muscle sprain to many months for a ruptured disc. Where surgery is required, hopefully the problem is corrected, and when healing is complete, the pain is gone.

When acute pain signals are sent through the normal pain pathways, the body has various neurological mechanisms to avoid, reduce, or tolerate the pain. Examples of adaptive mechanisms include:

1. **Reflexes.** Our nervous system commands us to perform a variety of complicated and protective reflexes when encountering pain. When you quickly withdraw your hand after touching a hot stove, you are performing an automatic motor reflex in response to the pain. If you move your hand quickly away from a painful source, the tissue damage can be minimized. If you step on a small pebble with your big foot, the nervous system commands the "pebble-pained" foot to quickly bend up while your opposite leg is told to straighten out so you avoid pain and keep from falling.

2. **Muscle spasms.** These often occur around a painful inflamed area. Protective muscle spasms act as a splint to "guard" the painful or unstable area and prevent further damage or movement. For example, someone with a low back disc herniation may develop protective spasms of the back muscles as an involuntary attempt to minimize movement and prevent damage of the inflamed disc area. As we very well know, these muscle spasms themselves are very painful. The body figures if it doesn't want a painful area to move, it will make that area even more painful so one will not even think about moving it!

3. **Accommodation.** As I indicated in the last chapter, this mechanism is one in which the body tries to tolerate persistent pain signals. The body releases its own pain medications—endorphins—which are chemicals that inhibit pain. This desensitization process makes it harder for pain signals to activate the pain pathways to the brain. The accommodation mechanism makes it more difficult for pain signals to reach the pain threshold (the minimum signal needed to activate the pain pathways). The "pain threshold" is the point of no return, when pain signals are "strong" enough to activate the pain pathways. The body has accommodated these pain signals by decreasing their intensity and therefore, decreasing the chance of reaching pain threshold.

Another example of accommodation occurs when you step into a hot tub. At first your skin actually hurts, but then the sensation becomes tolerable even though the water temperature hasn't changed. Another good example occurs when a husband ignores his wife's repeated request to take out the garbage. The words are still coming out of the wife's mouth, but the husband has been able to accommodate the words and not respond to them!

4. **Gate Mechanism.** The gate control theory of Melzack and Wall described a mechanism the body uses to inhibit pain. They observed that pain signals traveled in small diameter nerve fibers. Large diameter nerve fibers carry different types of sensory signals (touch and pressure) and can inhibit the signal transmissions of the smaller nerve fibers carrying pain. They proposed a gate mechanism in the spinal cord where the large and small nerve fibers converge. If signals from both the large fibers and small fibers arrive at the gate at the same time, the nerve signals from the large fiber will inhibit the small fibers, thus closing the gate for the small fiber transmission and opening the gate for the large fiber transmission. Only the large fiber signals—touch and pressure—are able to pass through the gate and travel upward to the brain. Small fiber signals, pain, are blocked at the closed gate.

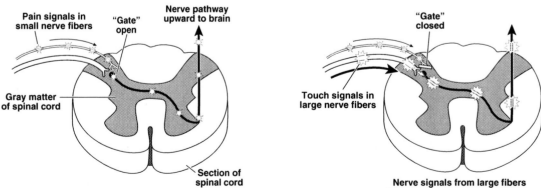

We can take advantage of this gate mechanism to control our persistent, acute pain. If we bruise or burn our hand, we will often blow on it or rub it. This blowing and rubbing sensation travels up the large nerve fibers and blocks out the pain signals traveling up the smaller fibers. If our legs are very painful from an injury, we may walk around to reduce the pain. The pressure and motion signals from walking will travel up the large nerve fibers and block the smaller fiber pain signals.

5. **"Fight or Flight" response.** This occurs when the body senses an injury and releases its adrenaline hormones (epinephrine and norepinephrine) to heighten the body's abilities to fight off the threat or take flight to evade it. The body and brain are put in a state of heightened awareness, and pain is lessened. If acute pain signals persist, the body can sustain this response for awhile before fatigue sets in.

   A good example of this response is the athlete who plays in spite of an injury. The pain from the injury may not be noticed because the athlete is in his "game mode" which is similar to this heightened awareness state. After the game, the painful injury is noticed much more as the adrenaline response wears off. The adrenaline temporarily blocked the acute pain.

6. **Brain Plasticity.** Plasticity is an adaptive capability of the brain where it can change its organization and function to adapt to a different environment. The mechanisms include sprouting (growing of new nerve fibers), unmasking (activating previously "quiet" nerve pathways), and hypersensitization (increasing the responsiveness of the nerve).

   An example of brain plasticity is the recovery that can occur in stroke victims. Brain damage resulting from lack of blood flow can lead to a stroke and cause paralysis on one side of the body. The damaged part of the brain cannot regenerate itself, but other unaffected parts of the brain may be able to "rewire" themselves from rehab therapies to help the weak parts of the body regain nerve signals and improve strength.

Chronic Pain ("Abnormal" Pain)

If there is a progression of tissue damage, or the pain signals persist even though the "acute" injury has subsided, chronic pain may result. Many conditions can give rise to chronic pain, and the key is that permanent changes occur in the pain pathways either from tissue damage or abnormal neurological changes. The pain pathways become abnormal, leading to persistent pain. Chronic pain can result at any part of the pain pathway: the nociceptors, neurotransmitters, nerves, spinal cord, or brain.

Nociceptors. Neuropathy, burns, inflammatory conditions (*e.g.*, rheumatoid arthritis), and causalgia (burning pain) are examples of conditions that cause damage to the nociceptors and increase pain signal transmission up through the pain pathway.

Neurotransmitters. Various neuromuscular disorders including myasthenia gravis, myotonia, and tetanus can cause chronic pain by interfering with the neurotransmitter mechanism.

Nerves. Carpal tunnel syndrome, radiculopathy (pinched nerve in neck or back), shingles, and thoracic outlet syndrome (pinched nerve in underarm) are some conditions that can cause chronic pain by irritating the nerves. Phantom limb pain can occur when a limb is amputated.

Spinal cord. Spinal cord injuries and spinal stenosis can cause chronic pain by damaging spinal cord pain pathways. Multiple sclerosis is an example of a condition that causes demyelination, or loss of the nerve's fatty insulation (myelin), which can lead to chronic pain.

A rare syndrome called congenital insensitivity to pain causes the person to be completely unresponsive to pain. This condition is felt to be related to problems in the spinal cord. Insensitivity to pain is not a good thing. In fact, people with this problem usually die young because of damage and complications to the body when pain was not perceived.

Brain. Brain problems that can cause chronic pain include multiple sclerosis, strokes, aneurysms, and brain tumors. These conditions can disrupt brain nerve signals and affect how pain is perceived.

A number of neurobiological changes occur at different parts of the nerve pathway when a chronic pain problem develops. The resultant chronic pain that is experienced is usually the result of 2 nervous system changes that occur:

1. The nervous system becomes hypersensitized to pain signals.

2. The nervous system is less able to inhibit pain signals.

This neuro "double whammy" is responsible for our fibromyalgia pain.

Fibromyalgia Pain

Many conditions can lead to permanent changes in the pain transmission mechanism and result in chronic pain that overwhelms the body's pain defense mechanisms. One such condition is near and dear to all of us, fibromyalgia. Fibromyalgia may not cause destruction along the pain pathways as other conditions I have mentioned can cause. However, fibromyalgia does cause chronic abnormal changes along all the pathway components and this results in chronic pain via both peripheral (from skin, muscles and nerves) and central (from spinal cord and brain) neurological mechanisms. The end result of fibromyalgia's abnormal changes appears to be a state of pain amplification that causes severe generalized pain. Fibromyalgia is ultimately a disease of amplified pain.

Dr. Robert Bennett has written and presented excellent information that explains why we hurt with fibromyalgia (*e.g.*, 1999 review article in *Mayo Clinical Proceedings*). If we trace the pain signals through the various parts of the pain pathway (from the nociceptors to the nerves to the spinal cord to the brain) in people with fibromyalgia, we find various abnormalities along the way. Many studies have shed light on different points along the complete pain pathway. I want to briefly summarize some of these different abnormalities and possible problems encountered by fibromyalgia pain signals on the path to the brain.

Nociceptors. Pain originates from the nociceptors (those specialized pain nerve endings). Trauma is a common trigger of fibromyalgia. Tissue injury, damage to the muscles and soft tissues, activates the nociceptors. Some studies have suggested that microscopic injury occurs in specific parts of the muscles (for those who aren't totally lost by now and want the medical names: muscle spindles, intrafusal fibers, and calcium pumps). Localized tissue injury probably activates arachidonic acid (a biological protein), which turns into "bad" prostaglandins (called Cox-II prostaglandins), and cause inflammation and pain.

In addition to trauma, autoimmune factors may be another pain nerve activator. Perhaps autoimmune processes create compounds which act as irritants and activate the nociceptors chronically to the point where they become "permanently" sensitized and irritated. As a result, biochemical, hormonal, and red blood cell changes occur that interfere with the cells' ability to receive adequate supplies of oxygen, glucose, and other nutrients. Blood flow, energy formation, and the cells' electrical and neurological harmonies are all disrupted. Since the nociceptors remain "faulty," the electrical and neurological balance remains abnormal, and the nociceptors continue to be activated. Pain-producing neurotransmitters are released and accumulate as long as the nociceptors stay activated at the peripheral level (skin and muscles, especially).

These persistent pain signals we experience may be interpreted as an itching, burning, swelling, or tingling at one end of the spectrum, or, at the other end, knife-stabbing, burning, or throbbing. One nociceptor can signal different pain signals and sensations depending on its level of irritation—the more irritated it is, the more severe the pain.

These changes can become permanent and cause the nerves to become sensitized to the point where they are easily activated to send pain, even in the absence of any noxious stimulus. In other words, persistent pain signals can *spontaneously* arise from peripheral nerve endings and bombard the rest of the pain pathway. So, instead of waiting for outside stimulation such as trauma, pressure, temperature, or touch to signal the nociceptors, these nociceptors send pain signals on their own, without any outside help. This "spontaneous" pain is what we complain about the most!

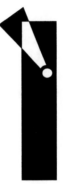

These changes can become permanent and cause the nerves to become sensitized to the point where they are easily activated to send pain, even in the absence of any noxious stimulus.

Nerves. The nerves, especially the sensory nerves and the autonomic nerves, "wonder what is happening" because they are getting bombarded by all of these signals from the nociceptors. At first, they try to diminish these painful signals by using accommodation and gate mechanisms. However, the signals persist and they, too, undergo a sensitization process. They become hypersensitized and react with an exaggerated response instead of a normal or diminishing response (accommodation). Now we get even more pain, numbness, swelling, burning, and other sensations. Some of the hypersensitization may be mediated by nerve growth factor, which has been found in higher levels in fibromyalgia. A high nerve growth factor may indicate the nerves are trying to regenerate or repair themselves. But instead of repairing the nerves so they act normal again, the opposite seems to happen. Nerve growth factor is probably enhancing the nerves' abilities to transmit pain to the spinal cord. More pain results, not less.

Spinal cord. At the spinal cord level, the fibromyalgia begins to take control. It is here that additional changes occur to perpetuate the pain and spread it to different levels. When pain generators first start firing, the spinal cord pain processing centers may act at first like a dry sponge and easily soak up all the signals. Our bodies may have many pain generators at any given time, but if they are slowly and intermittently firing, dry sponges can soak up the signals and not cause any bothersome symptoms. From time to time there may be an acute exacerbation of a problem leading to a lot of pain signals being generated, and if a lot of pain signals are dumped at once into the spinal cord sponge, only a little bit gets absorbed and a lot gets passed through and perceived as acute pain.

In fibromyalgia, however, the different pain generators continue to send signals and eventually the dry sponge becomes a wet sponge and it can't soak up anymore. The additional oncoming continuous signals will spill over the wet sponge, and this leads to persistent pain.

In fibromyalgia the different pain generators continue to send signals and eventually the dry sponge becomes a wet sponge and it can't soak up anymore. The additional oncoming continuous signals will spill over the wet sponge, and this leads to persistent pain.

The two main changes that occur at the spinal cord include pain amplification (by specialized nerves called NMDA receptors), and loss of pain filtering (by the diffuse noxious inhibitory control system). Spinal cord nerves are bombarded by continuous stimulation from the peripheral nerves, causing a progressive increase in electrical signals to be sent up to the brain. This phenomenon is called "wind-up," and is the neurological mechanism for the amplification of pain. Once this wind-up phenomenon occurs, a central sensitization results in which various types of sensory signals, not just pain, will arrive in the spinal cord, become amplified, and be sent to the brain as pain. The spinal cord becomes more sensitized to sending pain, lots of it. Once this happens, the spinal cord is not able to properly sort out and filter various sensory signals.

As a result, different sensory signals such as touch, pressure, temperature, and joint movement all become amplified and sent up the pain pathways, resulting in pain signals instead of the appropriate touch, pressure, temperature, or joint motion signals. This defect in pain transmission where there is increased sensitivity to all stimuli, even those which normally do not evoke pain, is called allodynia. Unfortunately for the person with fibromyalgia, the spinal cord is now "wired" to interpret nearly all sensory signals as pain, severe pain! We can still appreciate touch, pressure, temperature, joint movement, and other non-pain signals, but pain contaminates these signals, and we feel the pain.

Another key change at the spinal cord level is an increased formation of Substance P and other neurotransmitters (see Chapter 6). Substance P's primary role at the spinal cord level is to transmit pain signals and to sensitize the spinal cord so it is readily available to transmit pain. When Substance P reaches high concentrations (as it does in fibromyalgia), it can migrate up and down the spinal cord, away from the initial location of the pain signal. As a result, multiple levels of the spinal cord undergo sensitization and send increased pain signals, leading to a "generalization" of the fibromyalgia. This spreading of pain explains how one can develop generalized fibromyalgia from an initial regional area of pain. A common example of this occurs following a motor vehicle accident where a particular body part, such as the neck, was injured. Over time, the pain begins to involve the mid-back, low back, and ultimately the whole body, even though these areas were never injured. The substance P-induced spinal cord changes can explain this migration of pain from the neck to the entire body.

Brain. Our poor brains have no chance, do they? Any pain memory stored in the past will be re-awakened by this process. Fibromyalgia is notorious for causing previously injured areas to hurt more once it develops. This previously injured area may have settled down and become essentially pain-free, but the pain memories remained, although inactive. Thanks to the fibromyalgia pain amplification process, the inactive memories are reactivated. The pain centers of our brain, the limbic system and the cerebral cortex, are continuously fed these amplified signals from the spinal cord. Changes occur: serotonin levels decrease, brain waves change, sleep stages are affected, blood flow and glucose metabolism are affected.

The brain gets overwhelmed with these pain signals and spends a lot of attention and energy monitoring the pain. Fibrofog occurs. Emotional components are "attached" to pain, including fear, depression, anxiety, anger, hopelessness, and helplessness, which can further amplify the pain.

In patients with fibromyalgia, functional reorganization (brain plasticity) in both sensory and motor portions of the brain has been observed, and appears directly related to the chronicity of the pain (Dr. H. Flor, 2003). These brain changes may be viewed as pain memories that influence how painful and non-painful signals affect the body's sensory and motor responses. The brain makes these changes to enhance its ability to perceive pain, brain amplified pain.

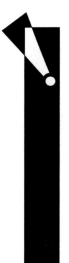

Fibromyalgia is notorious for causing previously injured areas to hurt more once it develops. This previously injured area may have settled down and become essentially pain-free, but the pain memories remained, although inactive. Thanks to the fibromyalgia pain amplification process, the inactive memories are reactivated.

This type of abnormal brain plasticity can be measured. As previously discussed, Dr. Gracely and Dr. Clauw published a study which demonstrated abnormal "hyperactive" areas of the brains and abnormal "quiet" areas of the brains in fibromyalgia test subjects who underwent functional MRIs. This provides objective evidence to support brain plasticity with both hypersensitive amplified pain, and turning off the ability to inhibit pain.

Fibromyalgia Pain Summary

To summarize, fibromyalgia changes our pain pathways. It may start off as a peripheral irritant, but eventually it becomes a self-perpetuating process that affects the entire pathway from the nociceptors to the brain. The main problem, in a nutshell, is amplified pain. The amplified pain is the result of our nervous system gaining the ability to magnify pain and losing the ability to inhibit pain. What comes in at a signal of a "1" does not end up in the brain as a signal of a "1" as it would in people without fibromyalgia. Our pain signal of a "1" gets amplified and magnified, and by the time it reaches our brain, it is a "10!" Other nonpainful signals get thrown into this pain amplification pathway and arrive at our brain as pain signals. Even tiny subconscious pain signals can get amplified, or the nerve pathways can automatically "fire away" without any obvious noxious stimulus to cause spontaneous pain.

These are not your everyday aches and pains, these are severe pains that cannot be ignored. This severe, chronic pain can completely disrupt one's life. And by the way, while all of this is happening, we continue to look completely normal on the outside.

To use the radio station analogy, we now have a Fibromyalgia (FM) station that plays continuously. This station picks up everything—rock and roll, country, R&B (representing different sensory signals) and plays these different types of music. But pain music is also played and it distorts the other sounds. The volume is stuck on high and you can't turn off the music. The result: an FM station that plays blaring pain music all day, all night, all the time!

Personal Snapshot

by Mark J. Pellegrino, M.D.

Here's a different way of explaining the dysfunctional neurobiological problems we have in fibromyalgia. I hope you enjoy it; don't be scared now!

Confessions of an N.E.O. (Neuron Executive Officer)

"Hi! I'm Gary Neuron of Central Nervous System Enterprises located at the corner of Brain and Spinal Cord Avenues. You might say I'm in the manufacturing business—I build pain pathways. I'm very good at what I do. I can take the tiniest of peripheral sensory signals, magnify their intensity tenfold, and route them straight to the brain. My company has grown so fast in the past ten years it's actually ridiculous. If they give awards for causing pain, I'd have to buy a planet just to hold them all."

"Did I mention that I was very good at what I do?"

"I must confess I have many talents and that's what makes me so successful. I'm like a jack-of-all-trades, or as we say in the neuro world, a depolarizer-of-all-synapses."

"I'm going to share with you what makes me so successful. You don't have to like me, but you probably want to hear what I have to say."

"First and foremost, I'm a great evaluator of potential recruits. Hey, if I'm going to build pain pathways, I need raw materials. I am constantly on the lookout for vulnerable candidates, people who are ripe to develop fibromyalgia. And I find them everywhere. I look for genetic patterns, a lot for major stresses, I follow the viral infections. I especially monitor whiplash victims and others with trauma. If your peripheral nerves are being challenged or struggling for any reason, I'm coming after you."

"Secondly, I'm a huge advocate of organized labor. I give individual peripheral nerve signals the opportunity to unite with a combined voice, a loud voice that you can't ignore. I promise them amplified voices in a beautiful central nervous system network. Pain signals are the easiest to work with, but I listen to all sensory signals: touch, pressure, positioning, and all the rest. I find a way to let them all be heard painfully."

"You see, before I came along, these sensory signals were crying out weakly. They were constantly sending signals from different tissues, all scattered about, with no real purpose or direction. But I heard them, and I found them and built them a nice pathway and gave them direction and purpose. I smiled at them, pointed to the brain and told them to make as much noise as possible on the way up (wink, wink!)."

"Once a pathway is built, it's like a paved highway that needs little maintenance. I'm proud of my engineering skills. It may take me many months, sometimes up to a couple of years, but my pain roads are a masterpiece once they are done. They hold up indefinitely and allow continuous traffic from all directions. Heck, I build roads to every part of the body, even places where you never thought fibromyalgia existed."

"Finding these remote locations is part of my Outreach Program. Why stop at the neck with a whiplash injury? I'll build those roads clear to your toes so they end up hurting just as much as your neck."

"I am a computer whiz too. I know how to press all your buttons to make you think of me all the time. I can amplify your pain. I can turn off your pain inhibitory circuits, I make your nerves hypersensitive. **'I TURN UP THE VOLUME!'**"

"I put the pain into ordinary non-painful signals. I put more pain in the painful signals. My favorite trick is to create spontaneous pain when you're not doing anything. I'm really good at that."

continued on next page...

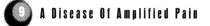

Personal Snapshot *continued from previous page...*

"Lastly, I'm very flexible and patient. Sure I have my specific patterns and unique style, but I go with the flow. I can wait a long time for the right opportunity to develop. I'm strong."

"I'm not invincible, I must admit. There are ways to try to beat me. You're probably wondering what they are. Well, I would be foolish to tell you, wouldn't I? I'm not stupid you know. In fact I'm very smart . . . did I mention that?"

"I have some advice for you though that I'll share: I work quietly so you can't hear me. If you're ever wondering whether you're getting fibromyalgia, stop what you are doing at once. Turn off any noises and listen very carefully. Do you hear anything? Anything at all? If not, you'd better be worried. Be very worried."

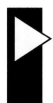

If You Want To Know More

1. Adams RD, Victor M. *Principles of neurology.* 7th ed. McGraw-Hill, 2001.

2. Bennett RM. *Emerging concepts in the neurobiology of chronic pain: evidence of abnormal sensory processing in fibromyalgia.* Mayo Clin Proc 1999; 74(4): 385–98.

3. Flor H. *Cortical reorganisation and chronic pain: implications for rehabilitation.* J Rehabil Med 2003 May; (41 Suppl): 66–72.

4. Gracely RH, Petzke F, Wolf JM, et al. *Functional magnetic resonance imaging evidence of augmented pain processing in fibromyalgia.* Arthritis Rheum 2002 May; 46(5): 1333–43.

5. Melzack R, Wall DP. *The challenge of pain.* Basic Books, 1983.

6. Rao SR. *The neuropharmacology of centrally-acting analgesic medications in fibromyalgia.* Rheum Dis Clin N Am 2002; 28(2): 235–59.

Causes Of Fibromyalgia

Top Ten Rejected Theories About The Cause Of Fibromyalgia

1. Oxygen allergy

2. Watching TV too close as a child

3. Firefly radiation

4. Eating too much microwave cooking

5. Microscopic defects in teeth enamel

6. Wet earthworm smells

7. Over exposure to sneezes from inconsiderate people who didn't cover their mouths

8. Too many refrigerator magnets

9. Mother overslept during pregnancy

10. Drinking too much water

In 1993, I wrote in my first book, *Fibromyalgia: Managing the Pain,* that "the exact cause of fibromyalgia is unknown." At that time, a lot of research had been done that shed light on various contributing factors. Since that time, additional research has uncovered significant clues to what causes fibromyalgia and how fibromyalgia develops. Areas such as genetics, trauma, infections, as well as autoimmune, biochemical, and neurobiological mechanisms, are helping us to refine our knowledge about what causes fibromyalgia. All of us involved with fibromyalgia, either by treating it or having it, have come to appreciate how complicated this condition is. Fibromyalgia has different types and subsets. More than one factor may be involved in causing it. Causes may be recognized, but the exact mechanism of how fibromyalgia develops from this cause is not fully known. Most importantly, there is more than one way to get fibromyalgia; it is an "end point" condition with multiple ways leading to it.

Think of fibromyalgia as a theme park, for example, the Magic Kingdom park in Orlando, Florida. The Magic Kingdom has various sections including Main Street, USA, Adventure Land, Frontier Land, Liberty Square, Fantasy Land, Tomorrow Land, and Mickey's Star Land. Think of these various sections as different subsets of fibromyalgia. However, with fibromyalgia you do not have lots of fun and adventure and meet famous cartoon characters! Now think of the different roads and highways that lead to this theme park. These represent the different ways that one can get to fibromyalgia; there are some direct paths via the main highways, and there are some back routes through smaller roads that represent indirect pathways. There are many direct and indirect ways to get to fibromyalgia, and once you are there, you may end up in a specific subset.

I think we can say a number of causes of fibromyalgia are known at the present time. Yet I continue to read in the scientific literature statements such as "the cause of fibromyalgia is not currently known … ," or "future research will hopefully discover the cause of fibromyalgia …" I think one of our inherent problems is that we try to be TOO scientific when we really need to be more practical and logical. We are allowed to use common sense along with our scientific research. A couple of inherent "problems" arise when talking about the cause of any condition, not just fibromyalgia. Let's review these "proof vs. probability" and "cause vs. mechanism" problems.

Proof vs. Probability

Causality is the relationship between a cause and its effect. In medicine, we speak of whether or not something causes a particular medical condition. We can ascribe a degree of causality. That is, at one end of the spectrum, we can say that a cause and effect relationship happens with absolute certainty. At the other extreme, the cause and effect relationship is only a remote possibility. Absolute certainty implies that scientific proof has been established with 100% certainty. However, scientific causality in medicine is rarely established to that degree. As Thomas Edison once said, "We do not know one millionth of one percent about anything."

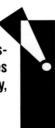

Probability means that the causality is more likely than not. It does not mean 100% absolute certainty, but 51% or more certain.

Much of the time, scientific discovery happens by accident. As an example, the drug Minoxidil was "accidentally" discovered to promote hair growth in balding people. The original use of this drug was to treat hypertension. A side effect was noted: hair growth. After further research proved Minoxidil causes hair growth, this product became available as a topical solution for treatment of hair loss. Minoxidil is still used in pill form to treat hypertension.

Most of what we treat in medicine does not have causes or treatment effects established with absolute certainty by scientific studies. If we waited for scientific proof to be established for everything we treated, doctors would not be able to treat most of the medical conditions known to us today. We have to recognize and acknowledge that our clinical practices are not based on absolute certainty principles, but rather on probability principles.

Sir William Gowers, the influential neurologist who first coined the term "fibrositis" in 1904, said this: "It is the balance of evidence that determines diagnosis. We must take probability as our guide, we have to act. We must deal with the probable as if it were certain. If we hesitate between two options we shall be powerless."

Probability means that the causality is more likely than not. It does not mean 100% absolute certainty, but 51% or more certain. Our clinical practices are based on principles of reasonable probability within a reasonable degree of medical certainty. We can't wait around for scientific proof to accidentally be discovered; we need to diagnose, treat, and determine causes now.

To use the argument that we do not have scientific proof, and therefore something cannot cause a condition such as fibromyalgia, is a ridiculous "defense." It may be difficult to establish scientific proof in medical research, but that does not mean we can't establish probable relationships between cause and effect with well-designed research studies. Dr. Muhammad Yunus, *et al*, reported a number of research techniques that can establish causality within a reasonable degree of medical certainty (*Fibromyalgia Consensus Report Additional Comments*, 1997). Examples of such research techniques include:

1. **Consistent clinical pattern.** This means that doctors who treat a condition regularly note a relationship between cause and effect.

2. **Case control studies.** These studies measure a response or outcome to a particular stimulus or treatment using a controlled subject population.

3. **Dose response relationships.** These studies measure a relationship between a specific quantity or dose and an outcome or response.

4. **Biologic plausibility.** This technique often relies on research of animals and use of a logical extrapolation to similar biologic human models. This also involves understanding biologic responses that can be measured at the present time, and then logically extrapolating what would happen over time.

There has been a lot of controversy regarding cigarette smoking and lung cancer. Is there a scientific causality? If we look at the different types of researches, it can be concluded that scientific causality has not been established with absolute certainty between cigarette smoking and lung cancer. Yet, there has been a consistent clinical pattern observed: doctors who treat people with lung cancer note that many of them are heavy cigarette smokers. There are case control studies and dose response relationships that suggest that the more one smokes, the more one is at risk for developing lung cancer. There is also biologic plausibility data that allows us to logically conclude, for example, that if there are over two dozen carcinogens in smoke, and carcinogens can cause cancer, then smoking can cause cancer. Even if it can't be proved that a single one carcinogen causes lung cancer consistently, it is plausible to assume that many carcinogens will do it.

With fibromyalgia, there are no scientific studies that establish causality with absolute certainty. There are many studies and patterns that establish scientific causality to within a reasonable probability. Doctors have to use the best of our clinical experience and research in evaluating and treating conditions. As Dr. Sackett said, "Good doctors use both individual clinical expertise and the best available external evidence, and neither alone is enough."

Cause vs. Mechanism

Another difficulty in determining cause is determining the difference between cause and pathological mechanism. In fibromyalgia, the cause would be WHY fibromyalgia developed. The pathologic mechanism would be HOW fibromyalgia developed. Let me give you a couple of examples to explain.

Someone throws a baseball and it accidentally hits your nose and breaks it (great example, huh?). The cause of your broken nose (the WHY) is the baseball hitting your nose and injuring it. The pathological mechanism of the injury (the HOW) is that high amounts of compressive force impacted the nasal bones, causing them to fracture. A fairly simple example, right?

Here is a more complicated example. You have allergies, and you are exposed to ragweed and develop a lot of congestion and sinus drainage. You then get a sinus infection and require an antibiotic. The pathologic mechanism (HOW) is that the body's allergic system was activated causing increased secretions. The increased secretions trapped more dirt and germs, and eventually a bacteria was able to establish itself in this sinus fluid and cause an infection. What was the cause (WHY)? The main overall cause was the ragweed which led to the problem to begin with, and the secondary cause was bacteria which directly led to the sinusitis. That particular sinusitis wouldn't have happened, however, without the ragweed.

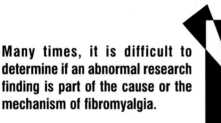

Many times, it is difficult to determine if an abnormal research finding is part of the cause or the mechanism of fibromyalgia.

Many times, it is difficult to determine if an abnormal research finding is part of the cause or the mechanism of fibromyalgia. Changes occur after fibromyalgia has developed, so an abnormality can be one of the consequences of fibromyalgia. It is like asking what came first, the chicken or the egg? The ongoing research challenge in fibromyalgia is to sort out the information into the proper categories and ultimately try to determine what comes first, and what happens after it develops. I often tell my patients that their fibromyalgia happened because "the sun, the moon, and the stars lined up just right for them!" Now that's pretty scientific, don't you think?

Probable Causes Of Fibromyalgia

I have compiled a list of probable causes of fibromyalgia. This list is based on my experiences and understanding of the current literature. My opinions on these probable causes may not be shared by everyone. My list of probable causes is as follows:

1. Genetics
2. Trauma
3. Connective tissue disease
4. Infection
5. Catastrophic stress
6. Chemical exposure

Genetics

Physicians who see patients with fibromyalgia can recall a number of patients who are relatives. I have seen numerous family members, mother-daughter, sister-sister, sister-brother, etc., who have the typical symptoms and findings of fibromyalgia. Several members of my family have fibromyalgia through four generations! I also see numerous patients who tell me they have family members known to have it (their family history is positive for fibromyalgia). Many adult patients state they had pain as a child. These observations support the notion that fibromyalgia can be inherited, or at least the tendency to develop fibromyalgia is inherited.

Several studies on the hereditary aspects of fibromyalgia have been published. Dr. George Waylonis and I published a study in 1989. We studied 17 families and as many first-degree relatives as we could gather up, and concluded that a number of family members had fibromyalgia in a pattern that suggested an autosomal dominant mode of inheritance. This means that if one parent has fibromyalgia, then 50% of the offspring has a chance of getting fibromyalgia, whether they are male or female. There appeared to be a variable latent stage which means that the fibromyalgia could develop at different ages in different offspring. There also appeared to be variable transmission (*i.e.*, it could "skip a generation"). My study found a high percentage of fibromyalgia in men with a positive family history, nearly equal to the women. This is much different than the people who present to the doctor's office, because more than six times as many women as men will be diagnosed with fibromyalgia. Men DO have fibromyalgia, but they take a different course than women. Sometimes we have to go out and look for them because they do not tend to come to us to be diagnosed.

Dr. Dan Buskila from Israel performed a study looking at 60 children of 21 mothers with fibromyalgia. He found a number (23%) of the offspring, most of them female, to have fibromyalgia. When he looked at the males with fibromyalgia, he found the ones who were under 18 had fibromyalgia almost as frequently as the women under 18. He concluded that fibromyalgia had a major genetic component that possibly fit the autosomal dominant mode of inheritance, especially among males and females under age 18. Dr. Buskila did another study looking at people with fibromyalgia and many of their relatives, and found that 45% of them reported widespread musculoskeletal pain resembling fibromyalgia.

Other studies have supported an inherited pattern to fibromyalgia. Dr. Muhammad Yunus performed Human Leukocyte Antigen (HLA) studies in fibromyalgia. HLAs are genetically determined molecules that are found in virtually all cells. HLA genes can be markers for certain diseases, and the results of Dr. Yunus' HLA study suggests a genetic role in fibromyalgia.

I believe that the current literature, combined with accumulated clinical experience, supports a genetic cause of fibromyalgia. A "common sense" approach would be to recognize that fibromyalgia is so common in the general population of the entire world that there must be some type of common genetic make-up that leads to it. Another logical conclusion from all of the available information is that people are genetically predisposed to getting fibromyalgia. I think a number of people are programmed genetically to develop fibromyalgia over time, probably independent of the environment. However, for a number of others, an environmental trigger must occur (*i.e.*, the other causes listed here) for the fibromyalgia to develop.

Who is at risk genetically to develop fibromyalgia? I think the following can be considered at risk:

1. A child with one or both parents with fibromyalgia

2. A child of one or both parents with a connective tissue disorder such as rheumatoid arthritis or lupus

3. A child with a sibling who has fibromyalgia

4. A child with a first-degree relative who has fibromyalgia

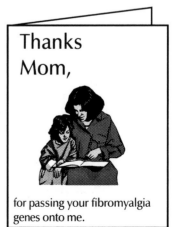

Thanks Mom, for passing your fibromyalgia genes onto me.

Just because someone is at risk does not mean he or she will automatically get fibromyalgia. The right "trigger" may never happen. If a child at risk does become symptomatic with fibromyalgia, there's a lot that can be done. Don't assume that someone will get fibromyalgia or that it will be bad if he or she does.

Genetics play a role in pain sensitivity. Dr. George Uhl found that differences in pain perception were due to variations on the surface of nerve cells, specifically on the molecule called the mu opiate receptor. The mu receptor works by bonding with natural chemicals called peptides that help diminish the sensation of pain. Individuals who have lots of these receptors have more ability to diminish pain; they have less pain. But those who have reduced mu receptors (too few mu's!) cannot diminish the pain as well, and even small stimuli can cause severe pain. The number of these receptors is controlled by the action of the mu opiate receptor gene. Those with fibromyalgia, or at risk for it, may be genetically mu deficient. I believe with additional research we will be able to further clarify specific genes causing pain, identify gene expression profiles of specific subtypes of fibromyalgia, and develop genetic-specific medicines to control pain and reduce the effects of fibromyalgia.

Trauma

Fibromyalgia caused by trauma is called post-traumatic fibromyalgia. Section 5 is devoted entirely to this sub-type of fibromyalgia. Trauma causes tissue injuries, and not everyone completely recovers from a trauma. In predisposed injuries, a physical trauma can trigger the development of fibromyalgia.

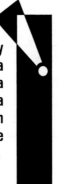

Physicians who treat fibromyalgia regularly report that the majority of fibromyalgia patients attribute the onset of fibromyalgia symptoms to a traumatic event. The trauma may be a sudden onset, *e.g.*, from a whiplash injury, or may be a repetitive cumulative-type trauma, *e.g.*, from years of typing or lifting.

Physicians who treat fibromyalgia regularly report that the majority of fibromyalgia patients attribute the onset of fibromyalgia symptoms to a traumatic event. The trauma may be a sudden onset, *e.g.*, from a whiplash injury, or may be a repetitive cumulative-type trauma, *e.g.*, from years of typing or lifting.

The story is always the same. Basically, a person is pain-free, then has a trauma, then develops pain that never disappears. Eventually that person is diagnosed with fibromyalgia. I've seen many people with no previous pain develop fibromyalgia right before my eyes following a trauma, despite my best treatment efforts to heal the trauma. This type of clinical experience screams for a logical conclusion based on common sense: Fibromyalgia must have been caused by the trauma.

The science of fibromyalgia and trauma is evolving. In 1996, a Vancouver fibromyalgia consensus group published a consensus report in the *Journal of Rheumatology*. The research that has been done so far uses scientific principles to support clinical probability. Let's review some of these techniques that support the probable relationship between fibromyalgia and trauma. Many studies have been published. I have reviewed a few of them here:

Consistent clinical pattern. Various researchers of fibromyalgia including Dr. Romano, Dr. Greenfield, Dr. Waylonis, Dr. Modolfsky, Dr. Wolfe, and others have published papers on clinical observations and clinical patterns of patients who developed post-traumatic fibromyalgia or post-traumatic myofascial pain syndrome.

Case control study. Dr. Dan Buskila (*J Rheumatol*, 1997) published case studies on patients who had whiplash injuries to the cervical spine and an injury to the lower extremity and found that fibromyalgia developed 13 times more in people who had a neck injury. This study showed a relationship between cervical spine injury and the onset of fibromyalgia, as well as showing that a regional injury can evolve into generalized fibromyalgia syndrome.

Biologic plausibility. Dr. Bennett has described how it is biologically plausible for a regional injury to lead to generalized fibromyalgia following a trauma. The mechanism by which trauma leads to fibromyalgia appears to be peripheral triggers from the trauma that mediate biochemical and neurological changes, first in the muscle and then in the central nervous system (spinal cord and brain). Once the trauma sets the process in motion, eventually it leads to fully developed fibromyalgia syndrome. The fibromyalgia may be regional where the injury occurred, or it may spread and become generalized over time and cause pain in areas that were never injured in the first place. There is a lot of controversy regarding trauma and fibromyalgia. To me, the clinical and scientific evidence support trauma as the second most common cause of fibromyalgia.

Rheumatic & Connective Tissue Diseases

Many people get fibromyalgia associated with another disease, particularly rheumatic and connective tissue diseases. After genetics and trauma, I believe this type of disease is the most common cause of fibromyalgia. Conditions in this category that can lead to reactive fibromyalgia include rheumatoid arthritis, lupus, polymyalgia rheumatica, and autoimmune disorders (thyroiditis, Sjögren's syndrome, and systemic reaction to silicone breast implants). Fibromyalgia does not turn into rheumatoid arthritis, lupus, or other inflammatory conditions, however.

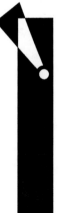

Fibromyalgia is common in patients with lupus. (Dr. Buskila, 2002). Fibromyalgia did not correlate with the lupus disease activity and has distinct clinical features. Sometimes the fibromyalgia symptoms may be confused with lupus activity, but despite its causative relationship with the lupus, the fibromyalgia becomes its own separate entity regardless of what the lupus is doing. I often see patients whose lupus (or other inflammatory condition) is in remission, but the fibromyalgia is flared-up and needs its own treatment.

All of the rheumatic and connective tissue diseases may actually be variations of auto-immune diseases. Autoimmune diseases can involve any system in the body, but the joints and connective tissue seem more vulnerable.

The immediate cause of the secondary or reactive fibromyalgia is the primary disease. However, the exact cause of most of these primary diseases is not fully understood. Theories for the cause of various rheumatic and connective tissue diseases include genetic susceptibility, infections, and certain stresses or exposures. The fact that the exact cause for the primary disease might not be known does not prevent one from stating that it is the cause of the secondary fibromyalgia. The cause should be the most immediate and direct one responsible and, in this case, the primary disease.

One could debate the "original" cause just as one could debate the theory of creation of the universe. What happened first? For example, we could say that fibromyalgia was caused by trauma. But what caused the trauma? It was a car that had run a stop sign. But what caused the car to run the stop sign? The driver was not paying attention. But what caused the driver not to pay attention? The driver was adjusting the radio dial. But why was the driver adjusting the radio dial? Because he didn't like country music. So is fibromyalgia caused by country music?

We can recognize more than one cause of a condition, and some are more direct than others. For the purposes of being very practical and logical, let's just say that the majority of the cause "weight" goes to the event closest to the development of the fibromyalgia. Rheumatic and connective tissue diseases in themselves cause specific symptoms and have specific measurable pathologies. Fibromyalgia, once it develops, becomes a separate entity and will often have a course independent of the original primary disease. For example, people with rheumatoid arthritis who have secondary fibromyalgia can have the rheumatoid arthritis in remission, but be in a severe fibromyalgia flare-up that is more disabling to them than the rheumatoid arthritis ever was.

All of the rheumatic and connective tissue diseases may actually be variations of autoimmune diseases. Autoimmune diseases can involve any system in the body, but the joints and connective tissue seem more vulnerable. Up to 5% of the adult population has an autoimmune disease; over two-thirds of those are women. Autoimmune disorders occur when the immune system begins to attack the body. Fibromyalgia can develop as a consequence of these primary diseases if the autoimmune/inflammatory mechanism sets off the "fibromyalgia cascade."

Many women with silicone breast implants develop symptoms and findings consistent with fibromyalgia. Various reports have been published which describe musculoskeletal manifestations following silicone breast implants. The APA described in Chapter 6 was initially detected in women who had developed musculoskeletal complaints following silicone breast implants. I have seen a number of women in my practice who got fibromyalgia secondary to implants. Whether the silicone caused an autoimmune-like condition which subsequently led to fibromyalgia, or whether the fibromyalgia resulted directly from the silicone exposure is not known for certain. Allergic-type reactions can be closely related to autoimmune reactions; either could lead to fibromyalgia.

Over the years, I have seen a consistent clinical association between fibromyalgia and the following rheumatic conditions: rheumatoid arthritis, lupus, polymyalgia rheumatica, sarcoidosis, Sjögren's syndrome, psoriatic arthritis, reaction to silicone breast implants, and autoimmune disease.

Infection

Like trauma, infection is one of those causes of fibromyalgia that just screams for common sense. I've seen hundreds and hundreds of people whose basic story goes like this: "I was fine, I got a virus, I developed fatigue and pain, and I've never been the same since." The logical thinking in this scenario is that fibromyalgia was not present before the viral infection. There may have been a hereditary predisposition or a vulnerability, but fibromyalgia was not present. The virus caused the condition to develop and it has been present since the virus and continues to be present. This is a straightforward infectious cause.

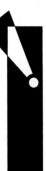

The mechanism by which an infection leads to fibromyalgia is probably related to inflammatory or autoimmune changes caused by the infection that starts the fibromyalgia cascade.

Not all infections are as straightforward. Many people who have fibromyalgia get a viral infection and find it worsens the fibromyalgia. People with active viral infections are at risk for additional infections, particularly bacterial infections which can create additional problems. Some people with fibromyalgia are more vulnerable to any type of infection because the fibromyalgia renders them more immunocompromised or more at risk for infection. The physician needs to sort out the various possibilities to determine whether an infection is the cause, a consequence, or an aggravator of the fibromyalgia.

The mechanism by which an infection leads to fibromyalgia is probably related to inflammatory or autoimmune changes caused by the infection that starts the fibromyalgia cascade. The actual clinical infection resolves and is long gone, yet fibromyalgia symptoms continue. Sometimes, the infecting virus or bacteria may hang around and create a persistent low grade infection which activates the autoimmune responses, thereby "triggering" the fibromyalgia. Many times, though, the infection has long disappeared, but permanent changes occurred in the body, and these changes caused fibromyalgia to develop.

Various viral infections can cause fibromyalgia. The Epstein-Barr virus which causes infectious mononucleosis is one. Cytomegalovirus causes a syndrome similar to infectious mononucleosis. Different strains of the influenza virus can also result in fibromyalgia. The adenoviruses, especially Type II, cause common colds, bronchitis, and various upper respiratory infections, and may lead to fibromyalgia. Human Herpes Virus 6 has also been implicated.

Reactive fibromyalgia has been described in patients with AIDS and hepatitis. Sometimes viral titers can be directly measured to demonstrate that an acute infection has occurred. This concentration can be correlated with the clinical development of fibromyalgia. Many times, though, the exact offending virus is not known, but we can still categorize the fibromyalgia as one that was caused by an infection, probably a viral infection, if it fits clinically.

Bacterial infections can also cause fibromyalgia. I have seen patients who have developed fibromyalgia after sepsis (blood infection) and salmonella infections, and one who, I felt, had gotten it from a *Listeria* infection. Some research studies found *Mycoplasma incognitus* and *Chlamydia pneumonia* in patients with fibromyalgia and chronic fatigue syndrome (Dr. Garth Nicolson and Dr. Darryl See). These infectious organisms may be causing some of the symptoms. Indeed, some of the patients improve with antibiotic therapy. Gulf War Syndrome, in part, may have been related to infections from one of these bacteria. Symptoms of Gulf War Syndrome include fatigue, headaches, depression, joint and muscle pain, sleep disorders, and poor memory (sound familiar?).

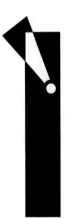

Fibromyalgia can be caused by yeast and parasite infections. I have seen some patients who developed it following a severe *Candida* yeast infection, and others following parasite infections such as *Giardia*.

Fibromyalgia can be caused by yeast and parasite infections. I have seen some patients who developed it following a severe *Candida* yeast infection, and others following parasite infections such as *Giardia*. Most of the time, yeast or parasite infections occur in patients after the fibromyalgia has already developed. These infections may aggravate the preexisting fibromyalgia or cause it to flare up. Fibromyalgia may predispose us to these infections by interfering with our immune function. On the other hand, these infections can sometimes cause the fibromyalgia by "triggering" the fibromyalgia cascade. Many of the symptoms of a chronic *Candida* yeast infection such as fatigue, irritable bowel syndrome, bloating, allergies, altered immune response, and skin conditions overlap with fibromyalgia symptoms. This can make it difficult to "separate" the two conditions and determine cause and effect relationships.

As I've mentioned, some infections come in, do their damage and disappear. The infectious agent is no longer present in the body and thus can't be detected at a later point in time. Other infectious agents may hang around in the body and establish a chronic infection, one that perhaps can be detected with blood tests. What remains to be seen is whether these chronic infections can be eradicated with antibiotic treatment and, if so, will the fibromyalgia symptoms disappear? Or has the fibromyalgia already established itself as a separate entity which does not disappear with the antibiotic treatment? Hopefully, we will have these answers in the near future.

Catastrophic Stresses

Catastrophic stresses are synonymous with emotional trauma. These are not your everyday stresses. Rather, they represent more severe stresses which can cause fibromyalgia. The mechanism is probably very similar to a physical trauma, only instead of a tissue injury, there is a stress injury that may disrupt the hypothalamic-pituitary-adrenal hormone regulation (the stress hormones). Dr. Leslie Crofford has described stress hormone abnormalities after a severe stress. Once fibromyalgia develops following such an emotionally stressful event, it can be exacerbated by additional stress. Catastrophic stresses or emotional traumas can include death of a loved one, serious illness in a loved one, history of abuse, severe illness, and more. A special type of stress that causes fibromyalgia is war. Researchers have evaluated war veterans with rheumatic conditions and have described conditions that appeared identical to fibromyalgia. Post-traumatic stress syndrome was commonly diagnosed in men who had fought in the Vietnam War. It is not surprising to find that many people who have been diagnosed with post-traumatic stress syndrome also meet the criteria for fibromyalgia.

Post-traumatic stress syndrome was commonly diagnosed in men who had fought in the Vietnam War. It is not surprising to find that many people who have been diagnosed with post-traumatic stress syndrome also meet the criteria for fibromyalgia.

Acute severe stresses can create changes in the hormones, behavior, sleep, and pain responses which ultimately establish a chronic feedback loop that amplifies pain and perpetuates fibromyalgia. The primary cause in this situation is the stress which leads to the fibromyalgia cascade.

Chemical Exposure

I've seen a number of patients who have developed fibromyalgia after chemical exposure. Usually they have inhaled fumes from offending chemicals which include petroleum oils, paint thinners, cleaning solvents, dyes, or gases/fumes from burning products. Most of the time, these patients are treated at the hospital, but have lingering symptoms and ultimately develop fibromyalgia. The mechanism whereby these chemical exposures cause fibromyalgia appears to be an allergic and/or autoimmune response that escalates and sets off the fibromyalgia cascade.

Many people with fibromyalgia are sensitive to chemicals, drugs, and environmental allergens like pollen, dust, and molds. A condition known as chemical sensitivity syndrome occurs when one becomes chronically fatigued and ill from exposures to various substances. An autoimmune mechanism is probably involved. Perhaps this condition is a subset of fibromyalgia. Various researchers have suggested that symptoms of Gulf War Syndrome (or Gulf War Illness) could have been triggered by various chemical exposures.

Tamara Liller, M.A., the Editor-in-Chief of *Fibromyalgia Frontiers* recently wrote an excellent summary of Gulf War Illness. She reviewed various possible culprits leading to Gulf War Illness (which is probably a form of fibromyalgia). Toxic chemical exposures have included vaccinations, anti-nerve agents, pesticides, chemical warfare agents, uranium (used in weapons and armor), petroleum, cleaning solvents, and even blowing sand could all have played a role or a combined role in triggering a chronic painful illness. Also, Gulf War veterans had a higher prevalence of an infectious micro-organism known as Mycoplasma fermentans, as reported by Dr. Garth Nicolson.

Dr. Daniel Clauw has advanced a new form of stress theory that argues that the majority of symptoms seen in Gulf War veterans were the result of a combination of external stress factors (trauma, infections, exposure to drugs or chemicals, and emotional stressors) combined with internal stress factors (tension, exhaustion, poor sleep, and physical symptoms such as headaches, pain, and fatigue). The bodies became overburdened with different stressors thereby adversely affecting the autonomic nervous system. These nerves affect the pain processing centers as well as the body's immune system and neuroendocrine systems. This Gulf War Illness stress theory model also describes how the general population can ultimately develop fibromyalgia.

Possible Causes/Probable Mechanisms Of Fibromyalgia

This group of conditions may be causes or mechanisms. They probably all have mechanisms in the development of fibromyalgia (the HOW). In addition, they could possibly be part of the cause of fibromyalgia (the WHY) or they may contribute indirectly to fibromyalgia. These entities include:

1. Hormonal disorders

2. Neurological conditions

3. Spinal conditions

4. Aging threshold

1. Hormonal Disorders

Various neuroendocrine dysfunctions (abnormalities of neurotransmitters and hormones) can cause problems. Concentrations of these substances are either too low or they are present in normal amounts but are not functioning properly. A number of people have low thyroid, low growth hormone, low cortisol, or low estrogen as reported by various researchers. Some people do better with thyroid, growth hormone, or cortisol replacement therapy. A subset of women experience aggravation of fibromyalgia symptoms when estrogen levels become relatively low as can occur during certain phases of the menstrual cycle and during menopause. Some of these women improve with estrogen supplementation even if the fibromyalgia does not disappear. Further research will hopefully answer a key question: Are the hormonal disturbances the result of fibromyalgia, or are they the cause of the ongoing problem?

2. Neurological Conditions

I see a number of people with multiple sclerosis, diabetic neuropathy, and postpolio syndrome who also meet the criteria for fibromyalgia syndrome. Did the neurological condition cause the fibromyalgia? Or is the fibromyalgia coincidentally present in addition to the neurological condition? A possible mechanism (or cause) is a neurological "trigger" that leads to pain amplification and, ultimately, fibromyalgia. In addition, neurological conditions cause weaknesses, muscle imbalances, and changes in muscle tone that create chronic mechanical stresses on the body tissues. These altered biomechanics, over time, can create a post-traumatic type of fibromyalgia.

3. Spinal Conditions

Some patients may be misdiagnosed with fibromyalgia when they actually have a neurological condition causing pain. Examples include Arnold-Chiari malformation, which is caused by inadequate development of the skull base; the cerebellum is crowded and compresses the brain stem. Another is cervical spinal stenosis (narrowing), which also may be developmental but can worsen due to aging, trauma or both. The spinal cord in the neck or at the base of the skull may be chronically compressed, which causes symptoms that include pain in the spine, torso and extremities, headaches, balance problems, weakness, numbness and abnormal reflexes. Many other symptoms such as bladder problems, bowel abnormalities, palpitations and hypotension may also occur. Dr. M.J. Rosner has reported a number of patients misdiagnosed with fibromyalgia who have been improved following decompressive surgery for Chiari malformation and/or cervical spine stenosis.

If surgery corrected all the symptoms, the person may not have had "true" fibromyalgia; rather, the patient had cervical cord compression from stenosis that caused symptoms mimicking fibromyalgia.

People who have neck injuries and neck arthritis may develop a "traffic jam" that causes more pressure in the cervical spinal cord and interferes with the Substance P distribution and pain control, ultimately causing fibromyalgia symptoms. More research is needed to clarify this.

It's certainly possible for fibromyalgia to coexist with a neck problem. It's also possible that a neck problem such as cervical spinal stenosis can lead to reactive fibromyalgia. We know that neck injuries can lead to fibromyalgia, so it is logical to conclude (biologic plausibility) that problems affecting the cervical spinal cord and nerves in the neck area could possibly cause the condition.

Dr. Thomas Milhorat and associates described an interesting Substance P abnormality in patients with a condition known as syringomyelia (a painful cyst in the spinal cord). They found that Substance P was increased in the spinal cord below the cyst, and decreased at the level of the cyst. This suggests that anything which puts a pressure on the cervical spinal cord can lead to changes in Substance P that increases pain (remember, people with fibromyalgia have high levels of Substance P).

People who have neck injuries and neck arthritis may develop a "traffic jam" that causes more pressure in the cervical spinal cord and interferes with the Substance P distribution and pain control, ultimately causing fibromyalgia symptoms. More research is needed to clarify this.

Other inherited conditions of the spine may increase one's risk for getting fibromyalgia, including idiopathic scoliosis, spondylolisthesis, and transitional vertebrae. These conditions, by themselves, are not usually painful. However, they may trigger the onset of fibromyalgia by causing altered spinal mechanics (which increases soft tissue sprain and strain) or neurological changes (which sensitizes the pain nerves). These "triggering" mechanisms could activate the fibromyalgia cascade and result in painful symptoms.

I see fibromyalgia commonly in individuals with scoliosis. The two conditions coexist, but I believe they are part of a genetic mechanism whereby a person inherits the tendency to have both. People who have fibromyalgia do not develop scoliosis as part of the fibromyalgia, but people with scoliosis are more at risk for developing fibromyalgia. Also, people with scoliosis may have a condition that causes neurological symptoms.

Nancy Allen, a Fibromyalgia Support Group Leader in California has shared with me her theory that an inherited condition of the spine known as spina bifida occulta may lead to fibromyalgia. Those with spina bifida occulta have a congenital defect in the lower spine that may lead to traction on the spinal cord (called tethered cord) in some resulting in pain, bladder dysfunction, other neurological symptoms, and even scoliosis. Nancy has a background in Biology and is approaching researchers with these ideas, hoping to stimulate interest in a project that will look for tethered cord in fibromyalgia patients.

I am impressed with Nancy's astute scientific reasoning and anticipate she will help find another piece of the fibromyalgia puzzle. If further research reveals a relationship between tethered cord and certain conditions such as fibromyalgia/spina bifida occulta, and scoliosis, then perhaps additional treatments may become available. Surgical sectioning of the filum terminale (the tethering ligament at the bottom of the spinal cord) is one accepted treatment for tethered cord complications. Perhaps someday this procedure may be considered to stop or even reverse neuromusculoskeletal complications in some patients who have both fibromyalgia and tethered cord.

Arthritis conditions of the spine such as osteoarthritis and osteoporosis need to be considered as well. Everyone gets osteoarthritis (wear and tear of the bones) with age, but not everyone gets fibromyalgia, so I don't think we can say osteoarthritis causes fibromyalgia. However, in people with fibromyalgia, osteoarthritis can cause it to worsen or flare-up. Both need to be treated.

Osteoporosis (thinning of the bones) can cause bone compression, ligament sprains, muscle strains and sprains, and biomechanical changes that are all likely to aggravate fibromyalgia.

4. Aging Threshold

A common story I hear from patients is that their pains gradually developed without any obvious precipitating event. We mentioned earlier in this chapter that genetics may cause some people's fibromyalgia to develop randomly at some point, and once the pain starts it's always there and can get worse over time. But is this process random, programmed, or subject to environmental factors? Probably a combination is involved.

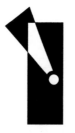

The aging threshold implies that as a person gets older, the threshold is lower for developing fibromyalgia.

I see many children and teenagers with fibromyalgia, but I see more adults in their 30's or older when they first developed fibromyalgia symptoms. If genetics were the only factor in developing fibromyalgia, I would expect more younger patients with chronic pain complaints. Genetic expression of a condition may take years to happen, so some people who first develop fibromyalgia symptoms in their 30's or later may have programmed genes causing the delayed expression. Although genetics are a factor, I think there might be additional factors contributing to the "delayed" development of fibromyalgia; factors that I refer to as the aging threshold.

The aging threshold implies that as a person gets older, the threshold is lower for developing fibromyalgia. The person may be more vulnerable to getting fibromyalgia from various causes as described earlier, but the aging process is also a risk for getting fibromyalgia, especially in women.

When we discussed pain mechanisms earlier in this book, I mentioned how both men and women were found to lose their ability to inhibit chronic pain signals as they got older, and that normal women already had a "defective" pain inhibitory system to begin with. Thus, any vulnerable person (who inherited fibromyalgia genes) would be less able to inhibit pain signals as he or she aged and would become more susceptible to developing amplified pain (women more than men).

Also, wear and tear changes on the body over time may contribute to the aging threshold. As we age, inevitably our muscles, tendons, ligaments, discs and joints show signs of deterioration from accumulated micro-trauma. These deteriorating tissues may form painful areas, *i.e.*, pain generators. In a vulnerable person, the development of painful areas may trigger the "amplified pain" cascade. Additionally, hormonal changes over time can increase the risk for developing pain. For example, early menopausal women are more likely to report increased fibromyalgia pain.

If we combine these different factors, we can appreciate how the pain/fibromyalgia threshold lowers as one ages, and it appears by the 4th or 5th decade (30's and 40's), the aging threshold has reached a "predictable" level where fibromyalgia can take hold, hence the increased frequency of fibromyalgia complaints in this age range (see diagram on next page). Once the pain threshold drops below the body's ability to inhibit potential/random chronic pain signals, the threshold is "breached." Now, chronic pain signals have a better chance of propagating the amplified pain cascade of changes and lead to fibromyalgia.

Diagram 10.1: Pain Threshold Changes with Age

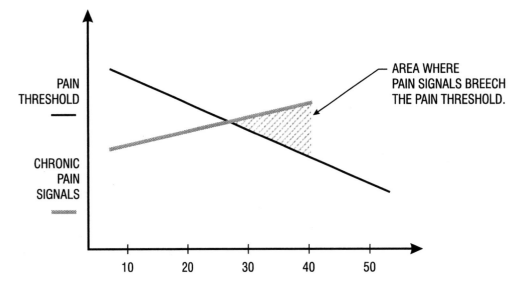

Drugs Causing Fibromyalgia-like Syndromes

Not all that appears to be fibromyalgia is always the case, thankfully! People can develop muscle pains, widespread aching and tenderness, joint pain, tendinitis pains, neuropathy-type pains and weakness from drug reactions. I have seen a number of patients with classic fibromyalgia symptoms who turned out to have a drug reaction. Once the drug was discontinued, the fibromyalgia-like illness completely reversed. In these situations, true fibromyalgia (irreversible) was not present.

Drugs that can cause reversible fibromyalgia-like syndromes are:

- Cholesterol Lowering Agents: Lovastatin (Mevacor), Fluvastatin (Lescol), Simvastatin (Zocor), Pravastatin (Pravachol), Atorvastatin (Lipitor)

- Anticonvulsants: Valproate, Ethsoximide, Carbamazepine, Hydantoins

- Antiarrhythmics: Procainamide, Quinidine

- Antibiotics: Minocycline, Isoniazid, Griseofulvin

- Hormonal Therapy: Leuprolide Acetate (Lupron)

- Antihypertensives: Hydralazine, Atenolol, Captopril, Methyldopa

- Anti-inflammatories: Penicillamine, Sulfasalazine, rarely NSAID's

- Antipsychotics: Chlorpromazine

- Antimalarials: Plaquenil

- Gout medicines: Colchicine

- Steroids

- Alcohol

- Cocaine

Some of the drugs are more apt to cause painless weakness rather than painful muscles and joints (*e.g.*, steroids, Colchicine, alcohol). Painful side effects of drugs are uncommon and are usually related to the dose of the drugs and duration of treatment. Cholesterol lowering agents, especially HMG-COA reductase inhibitors (also called statin drugs) are usually well tolerated but may cause myalgias in 1 to 7% of people. It is felt that these medicines disrupt muscle energy production by decreasing co-enzyme Q_{10} production (Ghirlanda *et al.*, 1993). Stopping the offending drug will usually result in complete reversal of the myalgias. Asking my patients what medicines they take, especially cholesterol medicines, is an important part of the clinical evaluation of myalgias.

If drug-induced muscle injury is suspected as a cause of a patient's painful complaints, certain labs may be ordered including creatine kinase (CK), a sensitive marker of muscle injury. Electrodiagnostic testing (EMG) may be helpful as well to look for muscle inflammation or neuropathy.

Some drugs can trigger an autoimmune reaction and cause drug-induced lupus. Individuals may have a genetic predisposition that makes them more vulnerable to this type of autoimmune reaction. Drugs that can cause a reversible form of lupus (with associated myalgias and arthralgias) include Penicillamine, Minocycline, anti-inflammatories, Atenolol and Sulfasalazine.

Some drugs can trigger an autoimmune reaction and cause drug-induced lupus. Individuals may have a genetic predisposition that makes them more vulnerable to this type of autoimmune reaction.

Another mechanism of drug-induced myalgia may be "unmasking" effects when a drug is discontinued. Instead of causing dose-dependent symptoms of myalgia, the drug is causing dose-dependent suppression of myalgia. An example of these medicines include hormone medicines such as thyroid medicines and especially estrogen medicines.

I have seen numerous patients whose pains FIRST started after reducing or discontinuing long- term medicines. One lady I saw developed myalgias after her gynecologist discontinued her Premarin which she had taken for 13 years. Her muscle exam revealed 14 of 18 positive painful tender points, so she met the 11 of 18 ACR-defined criteria for fibromyalgia. She resumed Premarin and her pains resolved, BUT she still had 12 of 18 positive painful tender points on exam. Perhaps she has true fibromyalgia that was in complete remission on the Premarin, and once the Premarin was discontinued, the fibromyalgia symptoms became unmasked.

Not everyone with fibromyalgia-like symptoms has true fibromyalgia, so the drug-induced symptoms are expected to be completely reversible. Some with fibromyalgia-like symptoms from a drug may actually have true fibromyalgia, and the drug aggravated the fibromyalgia symptoms. These people's fibromyalgia symptoms should settle down when the offending drug is removed, but may not be completely reversed. And finally, some may be vulnerable to getting fibromyalgia or have true fibromyalgia, and a prescribed medicine unrelated to fibromyalgia helps mask potential fibromyalgia symptoms that become noticeable only when the medicine is removed.

Unknown Causes Of Fibromyalgia

One of my pet peeves is the liberal use of the phrase, "the cause of fibromyalgia is unknown." This implies that we don't know anything about the causes. I have had some doctors and attorneys suggest to me that if the cause is unknown, then perhaps we are not even sure that fibromyalgia exists.

We know many causes, and I've described several in this chapter. We may not know the specific cause for a particular individual, but every single person with fibromyalgia has a cause, whether we know it or not. Just because we may not know the cause doesn't mean fibromyalgia isn't there. Fibromyalgia is a big world with many parts yet to be discovered. What knowledge we have empowers us, but let's not get too comfortable and arrogant about what we know, because we really know very little of the "big picture!"

Future Research

We have come a long way with fibromyalgia in the last 100 years. I don't mean that we feel like we are 100 years-old with fibromyalgia, although that's usually the case too! We are continuing to learn about the causes and mechanisms of fibromyalgia, and ongoing funding and research of this complicated condition will result in further understanding. Future research will continue to shed light on these factors:

1. More specific identification of fibromyalgia subgroups and better delineation of the overall fibromyalgia spectrum.

2. Better understanding of the actual pathological mechanism and learning what specifically triggers fibromyalgia from a microscopic or cellular level.

3. The ability to predict who will get fibromyalgia and what happens over time, and to understand the risks.

4. Additional genetic research to identify specific gene markers or specific neurobiological factors that contribute to fibromyalgia. Genetic research could also identify healing factors or specific gene therapy.

Controversies or not, causes or no causes, subsets or different conditions, or whatever the question, one thing is certain: we will continue to learn more about fibromyalgia in the future and understand it better.

▶ If You Want To Know More

1. Barrett, DH, Gray, GC, Doebbeling, BN, et al. *Prevalence of symptoms and symptom-based conditions among Gulf War veterans: current status of research findings.* Epidemiol Rev 2002; 24: 218–27.

2. Bennett RM, Cook DM, Clark SR, et al. *Hypothalamic-pituitary-insulin-like factor-1 axis dysfunction in patients with fibromyalgia.* J Rheumatol 1997; 24: 1384–9.

3. Bennett RM. *Emerging concepts in the neurobiology of chronic pain: evidence of abnormal sensory processing in fibromyalgia.* Mayo Clin Proc 1999; 74(4): 385-98.

4. Bridges AJ, Conley C, Wang G, et al. *A clinical and immunologic evaluation of women with silicone breast implants and symptoms of rheumatic disease.* Ann Intern Med 1993; 118: 929-36.

5. Buskila D, Neumann L, Vaisberg G, et al. *Increased rates of fibromyalgia following cervical spine injury. A controlled study of 161 cases of traumatic injury.* Arthritis Rheum 1997 Mar; 40(3): 446–52.

6. Buskila D, Press J, Abu-Shakra M. *Fibromyalgia in systemic lupus erythematosus: prevalence and clinical implications* Clin Rev Allergy Immunol 2003; 25(1): 25–8.

7. Cohen SB, Rohrich RJ. *Evaluation of the patient with silicone gel breast implants and rheumatic complaints.* Plast Reconstr Surg 1994; 94(1): 120–5.

8. Crofford LJ, Pillemer SR, Kalogeras KT, et al. *Hypothalamic-pituitary-adrenal axis perturbations in patients with fibromyalgia.* Arthritis Rheum 1994; 37(11): 1583–92.

9. Cuellar ML, Gluck O, Molina JF, et al. *Silicone breast implant: associated musculoskeletal manifestations.* Clin Rheumatol 1995; 14: 667–72.

10. Ghirlanda G, Oradei A, Manto A, et al. *Evidence of plasma CoQ10-lowering effect by HMG-CoA reductase inhibitors: a double-blind, placebo-controlled study.* J Clin Pharm 1993; 33: 226–9.

11. Greenfield S, Fitzcharles MA, Esdaile JM. *Reactive fibromyalgia syndrome.* Arthritis Rheum 1992; 35: 678–81.

12. Heffez DS, Ross RE, Shade-Zeldow Y, et al. *Clinical evidence for cervical myelopathy due to Chiari malformation and spinal stenosis in a non-randomized group of patients with the disagnosis of fibromyalgia.* Eur Spine J 2004 April 9; online: http://www.springerlink.com/app/home/issue.asp.

13. Iskandar BJ, Fulmer BB, Hadley MN, et al. *Congenital tethered spinal cord syndrome in adults.* Neurosurg Focus 2001; 10: 1–5.

14. Liller T. *Gulf War illness, the struggle continues.* Fibromyalgia Frontiers 2003; 11: 3–9.

15. Milhorat TH, Chou MW, Trinidad EM, et al. *Chiari I malformation redefined: clinical and radiographic findings for 364 symptomatic patients.* Neurosurg 1999; 44(5): 1005–17.

16. Mulholland RC. *Historical perspective: Sir William Gowers.* Spine 1996; 21: 1106–10.

17. Nicolson GL, Nasralla MY, De Meirleir K. *Evidence for bacterial (mycoplasma, chlamydia) and viral (HHV-6) co-infections in chronic fatigue syndrome patients.* J Chron Fat Synd 2003; 11(2): 7–20.

18. Pellegrino MJ, Waylonis GW, Sommer A. *Familial occurrence of primary fibromyalgia.* Arch Phys Med Rehabil 1989; 70: 61–3.

19. Romano TJ. *Clinical experiences with post-traumatic fibromyalgia syndrome.* W V Med J 1990 May; 86(5): 198–202.

20. Rosner MJ. *Decompression of craniovertebral stenosis leads to improvement in FMS and CFIDS symptoms.* New Dimensions in Fibromyalgia Symposium, Portland, Oregon, September 1997, http://www.nfra.net/Stenos3.htm

21. Sora I, Funada M, Uhl GR. *The mu-opioid receptor is necessary for [D-Pen2,D-Pen5]enkephalin-induced analgesia.* Eur J Pharmacol 1997; 324: R1–2.

22. Waylonis GW, Perkins RH. *Post-traumatic fibromyalgia. A long-term follow-up.* Am J Phys Med Rehabil 1994; 73: 403–12.

23. Wolfe F. *Post-traumatic fibromyalgia: a case report narrated by the patient.* Arthritis Care Res 1994; 7: 161–5.

24. Wolfe F. *Vancouver Fibromyalgia Consensus Group. The fibromyalgia syndrome: a consensus report of fibromyalgia and disability.* J Rheumatol 1996; 23: 534–9.

25. Yunus MB, Bennett RM, Romano TJ, et al. *Fibromyalgia consensus report: additional comments.* J Clin Rheumatol. 1997; 3: 324–7.

26. Yunus MB, Kahn MA, Rawling KK, et al. *Genetic linkage analysis of multicase families with fibromyalgia syndrome.* J Rheumatol 1999; 26(2): 408–12.

The Fibromyalgia Spectrum

As a senior resident at The Ohio State University in 1988, I gave a lecture on fibromyalgia at the Physical Medicine Grand Rounds. One of my lecture slides was entitled "Fibromyalgia, A Spectrum of Conditions?" I discussed how fibromyalgia appears to be a "broader" condition with specific subsets. Fibromyalgia was in that area between normal and disease, the "gray" area. Some of the subsets were closer to normal, involving regional pain only or milder symptoms without numerous associated conditions. Some subsets were closer to abnormal, with some features of connective tissue or rheumatic diseases but were not quite "there." Today I'm convinced fibromyalgia is indeed a "broader" condition with various subsets. I believe this information is helpful in explaining why everyone's symptoms are different even though they all have fibromyalgia. This chapter addresses how the fibromyalgia spectrum is part of the big picture in understanding fibromyalgia.

Fibromyalgia is a distinct medical entity, and appropriately so. We have long recognized, however, that many conditions overlap it, and various conditions exist that can lead to secondary fibromyalgia. Dr. Muhammad Yunus has developed the concept of Dysregulation Spectrum Syndrome (DSS) to describe how conditions overlap. Dr. Yunus describes DSS as representing various associated conditions that share similar clinical characteristics and pathologic mechanisms with fibromyalgia. Ten conditions are in the DSS umbrella: fibromyalgia, chronic fatigue syndrome, irritable bowel syndrome, tension headaches, migraine headaches, primary dysmenorrhea, periodic limb movement disorder, restless leg syndrome, temporomandibular pain syndrome, and myofascial pain syndrome. He predicts other entities will be added to this list in the future.

According to Dr. Yunus, conditions in DSS share a number of characteristics:

1. Patients with different conditions sharing similar profiles

2. Common shared symptoms, such as pain, poor sleep, fatigue, and female predominance

3. Hypersensitivity to pain

4. No "diagnostic" pathology that can be measured

5. Shared psychological complaints such as depression and anxiety

6. Shared common genetic factor likely

7. Common neurohormonal dysfunctions

8. Treatments directed at the central nervous system leading to improvement

9. TMJ dysfunction

Dr. Yunus' concept includes fibromyalgia as a member of a bigger DSS family.

I have discussed the fibromyalgia spectrum with my patients to help them understand the various subsets possible. I do not see fibromyalgia as a member of a bigger family, but as the main condition. It is the "founding father" and keeps its name. If fibromyalgia is the founding father, then the various overlapping conditions and subsets become the children. The name fibromyalgia remains, but different subsets have unique characteristics and together they become the fibromyalgia spectrum.

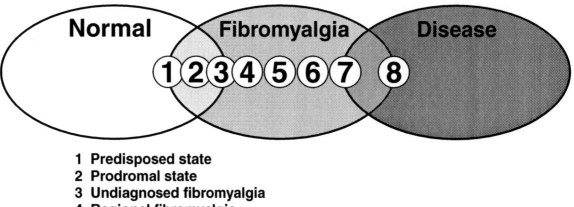

1 Predisposed state
2 Prodromal state
3 Undiagnosed fibromyalgia
4 Regional fibromyalgia
5 Generalized fibromyalgia
6 Fibromyalgia with particular associated conditions
7 Fibromyalgia with coexisting mild disease
8 Secondary fibromyalgia reactive to disease

The diagram above shows the concept of the fibromyalgia spectrum. The fibromyalgia entity partially overlaps with the normal entity on one side and the disease entity on the other side. Within the fibromyalgia entity are 8 subsets. The first subset is in the most "normal" portion of fibromyalgia, and the 8th subset is in the most "diseased" portion of fibromyalgia. Each number represents a distinct subset with distinct characteristics. The eight subsets of the fibromyalgia spectrum are:

1. Predisposed state

2. Prodromal state

3. Undiagnosed fibromyalgia

4. Regional fibromyalgia

5. Generalized fibromyalgia

6. Fibromyalgia with particular associated conditions

7. Fibromyalgia with coexisting mild disease

8. Secondary fibromyalgia reactive to disease

An individual can move up this spectrum—from a lower numbered subset to a higher numbered subset, but once in a particular subset, she/he does not return to a lower numbered subset. One can achieve a remission, but stays in that subset. In other words, there is no going back. Let's review the features of each subset.

Subset 1: Predisposed state. The individual is asymptomatic. Clinical fibromyalgia is not present in this state. The individual is at risk for developing fibromyalgia due to hereditary factors, which may include one or both parents with fibromyalgia or a rheumatic/connective tissue disease, or a sibling or first-degree relative with fibromyalgia.

Subset 2: Prodromal state. Prodromal means preceding, or the state leading to the condition. Clinical fibromyalgia is still not present. There is no widespread pain or painful tender points. The individual is not asymptomatic, however. Associated conditions common with fibromyalgia may be present in this stage, such as headaches, restless leg syndrome, fatigue or irritable bowel syndrome. Pain may be present at times, but intermittently (not chronic, persistent pains). Even though the individual may have one or more associated condition(s), widespread persistent pain is not present, so therefore fibromyalgia is not yet present. Typical fibromyalgia pain must be present before we can diagnose clinical fibromyalgia, no matter how many associated conditions may be present, but those who have numerous associated conditions are at risk.

Subset 3: Undiagnosed fibromyalgia. Chronic pain is now present, either regional or generalized in nature. This is the point of no return. The person has painful tender points which may or may not meet the American College of Rheumatology-defined 11 of 18 criteria. The person in this stage usually has milder symptoms and has not yet seen a doctor or been officially diagnosed with fibromyalgia. If this individual were to see a knowledgeable physician, that diagnosis would be made.

Subset 4: Regional fibromyalgia. Individuals in this stage have been diagnosed with fibromyalgia, but not generalized. Chronic pain is limited to one or a few areas such as the upper body or the low back. The symptoms may wax and wane. Usually, this subset is triggered by a trauma. I believe myofascial pain syndrome is part of this regional fibromyalgia, and both terms are essentially synonymous. Myofascial pain syndrome has become familiar through the work of Dr. Janet Travell and Dr. Robert Simons.

Myofascial pain syndrome is defined by painful muscles and the presence of trigger points and taut bands of muscle fibers which are ropey and painful when palpated. An involuntary shortening of the fibrous muscle band can create a local twitch response. Some of those who work with myofascial pain syndrome will argue that it is a separate distinct entity from fibromyalgia. I disagree. The similarities between myofascial pain syndrome and fibromyalgia are far greater than their differences. They both have trigger points, tender points, ropey muscles, sympathetic nerve dysfunction, ATP abnormalities, peripheral and central mechanisms, regional and generalized versions, and associated conditions. Sound familiar? The treatments are essentially the same. As our clinical experience has evolved and our knowledge and research have become more refined, I think it is clear that myofascial pain syndrome is a part of the overall fibromyalgia spectrum.

Individuals with regional fibromyalgia, over time, often develop generalized fibromyalgia. Or they can remain in this stage indefinitely. Identifying the regional stage early and treating it can definitely help to prevent progression.

Subset 5: Generalized fibromyalgia. Individuals in this stage have widespread pain and tender points. They will usually meet the American College of Rheumatology-defined 11 of 18 criteria, but as previously explained, one can still have generalized fibromyalgia with fewer tender points. Various associated conditions seen with fibromyalgia can be present—sleep disorder, irritable bowel syndrome, depression, fatigue, and so on, but these associated conditions are not taking on a life of their own so to speak, but are part of the whole and managed with the overall fibromyalgia treatment. Regional fibromyalgia can progress to this subset. Various causes of generalized fibromyalgia include genetic factors, trauma, infections, and more, but secondary fibromyalgia from a primary disease is not included in this subset.

Subset 6: Fibromyalgia with particular associated conditions. People in this group have developed associated conditions that are giving them particular problems which appear as "separate" entities requiring separate attention. Some of these particular associated conditions include irritable bowel syndrome, fatigue, tension/migraine headaches, and depression. None of these conditions in themselves have "classic" disease laboratory markers or cause tissue destruction, yet they may require treatments in addition to the overall fibromyalgia treatment. Another associated condition is dysautonomia (dysfunction of the small nerves) which can cause abnormalities such as hypoglycemia, hypotension, cardiac arrhythmia, irritable bowel syndrome, and vascular headaches.

Subset 7: Fibromyalgia with coexisting disease. Individuals in this category have a specific disease, and also have fibromyalgia. The disease doesn't necessarily cause fibromyalgia, but it can aggravate it if it's already present. Examples of diseases that can be present and worsen the fibromyalgia symptoms include:

- Hormonal problems (hypothyroidism, low estrogen, low growth hormone, and low cortisol).

- Infectious problems (yeast, parasite or viral infections).

- Low grade rheumatic or connective tissue disease (lupus, autoimmune disorders; dry eyes syndrome described by Dr. Don Goldenberg may be part of a low grade Sjögren's syndrome).

- Arthritic conditions (cervical spinal stenosis, osteoarthritis, osteoporosis, scoliosis).

- Neurological conditions (multiple sclerosis, polio sequelae, neuropathy, head injury residuals). For example, people who have both diabetes and fibromyalgia will often have more painful fibromyalgia because the diabetes caused the nerves to be more sensitive. Diabetes is a common cause of neuropathy, or damage to the small nerves, which is painful in itself and even more so with fibromyalgia. One needs to keep the diabetes under good control to help the pain.

- Lung conditions. I see a number of people who have fibromyalgia along with a lung problem such as emphysema, asthma, chronic bronchitis, or heavy tobacco use. Cigarette smoking can increase fibromyalgia pain. The nicotine in the smoke causes constriction of the blood vessels, decreasing blood flow, oxygen, and nutrients to the muscles, thereby increasing pain and spasms. Also, carbon monoxide in smoke enters the bloodstream and binds to the hemoglobin molecules in the blood. This blocks oxygen from binding to the hemoglobin, further decreasing oxygen availability to the muscles (and increasing pain). Stop smoking and your muscles will feel better!

These diseases exist concurrently with fibromyalgia but probably do not cause it. Any of these diseases can progress from a mild to a more severe state, and fibromyalgia worsens as the disease worsens. The physician determines if the disease is coexisting with and aggravating fibromyalgia (subset 7), or if a disease caused the fibromyalgia (subset 8).

Subset 8: Secondary fibromyalgia reactive to disease. Individuals in this category have secondary fibromyalgia. They have a primary disease (*e.g.*, lupus, rheumatoid arthritis) and fibromyalgia developed as a result of this disease. People in this subset probably wouldn't have fibromyalgia if they never had the primary disease. The primary disease requires treatment, and fibromyalgia may improve with this treatment. However, the fibromyalgia often requires its own treatment, and can continue to be a major problem even when the primary disease is treated or is in remission.

I find that the fibromyalgia spectrum provides a useful clinical model for me when evaluating and treating my patients. It helps me to "organize" them better! When I diagnose fibromyalgia, I try to be as specific as possible about what the cause is and what subset it fits. This helps me to better explain fibromyalgia to the patients and to individualize their treatment programs. Of course, if I've diagnosed fibromyalgia it would be subset 4 or greater. The patient wouldn't be seeking a medical consultation for subsets 3, 2, or 1. If possible, I note the cause. Each subset can have flare-ups or remissions within it, and I note that as well, if appropriate. Subsets 1, 2, and 3 are useful in appreciating the progression of fibromyalgia through the spectrum, and can be helpful when advising patients and family members who have specific concerns and questions.

Let's review some patient profiles to determine the subset they fit into in the fibromyalgia spectrum.

Patient #1. Mary is a 25-year-old receptionist with severe neck and shoulder pain. She had always been very active with aerobics and bicycling and had never had any pain requiring treatment until after a motor vehicle accident on April 7, 1998, when she was rear-ended and suffered a whiplash injury. The pain never went away, and when I saw her I found numerous painful tender points and trigger points with localized spasms in the neck and shoulder muscles.

Mary has regional fibromyalgia (subset 4). She was most likely predisposed to fibromyalgia and a traumatic event triggered the development of her regional fibromyalgia. She "leaped" from predisposed state (subset 1) to regional fibromyalgia (subset 4).

Patient #2. Martha is a 30-year-old housewife. She was diagnosed with fibromyalgia 5 years ago, and she was at a stable baseline with her home program of stretches, exercises, and using a hot tub. In the past year, she has been having increasing pain and fatigue and difficulty managing her fibromyalgia. She reports that in the past year she has been getting frequent yeast infections. She is on birth control pills and has had a couple of bladder infections requiring antibiotics in the past year. Her more recent history is otherwise unremarkable.

Martha has fibromyalgia with a coexisting disease, chronic yeast infection (subset 7). Her birth control pills, antibiotic treatment, and perhaps fibromyalgia have contributed to the chronic yeast infection. In turn, the yeast infection has aggravated her fibromyalgia.

Patient #3. Jamie is a 38-year-old school teacher. She has lupus, diagnosed when she was 13 years-old, and has been on various medications since then. She has been in remission for a number of years, but has developed widespread pain. Her sedimentation rate is not elevated to suggest active inflammation. Her clinical exam does not reveal any joint inflammation or active lupus findings, but she does have 16 of 18 positive painful tender points.

Jamie has secondary fibromyalgia from a disease (subset 8). In her case, the lupus is in remission, but her fibromyalgia is causing her problems and needs to be treated.

Patient #4. Jamie's 12-year-old son has been complaining of leg pains. The pains occur at nighttime, and Jamie has to rub the legs and use warm compresses. The pediatrician told her his pains were growing pains. Jamie's son gets occasional headaches, and sometimes he feels exhausted. He plays many sports, and if he works out a lot his muscles are very sore for several days. On exam, there are no areas of pain or painful tender points.

Jamie's son is probably in a prodromal state (subset 2). He is at risk because his mother has fibromyalgia and a connective tissue disease, and he has some associated conditions with intermittent pains, but has not developed the persistent widespread pain or painful tender points yet.

Patient #5. Bob is 42 years-old and has an awful lot of pain for his age. His pains are more severe than everyday pain, and sometimes he has had to miss work. He is an assembly line worker. He mentions this to his primary care doctor when he is there for his yearly physical. He is examined and found to have 12 of 18 positive painful tender points.

Bob had undiagnosed fibromyalgia (subset 3) until he became official, "entering the books" with generalized fibromyalgia (subset 5) after he saw his primary care doctor.

Fibromyalgia Spectrum Test

Let's see how well you have been paying attention in the chapter! I'm going to test your knowledge on the fibromyalgia spectrum. Below are 3 case histories for you to review and then determine which subtype of the fibromyalgia spectrum each case fits.

The answers follow.

Case 1: Peggy is 52 years-old and works as a secretary. For about ten years, she has been bothered by pains in her neck, shoulders, and upper back. In the past 2 years the pain has become more widespread. She has difficulty sleeping and has extreme fatigue. She also has irritable bowel syndrome. Recently she switched to a different computer at work and has been typing a lot more than usual. After a couple of weeks on this new computer, she noticed pain and numbness in her wrists and hands. This pain awakens her at night and she has to shake her hands to relieve the symptoms. She has noticed weakness in her hands, particularly when holding her coffee cup or trying to grip a pen. Since she developed these hand symptoms, she is noticing more pain throughout her arms, neck and shoulders.

Assuming this lady has fibromyalgia, what subtype does she have?

Case 2: Patty is a 32 year-old housewife. Eight years ago she was diagnosed with fibromyalgia syndrome and has managed this condition well with a regular program of stretching and exercises. She used to play tennis a lot, but since she developed fibromyalgia, she stopped playing regularly. Even before she was diagnosed with fibromyalgia, she was always prone to getting tendinitis or bursitis in various joints. Recently she accepted an invitation from a few of her friends to join a tennis league. She started playing tennis again once a week and within a few weeks noticed increased pains in her shoulders, forearms, hips, and knees. Her doctor diagnosed her with tendinitis and bursitis.

Based on this information, what subtype of fibromyalgia does Patty have?

Case 3: Tom is 39 years-old and started to hurt all over for the past several months. He has had various aches and pains in the past, but nothing like this. His wife thinks he is worried about turning 40. Tom thinks something else is going on because he never had this severe muscle pain before. He also has headaches and stomach cramps. He wakes up every night at 4:00 AM; he used to sleep through the night. He is also has a harder time concentrating at work, where he owns a printing company. He saw his doctor and his exam was normal except for various painful and sore muscles and 9 of 18 positive tender points. Laboratory studies were normal.

What is Tom's diagnosis? If he has fibromyalgia, what subset does he have?

Answers to Test Questions:

Case 1: Subset 7, fibromyalgia with co-existing disease. Peggy has fibromyalgia and carpal tunnel syndrome. When she developed carpal tunnel syndrome, this condition caused her fibromyalgia symptoms to flare up, causing neck, shoulder, and arm pain, as well as unique carpal tunnel symptoms (the hand numbness, pain, and weakness). Peggy's carpal tunnel syndrome was caused by repetitive typing. The carpal tunnel syndrome did not cause the fibromyalgia, nor did the fibromyalgia cause the carpal tunnel syndrome. These 2 conditions coexist.

Case 2: Subset 6, fibromyalgia with particular associated condition. Patty has fibromyalgia and a long history of tendinitis and bursitis, which are associated conditions in this case. Fibromyalgia can lead to painful tendons and bursas, particularly in the shoulders, forearms, hips, and knees. Usually the tendinitis and bursitis are not "true" inflammations, but they hurt just as bad. When Patty resumed playing tennis, she aggravated this tendinitis and bursitis, the associated conditions of her fibromyalgia.

Case 3: Subset 5, generalized fibromyalgia. This is a trick question! Even though Tom had fewer than 11 of 18 designated tender points as defined by the American College of Rheumatology, his history and exam are still consistent with generalized fibromyalgia. Remember, one can have fewer than 11 of 18 tender points and still have clinical fibromyalgia.

There is much disagreement and controversy among medical professionals and patients about categories and subsets of fibromyalgia or similar conditions. I'm not attempting to stir the waters with my version of the fibromyalgia spectrum, rather I'm trying to help you understand the fairly complicated nature of the condition and the different types I see. I find this model useful and practical in my everyday clinical practice. Remember one of my mottos: Keep things as simple as possible and make sure they make sense!

Up Close Patient Snapshot

by Mark J. Pellegrino, M.D.

Full Motor Recovery

Reprinted with permission from Cortlandt Forum

"When can I drive again, Doctor?" That Mrs. Smith could ask me such a question was remarkable in itself, considering that 8 weeks earlier she had been comatose and not expected to survive. She was baking cookies when she suddenly lost consciousness from a massive right intracerebral hemorrhage. Luckily, she was found within minutes by a neighbor, who summoned help.

By the time she reached the hospital, she was comatose and having seizures. She underwent emergency neurosurgery but failed to improve.

When I first saw her in rehabilitation consultation a week later, she was still unresponsive and on a ventilator. Previously, this 72-year-old widow had lived independently in her house and was an award-winning baker. At first, I thought substantial recovery was unlikely, since she had not improved neurologically despite early evidence on CT scan of resolution of her brain hemorrhage and swelling.

Even after she opened her eyes a few days later, I feared the long-term prognosis would be poor, since she had dense left hemiplegia and severe encephalopathy. I asked the social worker to investigate possible nursing home facilities.

However, Mrs. Smith had different ideas. As if a cerebral switch had been turned from off to on, she began making steady, significant progress. She regained some strength in her left arm and began to respond appropriately and follow simple commands. She was extubated and rapidly moved from ICU to acute therapy to inpatient rehabilitation.

I marveled at her progress. By the time she asked me about driving, her left-sided weakness had disappeared and she could walk without ambulatory aids. She remembered daily events but still needed supervision and verbal cues to safely perform her usual activities. Thus, I advised her not to drive. She was discharged to her sister's home, where Mrs. Smith would not be alone while she recovered further.

A month later, Mrs. Smith returned for a follow-up visit. As I drove into my office parking lot, I realized she was in front of me, driving her Lincoln Continental! During the visit, she gave me an update: she had stayed at her sister's for a few weeks before she was compelled to return home. She was happy and independent and had resumed her previous lifestyle, including housework, baking, and yes, driving. Neurologic and mental status exams were entirely normal!

She presented me with freshly baked cookies and thanked me for my help. As I watched her drive away, I realized how lucky she was to have beaten the odds on a miraculous recovery and was thankful that this special woman proved my first impression to be wrong.

If You Want To Know More

1. Dinerman H, Goldenberg DL, Felson DT. *A prospective evaluation of 118 patients with the fibromyalgia syndrome: prevalence of Raynaud's phenomenon, sicca symptoms, ANA, low complement, and Ig deposition at the dermal-epidermal junction.* J Rheumatol 1986; 13(2): 368–73.

2. Pellegrino MJ. *Fibromyalgia.* Lecture on physical medicine. Feb 1988.

3. Pellegrino MJ. *From whiplash to fibromyalgia.* ORC Publishing, 2002.

4. Pellegrino MJ. *Understanding post-traumatic fibromyalgia. A medical perspective.* Columbus, OH: Anadem Publishing, 1996.

5. Wolfe F, Smythe HA, Yunus MB, et al. *The American College of Rheumatology 1990 Criteria for the Classification of Fibromyalgia. Report of the Multi-Center Criteria Committee.* Arthritis Rheum 1990; 33(2): 160–72.

6. Yunus MB. *Central sensitivity syndrome.* JIRA 2000; 8: 27–33.

Fibromyalgia
Up Close & PERSONAL

12

Prognosis In Fibromyalgia

> An example of a personalized answering machine message of a person with fibromyalgia:
>
> (Digital computer voice) *"The person you have reached at 555-1234 has been changed. The new person has fibromyalgia and feels disconnected as if she is no longer in service."*

I am frequently asked what to expect; what is the prognosis regarding fibromyalgia? Determining a prognosis is one of the most important, yet most difficult, aspects in the practice of medicine. Prognosis is defined as a forecast of the probable outcome of a medical condition. Doctors try to determine whether there will be a recovery, a worsening, or complications by studying the nature and particular features of the medical condition. In determining any given prognosis, doctors must rely on knowledge of an individual's condition, symptoms, physical findings, natural progression of the pain, combined with his or her experience in treating individuals with fibromyalgia.

If a condition is expected to become worse over time, or if no cure is available, the prognosis may be "poor" or "guarded." If full recovery is expected, the prognosis would be "excellent." If improvement occurs, but the condition may persist, the prognosis may be "fair" or "good." Chronic conditions often have "poor" prognoses because there is no cure, even though they may not be life threatening.

Prognosis can be applied to different aspects of fibromyalgia. For example, we can talk about the prognosis of curing fibromyalgia, the prognosis of fibromyalgia's clinical course over time, the prognosis of successful response to treatment, the prognosis of whether fibromyalgia will cause disability, and more. For each component of fibromyalgia, we try to make a medical forecast or prediction based on the probability that a particular outcome will occur.

I have tried to determine the prognosis in fibromyalgia based upon my knowledge and experience combined with my understanding of the scientific literature (at least what I can remember of it!). Based on this, I will review prognosis for different components of fibromyalgia, from my point of view.

Will Fibromyalgia Ever Go Away? (Is there a cure?)

Fibromyalgia is a chronic and permanent condition. Once this condition has developed and is clinically measurable upon examination, it will be present for the remainder of the person's life. I am aware of no cure for fibromyalgia at the present time. Therefore, the prognosis is "poor" that a given individual's fibromyalgia will ever be completely cured. Even though the prognosis is "poor" for a cure, the prognosis is "good" that one can improve (or heal!).

Certainly we can feel better in spite of our fibromyalgia and some are lucky enough to get a complete remission, but the fibromyalgia doesn't go away. We are working on a cure, and I think we will find one someday, but in the meantime, let's live our lives to the fullest possible.

Will Fibromyalgia Get Worse Over Time? (What Is The Clinical Course Over Time?)

Fibromyalgia symptoms can improve. There may be less pain over time and sometimes fibromyalgia can go into remission. The prognosis for stabilization or improvement in most people over time is good, however, even though fibromyalgia is still present.

To explain what happens to a group of patients with fibromyalgia over time, I use the *1/3 Rule* to explain prognosis. In a group of people with fibromyalgia, the *1/3 Rule* means that:

1/3 of the people will do better over time

1/3 of the people will stay the same over time

1/3 of the people will do worse over time.

This means that at least 2/3 of the people will do better or not get worse over time; hence, the prognosis for most people with fibromyalgia to be stable or to improve is good. The *1/3 Rule* applies to a group of people with fibromyalgia. It is difficult to look at any one individual and accurately predict how that person will do over time. However, there are some characteristics that may help determine who would do more or less favorably over time.

Those who do better or at least not worse are most likely to have the following characteristics:

1. Early diagnosis of fibromyalgia after symptoms began
2. Younger age when diagnosed
3. Successful response to treatments
4. Few associated conditions
5. Have flexible job situations
6. Follow through with a home program

The 1/3 that get worse are more likely to have the following characteristics:

1. A delayed diagnosis after symptoms develop
2. No response to treatments or non-compliant with treatments
3. Numerous associated conditions that cause additional impairment
4. Stressful and physically demanding job
5. Men whose fibromyalgia came on rapidly and caused early disability

There are various reasons why the 1/3 group gets worse over time. Injuries or secondary conditions may have developed that caused an overall worsening of the fibromyalgia. For example, an individual with fibromyalgia may be involved in a motor vehicle accident and sustain a severe whiplash injury that permanently worsens the fibromyalgia and causes it to be more painful. Or a person may develop progressive osteoarthritis or an inflammatory arthritis, which causes fibromyalgia to worsen in addition to causing "separate" pain. I suspect some people are just "destined" to get worse with fibromyalgia regardless of whether or not intervening circumstances occur and whether or not the person had appropriate treatments.

Nearly everyone with fibromyalgia will experience flare-ups from time to time as part of the natural long-term course of fibromyalgia. In most, however, these flare-ups are a temporary aggravation of the baseline level that can last anywhere from days to weeks before the pain returns to the previous stable baseline. In some, however, flare-ups seem to lead to progressive worsening of the fibromyalgia and the previous stable baseline is never reached.

Although we know flare-ups will occur, we cannot predict when or how frequently. My patients have an average of 2 major flare-ups per year, and the average duration of each flare-up is about a month. These figures were determined by a retrospective review of patients, but there was a wide disparity among individual patients. Some people may have flare-ups every month, while others may not flare up for over a year.

Although a third of the people report that they get worse over time, I think everyone diagnosed with fibromyalgia who has had some opportunities for positive intervention with fibromyalgia treatments will have the potential to do better over time. Even those who report feeling worse pain over time may be more flexible and more functional than they were prior to their diagnosis. The patients may be more aware of the fibromyalgia and notice if the pain worsens. Yet they may still be successfully maintaining their functional abilities even with noticeably worse pain.

A way to understand how positive interventions can help one do better over time, compared to no treatment at all, is demonstrated in the following diagram. The diagram shows a patient's pain level over time with no treatment. You can see that the pain level became worse from the time of diagnosis and continues to get worse at a steady rate over time.

Now, suppose the same patient were treated for pain over time. She still became worse overall; however, she did not get as bad as she would have without treatment. So, if we compare the difference between the two, as noted in the diagram, we can see that the patient actually did a little better over time with treatment than without.

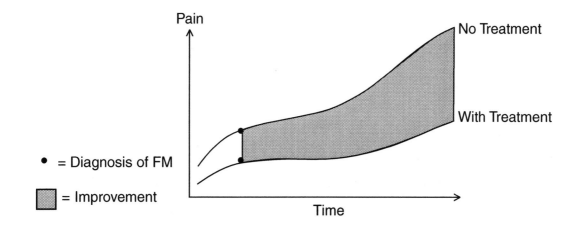

Thus, positive intervention did help this patient even though the pain got worse over time. So, hopefully we can say that the diagnosis and treatment of fibromyalgia will help a person over time, even if one feels worse. And if one feels worse, hopefully the functional abilities remain good despite the worsening pain.

Will Fibromyalgia Cause Disability?

Fibromyalgia causes impairment in everyone. An impairment is any abnormality of anatomic structure or physiological function. Tender points are impairments because they are soft tissue abnormalities in our bodies. Thus, everyone with fibromyalgia has an impairment.

Any restriction or lack of ability to perform a normal activity is considered a disability. The vast majority of people with fibromyalgia will have some type of disability or restriction as defined above. These restrictions include difficulty performing repetitive reaching, bending, twisting or standing, or difficulty with concentration and memory. By definition, fibromyalgia causes impairment in everyone and disabilities in almost everyone. Some people with fibromyalgia do not have any disabilities (and their last names aren't Ripley!).

Individuals whose fibromyalgia worsens over time have a higher probability (unfavorable prognosis) that they will have more functional impairment, disability or inability to perform various daily activities or job duties. I'll talk more about disability and fibromyalgia in Chapter 38.

Will Treatments Help Fibromyalgia?

Treatments DO help!

The next section in this book will tell you all about treatments for fibromyalgia. Treatments help reduce the pain, resolve a flare-up and return the condition to a stable baseline. The prognosis is good for getting some type of successful response to treatment. I am always reviewing treatment responses in patients to determine if they are improving and to make any changes needed in the program to achieve the best treatment response possible.

Treatments do not eliminate fibromyalgia, and they may only last a short while. I believe that a supervised medical treatment program which includes instruction on a home program can help control long-term symptoms. I do not encourage ongoing indefinite supervised medical treatment. Rather, I promote individual responsibility for following through with an independent, unsupervised home program to control chronic problems associated with fibromyalgia.

So, we're stuck with fibromyalgia, but we certainly have some control over how well we can do. We learn to accept the things we can control, but most importantly we also have to accept the things that we cannot control. As I look into my crystal ball to see what the future holds, I notice that there is a lot of … fog. Lots and lots of fog. Now isn't that typical?

▶ If You Want To Know More

Pellegrino MJ. *Inside fibromyalgia*. Columbus OH: Anadem Publishing, 2001.

SECTION III—TREATING FIBROMYALGIA

This section focuses on what I've learned about treating fibromyalgia. Many treatments are available and this section doesn't attempt to review every possible one, but rather, tries to give you the main ones. General treatment strategies with specific types of programs are introduced. Specific and detailed treatments directed by the doctor and personal "patient directed" treatment strategies that you can do are reviewed. Different doctors prefer different treatment approaches. I discuss my treatment styles and philosophies in this section and how I approach fibromyalgia patients.

Your goals with this lengthy section are to learn what can be done or what can be prescribed for your fibromyalgia. You should keep an open mind, and hopefully, you'll discover new ideas to incorporate into a successful ongoing home program.

Physical Medicine & Rehabilitation Philosophy

Numerous medical professionals and specialists treat fibromyalgia. One specialty in particular, Physical Medicine and Rehabilitation, is especially skilled at diagnosing and treating this chronic condition. A physician specializing in Physical Medicine and Rehabilitation is called a Physiatrist. I am a board certified Physiatrist.

The Physical Medicine and Rehabilitation specialty began in the 1930's to address musculoskeletal and neurological problems. Two historical events occurred to help shape and broaden this particular specialty. The first was the polio epidemic, which caused millions to suffer from acute pain and weakness and led to the physical medicine component of my specialty. Physical medicine modalities such as heat, electric stimulation, and water therapy, along with exercises to stretch, strengthen, and condition became important treatment approaches for acute polio, and ultimately for any problem that caused pain.

The second event that helped shape the rehabilitation component of my specialty occurred after World War II. Improved medical technology and techniques on the battlefield, plus the availability of penicillin, led to increased survival among injured soldiers. Many soldiers with head injuries, spinal cord injuries, infections, and amputations survived. Consequently, the number of disabled soldiers increased. Rehabilitation strategies were developed to help these disabled veterans improve functional and vocational skills, and ultimately help them return to civilian society as productive workers. Thus, the rehabilitation component was more focused on optimizing functional abilities and included retraining and an interdisciplinary team approach.

Physiatrists treat a wide range of problems from musculoskeletal pain to brain injuries. My specialty serves all age groups and treats problems that may affect all of the major systems in the body. The focus is on restoring function. A physiatrist diagnoses conditions that cause pain, weakness, and numbness, and may prescribe drugs, assistive devices, or a variety of therapies to improve functioning.

Specific philosophies unique to physiatry include a team approach involving various medical professionals, identifying rehabilitation goals to improve function, and focusing on improving one's quality of life. The word "habile," from which rehabilitation is derived, is Latin for "to make able again." This word is an embodiment of our unique treatment philosophies.

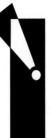

The Physical Medicine and Rehabilitation strategy empowers the fibromyalgia person with abilities to improve the quality of life, even if the condition is still present.

This approach applies naturally to the diagnosis and treatment of fibromyalgia because fibromyalgia affects all aspects of our lives and makes it difficult to function. The Physical Medicine and Rehabilitation strategy empowers the fibromyalgia person with abilities to improve the quality of life, even if the condition is still present. My private practice group adopted a motto some years back: Reclaim Your Life! I think this is an apt statement of our main treatment goal, especially in the fibromyalgia population.

Fibromyalgia Treatment Goals

It is a mistake to think of people with fibromyalgia as if we all have the same thing. Although we all have fibromyalgia, we certainly do not behave in the same manner, nor do we all respond the same to treatment. What works for one person may not work at all for another, because each of us is unique. We each need to be handled with special unique care, and each of us needs to identify our own specific treatment goals.

Specific fibromyalgia treatment goals that I identify for each individual include:

1. **Decreasing pain, even if pain is still present.** It would be great if everyone could go into remission and be pain-free, but this rarely happens. What usually happens is that the pain decreases, sometimes considerably, to a lower and more stable level. Some people achieve remissions where they feel hardly any pain.

2. **Improving function.** Even if the person is unable to resume activities enjoyed prior to developing fibromyalgia, one can improve by learning to focus on current abilities. That is why I like the word "habile," because it focuses on abilities, the positive. Too often, we tend to focus on the negative, our inabilities, by concentrating on things that we used to do. Remember habile!

3. **Learning a successful program to self-manage the condition.** Each of us with fibromyalgia has to live with this condition every day, so we should try to find out what works and learn to do it ourselves. We can't sling our doctors and therapists over our backs, carry them with us throughout the day, and pull them out when needed because of increased pain (this WOULD cause increased pain!). We must manage our pain as best we can by ourselves on a daily basis.

As I've said earlier, one does not have to be a physiatrist to diagnose and treat people with fibromyalgia. Many doctors and specialists want to help, will be open-minded, and use the best of all available treatment options to enable each individual to **achieve the highest quality of life with the least amount of pain possible.** YOUR qualifications are the most important: YOU are the one with fibromyalgia, and YOU must want to do better!

Evaluating The Patient

When I see a patient for the first time, I perform a comprehensive Physical Medicine and Rehabilitation evaluation. This includes a complete history and physical examination. I gather information on pain and various symptoms and particularly on how functional abilities have been impaired. Careful palpation is included as part of my physical examination. I examine the 18 designated tender point regions in addition to the rest of the musculoskeletal system to identify all areas that are particularly painful. I search for abnormalities that could help determine a diagnosis (spasms, weakness, swelling, etc.). Any abnormalities are documented.

If the evaluation is consistent with fibromyalgia, I document this diagnosis. I note any diagnosis that may apply to the individual's pain, even if it is different from fibromyalgia.

For example, there may be shoulder bursitis, rotator cuff tendinitis, spinal facet arthritis, lateral epicondylitis, hip sprain, or many other painful conditions. I don't simply put "fibromyalgia" as a diagnosis, but try to be as descriptive as possible. If a cause such as trauma or infection can be determined, I will note post-traumatic fibromyalgia or post-infection fibromyalgia. If the fibromyalgia is widespread, I will note generalized fibromyalgia. If it is more localized or regionalized, I will note regional fibromyalgia. If certain areas are particularly flared-up, or if particular associated conditions such as myofascial pain syndrome, sleep disorder, and irritable bowel syndrome are present, I will note those as well.

The following patient is an example of how I might approach my evaluation and conclusion. Mrs. Jones is a 36-year-old woman who reports pain throughout her body, particularly involving the muscles. She has a history of scoliosis. Her pains began in her early 30's and became generalized but fairly stable. In her late teens she was involved in a couple of motor vehicle accidents where she had whiplash injuries. She received some therapies for these whiplash injuries, and said her pains completely resolved within a few months of treatment.

In her early 30's she began to develop aches and pains that became more generalized and ultimately led to a diagnosis of fibromyalgia. A month ago she took a job as a librarian and has noticed increased pain and fatigue since starting this job.

Her mother has been diagnosed with fibromyalgia. Mrs. Jones has two children, a 17-year-old son who has frequent headaches and a 20-year-old daughter who has scoliosis. Mrs. Jones' examination revealed numerous painful tender points including 14 of the 18 positive designated tender points, but not the costochondral or medial knee areas bilaterally.

I would diagnose Mrs. Jones with generalized fibromyalgia. I note that there are various contributing factors to her fibromyalgia which include:

1. **Heredity.** Her mother has fibromyalgia and her two children may have prodromal symptoms

2. **Scoliosis.** This condition increases the risk of fibromyalgia, presumably due to increasing strain on the back muscles and alteration of the biomechanics. This may be a form of cumulative trauma.

3. **Trauma.** This includes both the cumulative trauma from scoliosis and the trauma from the motor vehicle accidents. The accidents did not appear to cause the fibromyalgia immediately because the pains disappeared after treatment, but they may have created pain memory and increased vulnerability that made it easier for fibromyalgia to involve these injured areas at a later date.

Mrs. Jones' fibromyalgia represents a good example of how the exact cause may be unknown, but more than one factor is known to be involved. I may not know exactly which factor(s) caused the fibromyalgia, but I know the cause is probably 1 or more of the three factors that I described. I would put Mrs. Jones' fibromyalgia in subset 5, generalized fibromyalgia. The new physical activities required of her librarian job has caused a flare-up of her fibromyalgia.

Treatment Recommendations

Different treatment recommendations for fibromyalgia include reassurance and explanation of the disorder, removing any mechanical stresses, analgesic drug treatment, physical exercises, and psychotherapeutic support in a multidisciplinary setting (Dr. Spratt, 2003). Each fibromyalgia patient requires an individualized program.

I review my findings and diagnosis with each patient. I discuss fibromyalgia in detail and make treatment recommendations. Sometimes, I recommend that other specialists be involved. For example, if I note my patient is clinically depressed, I may recommend a psychiatrist (specialist in depression) to specifically address the depression. I'll certainly treat the fibromyalgia, but I'm not a depression specialist. My fibromyalgia treatment recommendations will try to decrease pain, improve range of motion, decrease spasms, improve function, increase knowledge, develop a successful home program, improve interpersonal skills and relationships, and optimize quality of life. The first treatment (and the most important, I believe) is education.

Up Close Patient Snapshot

by Mark J. Pellegrino, M.D.

The Rodeo Roper's Rotator Woe

Mr. P's first words to me when he entered my office were "My left shoulder is killing me, Doc."

This was the major complaint of 42-year old Mr. P, a stocky mustached gentleman who wore blue jeans, a flannel shirt, and leather cowboy boots. As he told me of his gradually progressive shoulder pain, which worsened when he reached and lifted his left arm, I immediately suspected a rotator cuff problem. He had worked in a factory for 20 years and could have a cumulative trauma disorder commonly seen with overuse of the arms. However, Mr. P's managerial job did not require repetitive motion of the left arm and shoulder.

On further questioning, Mr. P revealed that he was a cowboy. More specifically, he was a professional steer roper. Having never met a "real" cowboy, I listened intently as he educated me about his hobby.

Steer roping requires a team of 2 riders, a "header" to rope the steer's head and a "heeler" who ropes the steer's hind legs. Being a left roper, Mr. P had to be a heeler. He could release the lariat faster from the left side, giving him a competitive advantage. He competed in at least 2 contests each weekend and had several evening practices during the week.

Recently his performance had been hindered by his shoulder pain. Years of repetitive, strenuous roping had led to rotator cuff inflammation. His condition was confirmed on physical exam by the presence of left shoulder pain and weakness, made worse by resisted shoulder abduction. A shoulder X-ray revealed a large calcium deposit on the left cuff region.

Fearing a rotator cuff tear, I recommended both magnetic resonance imaging of the shoulder and a cortisone injection into the shoulder. Mr. P confided in me that he couldn't have these done because he was terribly afraid of closed spaces and needles. He was also concerned that his shoulder problems would permanently end his roping career.

We embarked on a treatment program that included oral antiinflammatory medications, physical therapy, reduction of his weekly practice time, and warm-up shoulder stretching exercises before his roping activities. Fortunately, he made considerable improvement with these measures. His shoulder pain subsided, his roping improved and he began winning more contests. He was most appreciative of my help and invited me to see him in action.

I took my six-year-old son with me to pay an "unofficial" house call to watch Mr. P at a steer-roping rodeo. Not only did I enjoy watching his pain-free acquisition of first place, but my son was even treated to a memorable ride on Mr. P's horse.

▶ If You Want To Know More

Pellegrino MJ. *Inside fibromyalgia*. Columbus, OH: Anadem Publishing, 2001.

Education

As I said earlier, the single most important treatment is education. Learning about fibromyalgia and understanding it is half the battle. John Patrick has a memorable quote in which he said, "Pain makes man think. Thought makes man wise. Wisdom makes life endurable." Education is the first step to making your fibromyalgia more manageable.

Once your doctor has diagnosed your fibromyalgia, he or she will need to review some important points:

1. **It is a real condition.** You are validated with this diagnosis. This confirms once and for all that you are not crazy. You have a definite unique condition called fibromyalgia.

2. **Fibromyalgia is not life threatening.** You will not die from it. You may feel miserable and scared, but it is not fatal. Even if it's not life-threatening, it can be life-dreadening. You need to find ways to improve your quality of life with fibromyalgia.

3. **Fibromyalgia is not deforming or paralyzing.** It can cause joint pain and weakness, but it does not cause destruction of joints or paralysis like certain rheumatological or neurological conditions.

4. **Fibromyalgia does not turn into a life-threatening, deforming or paralyzing condition.** You will not get lupus or rheumatoid arthritis from your fibromyalgia. Some people have fibromyalgia in addition to these conditions, but fibromyalgia doesn't turn into them. You may be stuck with fibromyalgia, however.

5. **Fibromyalgia is a treatable disorder.** It can improve. It can go into remission. It can be healed even if it can't be cured.

6. **It will not be easy having fibromyalgia.** Everyone knows that good things never come easily! Fibromyalgia is a nuisance and can be debilitating. Not everyone achieves the hoped-for pain reduction or improved abilities. You have to work hard to keep fibromyalgia under control, and you have to continue to work hard to maintain a stable baseline.

I educate all of my patients about my treatment philosophy, which uses a multidisciplinary approach to achieve two general goals: 1. find out what works; 2. teach the person a successful home program. The patient needs to understand that she/he is an active member of the multidisciplinary team approach. There are numerous health professionals who treat fibromyalgia, and I explain my role as a team member, primarily the "coach," while the patient is the team "captain." I try to guide the patient to consistent "winning" strategies.

Realistic Goals

Part of the education process is establishing realistic goals. We live in a time when we expect perfection, and we expect results. We are used to custom-ordering and getting what we order. For example, we go into a restaurant and we say, "I'd like my steak well done," "Put some lemon in my water," and "Please bring me the ketchup." Or we go to a hair stylist and say, "That looks good, but take a little more off on the right." We expect our requests to get done, and done well!

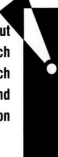

I educate all of my patients about my treatment philosophy, which uses a multidisciplinary approach to achieve 2 general goals: 1. find out what works; 2. teach the person a successful home program.

So we go to the doctor and expect the same custom-order results. We say, "Doctor, I would like to be pain-free," or "I would like to play sports again like I did in high school."

I explain to the patient with fibromyalgia that we need to set goals that are realistic. We may not be pain-free, but we can try to decrease the pain, make it more stable, or get it into a remission. Perhaps we cannot do sports like we did in high school; we can never do what we did in high school because we have gotten older. But we can learn to increase our activity level and quality of living in spite of having fibromyalgia. Even if we can't do a particular sport, we can find other activities that are enjoyable.

By gently guiding patients towards realistic expectations, I try to ease the burden of perfection. It is okay to change our expectations to something that may be less than perfect, but much more easily accomplished.

Self-Responsibility

I encourage all patients with fibromyalgia to learn everything they can about the condition and how it affects them. I emphasize the importance of self-responsibility: learning to take control of fibromyalgia and striving to cope successfully with this condition each and every day. It is your responsibility to actively discover what works best for you. The more you know and understand, the less frightening or unbearable it becomes and the more "normal" you will feel again. Being self-responsible means that you recognize and accept fibromyalgia as part of you, and you learn how to adjust your lifestyle to best control your symptoms. Part of being self-responsible is increasing others' awareness, particularly your family, friends, and employers. We need to help others understand what we are going through.

Another key part of self-responsibility is following through with your treatment program. This takes daily work on your part. Your doctor and medical team can give you a lot of recommendations and ideas, but it is up to you to carry out the recommendations and find the right program and right balance for you and your everyday life. Medical professionals are here to help and to point you in the right direction, but you have to live your own life.

Learning About Fibromyalgia

You need to take an active role in becoming an informed fibromyalgia patient. The more you understand your diagnosis, the more qualified you become, and the easier it is for you to make a decision regarding your condition. You can also learn what specific questions to ask your healthcare professionals.

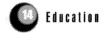

Information therapy is a term for supplying patients with health information, enabling them to make informed decisions about their health and care, to participate in their own well-being, and thus to decrease the use of healthcare resources (Donna J. Mitchell, 1994). By increasing your knowledge, you will increase your confidence in your abilities to responsibly manage fibromyalgia. I provide patients with a brochure on fibromyalgia and keep them updated.

Libraries

Libraries are a great resource for people with fibromyalgia. Personally, I think I've spent a third of my life at various libraries at The Ohio State University. There are many types of libraries that have a wealth of information via books, magazine articles, videos, and computer technology. Types of libraries include public libraries, academic libraries, medical libraries/health sciences libraries, hospital libraries, or patient/consumer health libraries. Find a library that can accommodate your specific needs that include a physically accessible building, well-trained staff, technology assistance, and guidance to specialized resources.

Ask for help! Try to find library workers who have a special interest in medical research. These people are good contacts for fibromyalgia networking. If you want a specific article or book, try to have the most complete information possible regarding the title, author, journal name, publishing company, date of publication, etc. The library worker can help you search databases using key words. 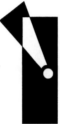 **The more you understand your diagnosis, the more qualified you become, and the easier it is for you to make a decision regarding your condition.**

Remember to write down the information while you are reviewing the material. Don't trust yourself to remember this a month later (or even an hour later or in my case…what were we talking about?). Keep your information organized so you can easily track down the necessary information when you need it. Library research can be confusing and overwhelming, but research will be easier once you understand the system and identify a knowledgeable library worker. Remember, learning is supposed to be fun. And also remember, libraries are big, so don't get lost. Wear bright clothing so it can easily be spotted by the night cleaning crew!

Internet

Internet resources on fibromyalgia provide an endless learning opportunity. Information on fibromyalgia as well as discussion groups are available, so the Internet can be both educational and supportive. Numerous websites are available for information both from medical university centers and from patient support and consumer standpoints.

A wealth of fibromyalgia information is available on the Internet, and many patients take advantage of this remarkable resource. I advise people to be cautious when gathering information and advice on the Internet and to be aware of potential pitfalls as well as benefits.

The benefits include a readily available "encyclopedia" on fibromyalgia and a good place to get basic overview information. There are also numerous fibromyalgia discussion groups and support groups that can provide valuable support and bonding experiences. Many friendships have been established via these cyber support groups. Many reputable hospitals, universities, and organizations have websites that provide reliable and helpful information on fibromyalgia. Various fibromyalgia newsletters have web pages and online information available.

POPULAR WEBSITES FOR FIBROMYALGIA

The Oregon Foundation: www.myalgia.com

Fibromyalgia Information: www.ncf.carleton.ca/fibromyalgia/

National Fibromyalgia Association: www.fmaware.org

National Fibromyalgia Partnership: www.fmpartnership.org

Fibromyalgia Network: www.fmnetnews.com

National Fibromyalgia Research Association: www.nfra.net

Medline is an example of an Internet site that provides accurate, up-to-date medical research information. Most articles referenced in Medline are written by and for health professionals, but they can prove extremely helpful for consumers. Medline searches can be done by subject, author, journal title, and text word, and there are citations from nearly 4,000 biomedical journals from around the globe.

To access the Medline, at no cost, 24 hours a day, 7 days a week, all that is required is a computer with Internet access. First, users should go to the National Library of Medicine home page (www.nlm.nih.gov) and click on the "Free Medline." The resulting screens will guide you to citations of articles from medical journals. Library staff who are trained to use the Internet can assist you in finding information on healthcare issues. You can know what your doctors know!

The possible pitfalls of the Internet include the potential for overwhelming, complicated, and confusing information from a variety of sources. Invariably, if you talk to a hundred people, you will get a hundred different recommendations on how to best manage your fibromyalgia. A lot of good advice can be obtained from caring individuals, but the reality is that there are a lot of people on the Internet who provide medical advice but have no medical license or medical background. This is often done to try to sell a particular product or solicit something from unsuspecting individuals. This can be dangerous because if an unsuspecting individual follows what is believed to be medical advice from a fraudulent person, that unsuspecting person could sustain injury or harm.

I instruct people to be careful when interpreting information. The best strategy is to gather the information and share it with your knowledgeable medical professional and come up with a mutually agreeable treatment plan.

Support Group

A support group can be a valuable means of both education and treatment in fibromyalgia. Having the opportunity to share experiences with someone who has the same condition can be a powerful therapeutic tool. The Internet can be a place to meet people and participate in a support group. There are various Internet fibromyalgia support groups, so you don't ever have to leave your house. This may be a good option for patients with limited outdoor mobility or those who may be more comfortable remaining "anonymous."

"Real life" support groups can provide a unique treatment dimension. A support group consists of individuals who share a common problem—fibromyalgia—and who are interested in meeting on a regular basis to share information and experiences (and donuts!). A successful support group can consist of as few as 5 members, but usually has between 10 and 20 members. Of that group, there are individuals with newly diagnosed fibromyalgia who are in the early stages of accepting and coping with their condition and need guidance and support from more experienced members. Those with more experience can relate to the newer members, yet still learn new things themselves.

About 12 years ago, many of my fibromyalgia patients expressed an interest in forming a group. With the help of a facilitator, we organized and have been meeting on a monthly basis ever since. My interests are both personal and professional; my involvement with the support group includes being both an active participant and a professional advisor. Our group has been fortunate to have wonderful people who are committed to helping each other.

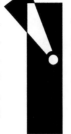

A support group can be a valuable means of both education and treatment in fibromyalgia. Having the opportunity to share experiences with someone who has the same condition can be a powerful therapeutic tool.

Try to find a support group in your area. There are different kinds of groups, but the usual one would meet on a monthly basis for a couple of hours, with perhaps one hour being devoted to education and the second hour being devoted to support. Self-help groups that are run by patients can focus on more "personal" issues. Educational sessions could include having guest speakers on different topics involving fibromyalgia. One meeting a year, members could perform a literature review and discuss different aspects of fibromyalgia. Support can take the form of helping a member resolve a difficult situation; discussing issues such as anger, depression, and stress management; and sharing strategies.

I emphasize involving the patient's significant others in the education process. Fibromyalgia doesn't just affect the patient. It involves the spouse, family members, co-workers, and more. Education helps the patient's significant others understand the condition and provide support and encouragement. I have made my office facilities available for regular support group meetings, and we have a big bulletin board with fibromyalgia information about seminars, books, articles and other pertinent information available.

Beware Of Misinformation

Not all information is medically accurate or helpful, especially Internet information. You need to be careful how you use it. As a group, we are more vulnerable to misinformation. Because of our severe chronic pain, we may: be more desperate for help; feel overwhelmed; have difficulty concentrating and processing information; be more emotional and easily influenced; and be more easily convinced to try new products. Unfortunately, there are companies out there waiting to take advantage of us. They try to entice us with products that they claim will help us—help us spend our money, that is!

Here are 13 things to watch for to avoid being unlucky:

1. **It sounds too good to be true**. Like the old adage in investments, if it sounds too good to be true, it probably is. Trust your fibromyalgia knowledge, and don't let your hope override good common sense.

2. **It will cure fibromyalgia**. There is no cure for fibromyalgia at this time. There are a lot of treatments for fibromyalgia, but if the proposed treatment uses the word "cure," stay away from it.

3. **The product involves multilevel marketing**. The main reason to avoid these is that they are expensive. You had to pay five other people's profits when you purchase your product.

4. **The product involves a secret technique or formula**. If the promoter fails to disclose specific information about the product or how it works, stay away from it. I know a massotherapist who promoted a unique technique that gave great results but would not disclose the technique; you have to pay $2,000 to join this "special program." It turns out that the techniques used are commonly used by massotherapists.

5. **The product is supported by personal testimonies only.** Consider this typical story for a product: "Poor Michael used to be so active, but then he developed fibromyalgia and couldn't even get out of bed. Then one day, he discovered *Fibro-Be-Gone* and began taking it. Within one week, his fibromyalgia symptoms were all gone. Now he is running three miles a day, skiing on weekends, and working full-time as the owner of a company that sells *Fibro-Be-Gone*."

   This type of sensational advertising based on personal testimony is designed only to sell you a product. Maybe a particular product worked for a particular person, but everyone is a unique individual who responds differently to treatments.

6. **Questionable medical qualifications**. Many times, the supposed "medical professional" has no actual medical credentials. On the Internet, anyone can be a medical professional. Individuals can mislead you by putting M.D. after a name. There is no law that prohibits someone from putting initials, including M.D., D.O., or D.C., after a name. The M.D. can mean macarena dancer! To avoid becoming a victim of fraud or misrepresentation, ask about credentials and do research. If the person says he or she is a medical doctor but won't disclose what medical school was attended or give any specific information about medical training, then this person is probably a fraud.

7. **Medical recommendations are made by non-medical professionals**. Unfortunately, many non-physicians try to make medical diagnoses and medical treatment recommendations to people with medical conditions such as fibromyalgia. This is illegal. If the person giving the advice is misrepresenting that he or she is a licensed physician, this is fraud. The privilege of making medical diagnoses and treatment recommendations should be reserved for those who dedicated many years of their life to obtaining medical knowledge and training and who maintain current medical license. If you follow fraudulent medical advice, you could be injured. Check qualifications before you deem a source credible, no matter how good this person sounds. Call the AMA, the State Medical Board, or the local medical society office if you have a question about a doctor's qualifications.

8. **The promoter has a vested financial interest in the product**. I recently received a flyer in the mail that said, "A very special workshop is about to take place in your area." The flyer then described a doctor who was experiencing great results with fibromyalgia patients using a new product. It reported, "In just 11 weeks, he has increased his monthly revenue by $4,000, and is enjoying his practice like never before." The promoter of this product was trying to entice me to pay for the workshop, become a distributor, and try to encourage my patients to use this product. The promoters benefit financially from this arrangement, thus they have a vested financial interest. How can you trust the promoters of this product to be unbiased when giving you information?

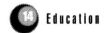

9. **The promoter of the product has a painful condition—fibromyalgia**. Beware of the person who knows exactly how you feel because he or she claims to have the condition and has just the product for you to get rid of the condition.

10. **High pressure marketing system**. What better way to get our money than to use fancy sales pitches, brightly colored literature, catchy slogans, and so forth and so on. If you feel that you are being presented with a heavy marketing pitch, you are. Don't buy things because you feel pressured into doing so.

11. **A video tape, DVD or audio cassette tape comes with the marketing kit**. I've learned to stay away from products that have any type of tape that comes with the marketing kit!

12. **The product is unavailable anywhere else**. Two problems with this. If it is not available anywhere else, they usually charge an arm and a leg for it. Also, if it is not available anywhere else, maybe it is not really a good product. If you can't compare this product with something else, stay away from it.

13. **Your doctor won't know anything about this product**. This is a double whammy. Not only does the promoter try to convince you that your physician is misinformed, but he also tries to qualify himself as a knowledgeable person who will inform you (instead of your doctor). Don't get suckered in by this technique.

I'm not saying that no product can be helpful if one of the 13 red flags above is raised. Nor am I saying that someone who has fibromyalgia can't give you helpful advice or recommend products. I know many caring credible business people who sell products or services for people with fibromyalgia. I am simply telling you to be cautious, and don't act upon your emotions or a pressure market sell. If a red flag goes up, STOP, and agree that you are going to take the pressure off yourself and defer any decision until a later time after you have done some research. Spur of the moment decisions are costly ones, so make your decision LATER.

I have some strong feelings about those who prey on people with fibromyalgia. I can be diplomatic, though, and say simply that it is your responsibility to avoid being an unsuspecting victim.

Work With Your Doctor

Your goal is to interact with your physician to become as informed as possible, and to feel as well as possible. Some physicians are more comfortable with knowledgeable patients than others. (This may be an understatement!)

Try to approach your physician in a way that does not seem confrontational. If you walk into your doctor's office with a list of 50 questions and a stack of ten articles, you may overwhelm a doctor who has 15 minutes scheduled to see you. Ask your most important questions and work together on strategies for increasing your knowledge.

Learning is an ongoing process. You can't learn everything about fibromyalgia in a day. My body of medical knowledge didn't stop when I finished my residency. I need to continue to learn by experience, by reviewing literature, and by interacting with you. You are doing the same. Together, we become even smarter!

Pledge For Fridge

Cut out at dotted line and tape to refrigerator

Fibromyalgia Patient Affirmation

1. I have a real condition called fibromyalgia.

2. My fibromyalgia is not life threatening and I am not going to die from fibromyalgia.

3. My condition is not deforming or paralyzing.

4. Fibromyalgia does not turn into a life-threatening, deforming, or paralyzing disease.

5. I can do many things to "heal" my fibromyalgia even if it can't be cured right now.

6. It won't be easy having fibromyalgia, but I will learn as much as I can about my condition.

7. I will use that knowledge to manage my condition and gain control of my life with fibromyalgia.

Fibronomics

With fibromyalgia, we have to pay extra attention to our bodies so our pain doesn't flare up so often. I believe the first step in any exercise or home program is observing proper posture and body mechanics. We can make time to stretch and exercise, but observing proper posture and body mechanics needs to be continuous and automatic.

All of us have experience with trying to achieve proper posture. We may remember Grandma reminding us to "sit up straight." I still remember the grade school nuns telling me, "Don't slouch!" It was as if somehow sitting properly at all times would prevent our spines from bending and curving or freezing in some abnormal position.

We learned how to lift heavy objects using our legs and not bending over at the waist to prevent back injury. As we became more sophisticated, we learned ways to maneuver our bodies to avoid causing injuries or pain, yet still complete the functional task at hand.

Ergonomics is a scientific study of posture and body mechanics and its relationship to various tasks. Ergonomics specifically involves designing equipment for work to fit the capabilities of the human body in order to minimize the risk of injury. Examples of ergonomic applications include tools that minimize strain on the wrist, keyboards that are curved and slanted to fit the hand better, and secretarial chairs with armrests and back support. A key goal in ergonomics is to achieve a natural position for the human body where there is minimal or no strain on the joints and soft tissues.

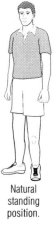

The natural standing position of the human body is when the head is relaxed and slightly bent forward, the arms are loosely hanging down at the sides with the elbows bent to a 90 degree angle, the wrists straight, fingers relaxed and slightly curled in, the back in a natural lordotic curve, the knees slightly bent, and the feet about 12 inches apart.

If an unnatural or awkward position occurs, more strain is placed on the joints and soft tissues. Examples of unnatural positions include: head turned to the side or looking up, arms outstretched or overhead, elbows away from the body, wrists bent, palms up, body leaning forward and bending.

Natural standing position.

One cannot maintain natural body positions all day long. On the other hand, if we put a lot of strain on our tissues by repeated unnatural positions, we are at risk for injury or pain. A strategy: promote proper posture to prevent painful people!

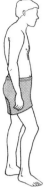

With fibromyalgia, we have to develop a different concept of what is considered proper posture. All of the stuff that Grandmother told us just doesn't work. When we try to sit up straight for a long time, we hurt more. Slouching is actually comfortable. And, let's face it, we are not trying for modeling careers. We just want to be comfortable. Many of us who have had fibromyalgia for years develop a characteristic fibromyalgia posture that results from countless hours in a comfortable but less than perfect posture.

A different set of rules apply to fibromyalgia posture. We need to reprogram our minds and muscles for these fibromyalgia posture and body mechanic rules. We need to learn Fibronomics.

Fibromyalgia
posture.

Fibronomics is defined as *the art of properly manipulating our fibromyalgia bodies in the environment to enable completion of an activity with minimal pain.* Fibronomics can be applied to everything we do in life, no matter how simple it is. There are four easy rules of fibronomics, and once these are learned and applied, our bodies will automatically follow them.

The Four Rules To Fibronomics Are:

1. Arms stay home

2. Unload the back

3. Support always welcome

4. Be naturally shifty

Rule #1: Arms Stay Home

Fibromyalgia muscles in the neck, shoulders and upper back area do not like activity that involves reaching or overhead use of the arms. Isometric contractions occur when muscles stay continuously contracted. This causes decreased blood flow, decreased muscle oxygen, and increased pain. Any time the arms are away from the body, the trapezial, scapular, shoulder and upper back muscles all go into sustained isometric contractions, which usually causes increased pain after only a few seconds. Many will notice immediate increased pain or feelings of weakness in the arms when we reach. Sometimes we are so focused on what we are doing that we may not notice the early pain signals arising from our neck, shoulders, and upper back until it is too late.

The favorite position of our arms is at the sides with our elbows touching our sides and bent at a 90 degree angle. Our arms stay home (with the rest of the body) and do not reach away while performing a particular task. We should try to maintain this position as much as possible, so we need to move our whole body, not just our arms, when we want to confront each specific task.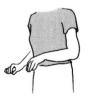

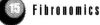

Examples of using Rule #1: Arms stay home.

1. **Problem**: Reaching up to write on chalkboard.

    Solution: Move body closer to board and write only in the mid to low portions of the board, not at the top of the board.

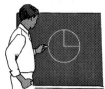

2. **Problem**: Reaching forward to type on a keyboard.

    Solution: Raise chair, lower the keyboard by installing a drop keyboard mechanism into the desk, move chair as close to keyboard as possible. You might also place keyboard on lap. Enlarge the screen so you can see better.

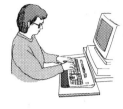

3. **Problem**: Washing windows by reaching.

    Solution: Get closer to the wall, use a long-handled tool such as a squeegee.

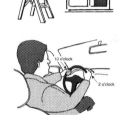

4. **Problem**: Prolonged driving with arms at the 10 o'clock and 2 o'clock wheel position.

    Solution: Move seat closer to steering wheel, place hands in 4 o'clock and 8 o'clock positions.

Rule #2: Unload The Back

The back actually includes the entire spine, pelvic, and hip areas with particular emphasis on the lower back and sacroiliac region. Many back and pelvic muscles interact with each other to maintain proper alignment. Anything that causes a shift in this alignment can create mechanical imbalance and/or a misalignment. Pain occurs, whether it be from bones, ligaments, nerves or muscles. Activities that increase the load on the back are bending forward, prolonged standing, bending at the waist to pick up an object, or arching the back. All of these will increase the potential for mechanical imbalance and pain in our fibromyalgia muscles. We need to learn how to unload the back.

Ways to unload the back include:

- Avoid bending forward at the waist; maintain a natural lordotic (arched) curvature.

- Cross legs or put feet up on a foot rest when seated.

- Lie in a fetal position on your side with a pillow between your knees.

- Avoid bending over and picking up heavy objects; bend your knees and lift with your legs, keeping your back straight.

- Wear sensible shoes; no heels!

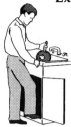

Examples of using Rule #2: Unload the back.

1. **Problem**: Leaning forward at the kitchen sink.

   Solution: Keep back straight, open cupboard door under sink and lift leg into cupboard. Use long-handled sponges.

2. **Problem**: Riding sports bike bent forward.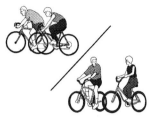

   Solution: Avoid rams horn style handle bars. Use a wider comfortable seat that places the back in a more natural position.

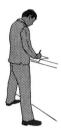

3. **Problem**: Leaning forward at the waist over a counter to sign papers.

   Solution: Spread legs to lower body but maintain good back posture, then sign papers without bending forward.

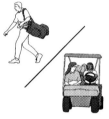

4. **Problem**: Carrying heavy golf clubs puts strain on the back.

   Solution: Play 9 holes instead of 18, ride a cart or use a pull-cart, or use a caddy.

5. **Problem**: Applying make-up by tilting head back and looking into a wall mirror puts strain on the neck.

   Solution: Look down into a magnifying mirror.

6. **Problem**: Bending and lifting at work causes low back pain.

   Solution: Here are four techniques for lifting:

Modified Diagonal Lift:

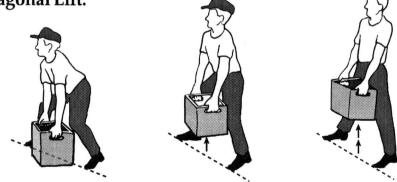

The modified diagonal lift is used for lifting heavy items which are 1 or 2 feet off the floor. Establish a wide stance with one foot in front of the other. Placing yourself slightly over the item, bend at the hips and at the knees. With the head and shoulders up, straighten the knees and hips to lift the object off the ground.

One Knee Lift:

Place one foot beside the front portion of the object to be lifted; drop slowly to other knee. Grip the object firmly at near and far corners with head and shoulders up and lower back arched, then lift or roll the object onto top of thigh. Maintaining same posture, stand with object cradled. (Avoid this lift if you have knee problems.)

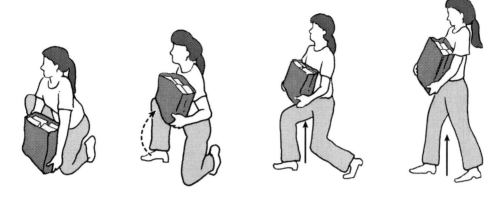

Golfer's Lift:

This lift can be used by people with knee problems, decreased leg strength, or when they must lift where there is a barrier in front of the item (such as a railing or deep storage container). Place one hand on table or other fixed object to support the upper body; arch the back, bend at the hips, and raise one leg behind yourself. By raising one leg, the upper body weight is counterbalanced and bending forward from the low back is reduced. To pick up item, the individual should look up, push off with free hand, and lower the raised leg.

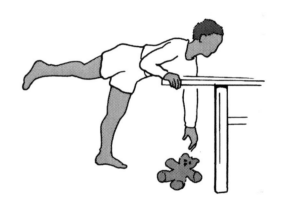

Straight Leg Lift:

This lift is used when knees and waist cannot be bent. Position body as close to the object as possible. If you are reaching over something into a lower work area, press your legs forward against the object over which you are reaching. While bending slowly at hips (not the waist), you should firmly grasp item and bring it closer if necessary. With the low back arched and head up, complete the lift by rotating hips backward to a full standing position.

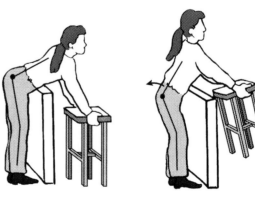

Rule #3: Support Always Welcome

We should take advantage of existing environmental structures to relieve some of the force on our bodies. Our muscles work hard every day to support us and get us from one place to another. We expect that our muscles will get tired, and usually when they get tired, they hurt more. It is okay to use extra support to relieve our muscles whenever we can. Our muscles won't deteriorate or atrophy if we are responsibly using additional support.

Examples of using Rule #3: Support always welcome.

1. **Problem**: Arms become tired and hurt.

   Solution: Use armrests, pillows, or furniture (table, desk, or countertop) to rest arms. Cross arms or rest on head, lap, or body. Hold one arm with the other. Put arms in pockets, muffs, or slings.

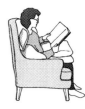

2. **Problem**: Back is tired and hurts.

   Solution: Sit in a chair, particularly one with a good seat and back. Lean against a wall or other object. Use a footstool or pillow for additional support. Use a brace or a belt.

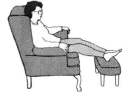

3. **Problem**: Neck is tired and hurts.

   Solution: Use pillows to support the head and neck. Hold your head in your hands. Wear a soft cervical collar when driving/riding on long trips or bumpy roads.

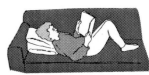

4. **Problem**: Whole body feels tired and hurts.

   Solution: Lay down. Use various pillows and cushions. Sit in a recliner.

Rule #4: Be Naturally Shifty

This rule emphasizes maintaining natural or neutral body and joint positions, and periodically moving the muscles. If we keep our muscles in one position for too long, we tend to get painful tightening and spasms. To counteract this, keep moving the muscles regularly. Some people have more tolerance than others, but we all have our limit, and if we spend too much time in one particular position, we will experience increased pain. We must learn to automatically alternate between positions such as sitting, standing, and walking. This strategy will enable various muscle groups to relax and stretch regularly.

Examples of Rule #4: Be naturally shifty.

1. **Problem**: Sitting up straight hurts.
   Solution: Slouch at times; alternate this with sitting up straight.

2. **Problem**: Standing in line hurts.
   Solution: Shift weight from side to side, walk around in your place.

3. **Problem**: Sitting in a hard chair for a long time causes the back and legs to hurt.
   Solution: Be fidgety, shift around in the chair, move the legs, frequently stand up and stretch. Take a cushion with you!

Applied Fibronomics!

Use fibronomics to examine everything you do. First, determine why an activity may be causing pain by identifying the fibronomic rules that are violated. Sometimes the activity may be obvious, other times it may be subtle, but think about the rules and analyze every single thing that you do no matter how automatic it is. Correct these violations and practice these new strategies until they become automatic additions to your body mechanics. At first, you must consciously think about these violations and take steps to correct them. After a while, your subconscious takes over and the techniques will become automatic.

The following are some more examples of daily problems where proper application of fibronomics can be helpful.

Example 1—Problem: Sitting on bleachers at a sporting event causes significantly increased back pain.

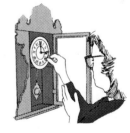

Fibronomics rules are violated by prolonged sitting without alternating positions and unsupported sitting, which increases the load on the back.

Solutions: Bring a folding chair with you to the bleachers and use it, allowing the back to be supported. Take frequent standing and walking breaks, averaging at least a minute of standing/walking for every 15 minutes sitting.

Example 2—Problem: The clock collection is posing a problem since winding up clocks once a week causes increased neck and shoulder pain and causes arm fatigue. (Isn't clock collection common in people with fibromyalgia!?)

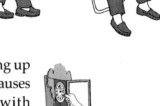

Fibronomics rules are violated by reaching your arms out to try to wind the clock. This increases isometric contractions in the neck, shoulders and back (causes timely PAIN!).

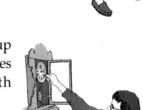

Solutions: Stand on a stool to lower the arms to a more natural position. Move closer to the clocks so the arms stay in, then wind, taking no more than 10 winds before stopping to drop the arms to the side for a few seconds; then resume the winding. Arms stay home when whining—I mean winding!

Example 3—Problem: Getting the hair ready in the morning can cause a lot of pain, yet we have to look presentable for the day.

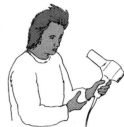

Fibronomics rules are violated by arms reaching up over your head and leaning forward over the sink, which puts an increased load on the back, and not taking advantage of any available support.

Solutions: Use the other arm to hold the arm used to fix the hair or hold the blow dryer. Hold hair dryer lower (arms more at sides) and direct air upwards. Bend head down so it is closer to the air. Obtain a folding director's chair to sit on in the bathroom and perform morning duties in a more favorable position. Consider a new hairstyle that is more fibro-friendly. Remember, you look beautiful just as you are!

Example 4—Problem: Reading and studying causes considerable increased neck pain and headache.

Fibronomics rules are violated by the sustained positioning of the head and neck which causes painful tightening, and the lack of neck support while maintaining the studying position. When studying, we are so focused on the material that we don't notice the early clues our neck, head and shoulders may be giving about increased pain . . . until it's too late!

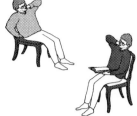

Solutions: Alternate positions every 30 minutes from sitting at a desk to lying in bed with a pillow propped behind the head. Set a timer to remind you when it's time to change positions. Use a pillow or book holder to prop up the book and allow you to more comfortably adjust your head position. Lean back in the chair so head and neck are more supported. Lie on the bed with neck and head supported with a pillow, bend knees, and put the book on your lap.

Example 5—Problem: Sitting in a chair is painful to the lower back, and when standing up after sitting in a chair for a while, spasms and stiffness in the back make it difficult to get out of a chair and stand up straight.

Fibronomics rules are violated by prolonged sitting without alternating positions, and lack of adequate support for the back due to poor chair design increases strain on the back.

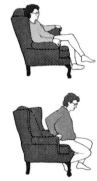

Solutions: Crossing the legs is an excellent way to unload the back and pelvis. Remember to alternate the legs crossed. Use a footstool to rest both legs and raise the knees. Sit in a good chair that has a sturdy back and arms to maintain proper body alignment; use a lumbar cushion or pillow to support the natural low back curvature. When getting out of a chair, use the "back pedal technique." First, scoot forward to the front edge of the chair. Then plant one foot behind the chair as far as possible. With the arms pushing off the armrests, stand up while maintaining a natural back position without bending forward.

Example 6—Problem: Getting out of bed or off the couch causes severe back pain.

Fibronomics rules are violated because the back is under extreme stress when a "sit-up" is performed to get up. Also, the upper body is trying to raise up unsupported before the legs swing over.

Solution: Transfer out of bed using a log roll technique. First, roll your body, log roll style, onto your side, then curl up your legs so your knees come forward and over the edge of the bed. Use the arm opposite the side on the bed to push on the surface near your waist level at the same time you swing your legs off the edge to allow a quick yet smooth sitting up motion. This avoids undue stress on the back.

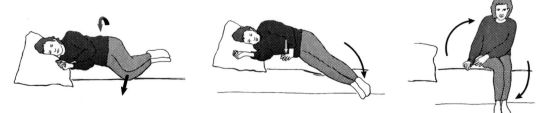

Wear A Mental Seat Belt

I pay particular attention to fibronomics in my everyday activities. In fact, I tend to be a little paranoid at all times. I don't want to do anything that will cause my fibromyalgia to flare up, so I try to be extra cautious to make sure I am following proper fibronomics!

We wear a car seat belt as a protective device to prevent injury in case of an accident. I say we should wear a mental seat belt at all times to help prevent a fibromyalgia flare-up and remind us not to be careless. Not only do we need to follow proper fibronomics, but we have to remind ourselves that every situation is a flare-up waiting to happen. One of the most common causes of flare-up is a body injury, so we need to avoid any potential harm or injury to our body as part of controlling our fibromyalgia.

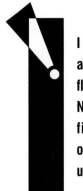

I say we should wear a mental seat belt at all times to help prevent a fibromyalgia flare-up and remind us not to be careless. Not only do we need to follow proper fibronomics, but we have to remind ourselves that every situation is a flare-up waiting to happen.

Here are some examples of how I wear a mental seat belt at all times:

- Whenever I'm going up or down steps, I always hold onto the rail. I've gone up and down steps a million times, and I know what it is to slip and fall. My last great stair wipeout occurred in college. I slipped on the top step on the way down, and slid or bounced down 10 steps. My books went flying. I knocked books out of the hands of two girls walking up the steps. Luckily, only my ego was bruised.

- By holding onto a rail at all times when I am on the steps, I not only remind myself not to fall, but I am physically preventing myself from falling should I lose my balance.

- Whenever I am walking on icy ground, I assume I will fall and break a bone. No matter how close my car is or how much I'm in a hurry, I always walk slowly and carefully on ice. I make sure that my balance is stable at all times, and I avoid lifting one foot too far off the ground when taking steps to minimize the chance of losing my balance.

- Whenever I am picking up something off the floor, I pretend it weighs 100 pounds. We usually don't hurt ourselves when we bend over to pick up something heavy because we know the object is heavy and take extra care in following proper posture. We get into trouble when we bend over quickly and twist to pick up something small like a little piece of paper. More often than not, this is the way we sprain our backs. I pretend that the little piece of paper weighs 100 pounds to remind myself to follow proper body mechanics and pick up the paper slowly so as not to catch my back off guard.

- Whenever I feel a sneeze coming on, I make certain I assume the proper sneezing position: arms tucked tightly to the sides and bent, head and back slightly bent forward in a braced position, and knees slightly bent. I've had too many flare-ups in the past from "unprotected" sneezes. Now I am paranoid—and careful with my sneezes.

Remember to wear your mental seat belt at all times. It is a fibro law! Be especially careful on steps; wet, icy, slippery surfaces; or gravel, grass, hilly, bumpy surfaces. Be careful when you are carrying packages, and—all of the time! Remember to use your fibronomics.

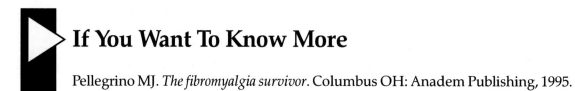

If You Want To Know More

Pellegrino MJ. *The fibromyalgia survivor.* Columbus OH: Anadem Publishing, 1995.

Fibromyalgia
Up Close & Personal
16

Medications & Injections For Fibromyalgia

Certain drugs may reduce pain and improve overall feelings of well-being. No one type of medication works for everyone, and no one medication causes 100% improvement. You and your doctor need to experiment and work together to find out what is best for you. Pain relief, improved sleep, and improved mood are examples of goals that prescription medicines can help you reach.

As a group, those of us with fibromyalgia do not tolerate medicines well. We are very sensitive to medicines and often experience side effects such as nausea, drowsiness, or light-headedness. People with fibromyalgia are similar to the geriatric population in that both groups usually require smaller doses of medicines because "regular" doses are more apt to cause side effects. We may have side effects that the drug companies never realize could happen with their medicines! One person may tolerate a particular medicine, but the next person will get sick on it. I am particularly sensitive to medicines, and I always joke that the day they discover a pill to cure fibromyalgia, I'll take it and within seconds will get sick! Prescribed medicines can provide great benefits to many, however.

Categories of drugs used in the treatment of fibromyalgia include:

1. Analgesics
2. Anti-inflammatory drugs
3. Antidepressant medicines (tricyclics and selective serotonin reuptake inhibitors)
4. Muscle relaxants
5. Sleep modifiers
6. Anti-anxiety medicines
7. Anticonvulsants
8. Antibiotics
9. "Other" medicines
10. Topical medications
11. Over-the-counter medications

We'll review each category briefly.

Analgesics

Analgesics are pain killers and can include over-the-counter medicines such as Aspirin and Acetaminophen, or prescription-strength pain pills like narcotics or opiates (*e.g.*, Codeine, Vicodin, Darvocet, OxyContin and Percocet). Ultram and Ultracet are pain relievers that differ from narcotics in their action on the central nervous system.

These medicines do not alter the fibromyalgia, but they can help take the edge off pain. Narcotic medicines have potential for adverse side effects including drowsiness, difficulty with concentrating, and addiction, so they should be used carefully. Many people with fibromyalgia are sensitive to codeine medicines, which can cause nausea or an allergic reaction. Ultram and Ultracet can cause allergic reactions in people sensitive to codeine, and a small number of people taking these medicines have seizures (Ortho-McNeil pharmaceutical letter to healthcare professionals, March 20, 1986). As a pain specialist I will frequently prescribe analgesics, including narcotics, for patients experiencing severe pain.

Currently no medicines are approved by the FDA for treatment of fibromyalgia in the United States, although doctors prescribe pain medicines all the time for fibromyalgia. A recent study (Dr. Bennett, 2003) reported that Ultracet (Tramadol HCL/Acetaminophen) is effective in reducing pain in people with fibromyalgia. This study's findings provide encouragement for eventually getting FDA approval for a specific drug treatment for fibromyalgia.

Anti-inflammatory Drugs

Anti-inflammatory medicines include aspirin, nonsteroidal anti-inflammatory drugs (NSAIDs for short) such as Cox-I inhibitors and the newer Cox-II inhibitors, and corticosteroids such as Prednisone or Dexamethasone. These medications are both anti-inflammatory and analgesic. Some of these medicines such as Ibuprofen are available both over-the-counter and by prescription.

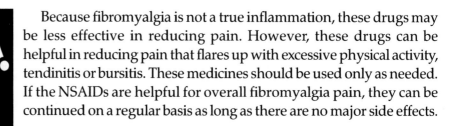

Because fibromyalgia is not a true inflammation, these drugs may be less effective in reducing pain. However, these drugs can be helpful in reducing pain that flares up with excessive physical activity, tendinitis or bursitis.

Because fibromyalgia is not a true inflammation, these drugs may be less effective in reducing pain. However, these drugs can be helpful in reducing pain that flares up with excessive physical activity, tendinitis or bursitis. These medicines should be used only as needed. If the NSAIDs are helpful for overall fibromyalgia pain, they can be continued on a regular basis as long as there are no major side effects.

The major side effect of the anti-inflammatories (*e.g.*, Ibuprofen, Naproxen, Lodine, Daypro) is bleeding from gastrointestinal ulcers. This problem is more common the longer the medicine is taken. However, a new medication class is available, Cox-II inhibitors, which include Celebrex and Bextra (Searle Pharmaceuticals), and Vioxx (Merck). This new form of NSAID selectively blocks only the Cox-II enzymes, which control the production of chemicals that cause inflammation and pain; these chemicals are known as prostaglandins. Good prostaglandins that help the stomach lining, kidneys, and platelets are formed by the Cox-I enzyme system and are not affected by the Cox-II inhibitors, thus avoiding gastrointestinal bleeding.

I prescribe various types of anti-inflammatories on a regular basis, and sometimes patients will respond very nicely to these medicines. To avoid risk of bleeding or other side effects, patients should not take over-the-counter anti-inflammatory medicines in addition to the prescribed ones.

Antidepressant Medicines

The antidepressant medicines include tricyclics (*e.g.*, Amitriptyline, Nortriptyline, Doxepin, and Trazodone), and selective serotonin reuptake inhibitors (*e.g.*, Prozac, Zoloft, Paxil, Effexor, Serzone, and Lexapro). These medicines can treat pain, altered sleep and mood disturbances seen in fibromyalgia. The tricyclic medicines are helpful, but frequent side effects include dry mouth, drowsiness and weight gain. Sleep disturbances can be reduced by using low doses. Carefully controlled studies have shown that low doses of tricyclic antidepressants can benefit fibromyalgia patients (Carette et al., 1986, Goldenberg et al., 1986).

A recent study presented at the annual meeting of the American Psychiatric Association was the first to look at the benefits of a controlled-release selective serotonin reuptake inhibitor, Paxil CR (made by GlaxoSmithKline) in treating fibromyalgia. This placebo-controlled double blind study found that Paxil CR decreased the symptoms of fibromyalgia significantly in patients compared to the controls.

Amitriptyline can cause extreme sedation and a morning hangover, even at low doses. I've found that Nortriptyline or Trazodone has fewer side effects but give the same benefit. Even though the sedation side effect of the tricyclic medicine may have worn off by morning, the other benefits of the drugs (decreased pain, muscle relaxation, and improved mood) can continue throughout the day. Because the tricyclics can provide more than one beneficial effect, I think these medicines are handy in fibromyalgia treatment. It is like using one pill to do the work of several.

The selective serotonin reuptake inhibitors work well in treating depression. They also block the breakdown of serotonin, the brain hormone that is low in people with fibromyalgia and depression. Serotonin is important in the brain's regulation of pain and sleep. By selectively inhibiting the breakdown of serotonin, these medicines increase the serotonin concentration in the body and are effective in treating central pain.

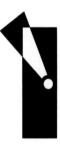

Using a combination of a serotonin reuptake inhibitor during the day and a tricyclic at nighttime can be an effective combination medicinal approach.

These medicines have fewer side effects than the tricyclics, although they can cause sexual dysfunction and weight gain. Liver complications have been reported in some patients, so these medicines must be monitored by the physician. Using a combination of a serotonin reuptake inhibitor during the day and a tricyclic at nighttime can be an effective combination medicinal approach (Goldenberg, 1996).

Muscle Relaxants

Muscle relaxants can decrease pain in people with fibromyalgia. Medicines in this family include Flexeril, Soma, Skelaxin, and Robaxin. The most common side effect is drowsiness. I have found that muscle relaxants do not really decrease muscle spasms or truly "relax" muscles, because the painful area still has palpable spasms. Rather, the medicine appears to help by a central neurological mechanism that reduces muscle pain. If drowsiness is a side effect, this medicine should only be taken in the evening so it doesn't interfere with driving or concentration. The drowsiness side effect may be useful at night if it helps improve sleep.

Medicines in the antispasticity category can be used to treat muscle spasms. Two of these medicines, Zanaflex and Baclofen, have been shown to help reduce back muscle spasms and pain. Antispasticity medicines are primarily intended for people who have neurological conditions causing involuntary muscle spasms (such as spinal cord injuries, multiple sclerosis, or strokes). However, they may have a role in patients with fibromyalgia who have muscle spasms, headaches and pain.

Sleep Modifiers

Various medicines including some already mentioned (analgesics, antidepressants, and muscle relaxants) can treat insomnia. True sleep modifiers include benzodiazepines like Restoril and the hypnotic non-benzodiazepines such as Ambien. The most common reported concern about using sleep modifiers, especially benzodiazepines, is the habit-forming potential. Ambien is reported to be less habit-forming but can cause rebound insomnia when it's stopped. Sonata is a newer sleep modifier that is not habit-forming and doesn't cause rebound insomnia. Sometimes sleep modifiers are prescribed in short intervals only.

I have found that sleep modifiers improve deep sleep, and particularly improve the morning perception of a good night's sleep. This improved sleep can carry over into a better day.

I have found that sleep modifiers improve deep sleep, and particularly improve the morning perception of a good night's sleep. This improved sleep can carry over into a better day. Sleep modifiers are short-acting medicines, so they work during the night and are usually eliminated from the body by morning, hence the low chance of a morning hangover. Some people report nightmares with these medicines, but usually these medicines are "silent;" that is, one doesn't realize any medicine was taken, other than knowing that sleep was better. I've devoted a chapter (see Chapter 22) to review the sleep problem so many of us have.

Anti-anxiety Medicines

Anxiety is a common problem in fibromyalgia and contributes to pain, muscle tension, and irritability. It can make depression and insomnia worse. Various medicines, including antidepressants and muscle relaxants, treat anxiety. Benzodiazepines such as Klonopin, Ativan, and Xanax are commonly used medicines. These medicines also cause sedation and thus can improve sleep. Possible side effects include depression and decreased memory. Sometimes it is difficult to determine whether symptoms are due to fibromyalgia or are side effects of medication.

I have found Klonopin to be a particularly useful medicine in the evening, especially when there are leg symptoms (pain, restless leg syndrome, jerking of the legs called myoclonus) that interfere with sleep. Low dose Klonopin therapy is one way to improve the balance of the inhibitory receptors (GABA) and excitatory receptors (MMDA) in the central nervous system. Most fibromyalgia patients have too much activity in the excitatory receptors (MMDA receptors), and Klonopin can increase the pain inhibitors' activity to achieve a more normal balance, improving sleep and reducing pain.

Anticonvulsants

Anticonvulsant medicines were originally developed to treat seizure disorders and epilepsy. A number of medicines in this class have also been found to be helpful in treating pain, particularly neuropathic pain. People with fibromyalgia who have a lot of burning or electric-shock feelings in their hands and feet may improve from a trial of anticonvulsant medicines. Examples of medicines in this category include Neurontin, Dilantin, Depakote, Tegretol, Gabitril and Keppra. Sedation is a common side effect especially if higher doses have to be used to control pain.

Antibiotics

Antibiotics can have a role in treating fibromyalgia. Dr. Garth Nicolson has isolated a microorganism, *Mycoplasma fermentans*, as a possible infectious cause of Gulf War Syndrome (remember, this may be a type of fibromyalgia). Some patients had less pain and fatigue after taking antibiotics (*e.g.*, Doxycycline, Erythromycin and Zithromax), presumably due to the eradication of the *Mycoplasma*. Antibiotics may also inhibit certain enzymes that cause inflammation (anti-inflammatory mechanisms) rather than acting via an anti-infection mechanism.

Zovirax is an example of an antiviral antibiotic that can be used in some patients whose symptoms or flare-ups are felt to be related to a virus (mono, for example). An example of a natural antibiotic is olive leaf extract (Oleuropein).

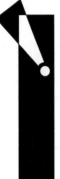

I have had some patients who improved after a course of antibiotics. For example, I have a few patients who get flare-ups of leg pains that seem to respond only to the antibiotic Erythromycin. Other patients with chronic fatigue flare-ups have responded to broad spectrum antibiotics.

I have had some patients who improved after a course of antibiotics. For example, I have a few patients who get flare-ups of leg pains that seem to respond only to the antibiotic Erythromycin. Other patients with chronic fatigue flare-ups have responded to broad spectrum antibiotics. Lately, I have been recommending olive leaf extract as a natural alternative to the flu vaccine in those who previously flared-up after receiving the vaccine.

Antibiotic use increases one's chance of getting a *Candida* yeast infection, which can increase fibromyalgia symptoms. Yeast antibiotics (Nystatin, Diflucan) may be indicated in fibromyalgia if there is a *Candida* infection that is causing increased pain and other symptoms (see Chapter 25). Over time we may identify a specific subgroup of fibromyalgia patients who have antibiotic-responsive symptoms.

"Other" Medicines

Other medicines can be used to treat chronic pain. Some medicines are developed specifically for a pain problem, *i.e.*, migraine headaches. Other medicines were originally developed for a different purpose and were subsequently found to be helpful in treatment of painful problems. Examples of "other" medicines include:

Migraine medicines. Headaches are a common problem with fibromyalgia, including migraine headaches, and various headache medicines are available. Specific migraine medicines include the 5-HTP receptor agonists (Amerge, Axert, Frova, Imitrex, Maxalt, Relpax, Zomig) and Midrin (isometheptene derivative). Beta-blockers such as Inderal can be helpful in preventing migraines. Treatment of migraine headaches is reviewed in more detail in Chapter 26.

Antispasmodic Medicines. This category of medicine can be helpful in treating severe cramping pain as often seen with irritable bowel syndrome and irritable bladder. Bowel spasms can be treated with medicines such as Levsin and Levbid. Bladder spasms can be treated with medicines such as

Ditropan, Urimax and Detrol. I'll review treatment of irritable bowel syndrome and irritable bladder in more detail in Section IV.

Guaifenesin. Guaifenesin is used in over-the-counter cough and cold preparations and can be prescribed in tablet form. Dr. R. Paul St. Amand has championed the use of Guaifenesin for treatment of fibromyalgia. He hypothesizes that an accumulation of phosphate occurs at a cellular level in those with fibromyalgia and this defect interferes with the muscle calcium pumps and causes them to malfunction, resulting in muscle spasms and pain. Guaifenesin helps increase the excretion of phosphate and Dr. St. Amand has treated many people in his practice with this medicine and has reported good results.

A double-blinded study was done in 1996 to evaluate the effects of Guaifenesin in treating fibromyalgia. The authors of that study concluded that there was no difference in the response between the placebo and Guaifenesin group. A number of patients with fibromyalgia have reported decreased pain when taking Guaifenesin, however. There has not been any reported toxicity or long-term side effects with Guaifenesin that I'm aware of.

Dextromethorphan. Dextromethorphan is also a cough suppressant, like Guaifenesin. This medicine is an NMDA receptor antagonist. As we discussed in Chapter 8, "Normal Pain," the NMDA receptors are responsible for amplifying and enhancing chronic pain signals at the spinal cord level. A medicine that is an antagonist is one that inhibits the nerve activity. Dr. K. A. Nelson performed a study in 1997 (*Neurology*) in which he showed that Dextromethorphan can be used successfully in the treatment of shingles pain.

Dr. Robert Bennett published an abstract in 2000 showing 18% of those with fibromyalgia in this study experienced a significant and impressive improvement in pain with Dextromethorphan compared to placebo. Thus, taking Dextromethorphan (prescribed or over-the-counter) may have a therapeutic role in a subset of fibromyalgia patients. If you are taking a pain medicine, then taking a small dose of Dextromethorphan along with this medicine could boost the pain-relieving powers.

Topical Medicines

I use several types of topical medicines in the treatment of fibromyalgia pain. Prescribed topical medicines include Lidoderm patches, Duragesic patches and compounded pain creams. Lidoderm patches contain 5% Lidocaine in a rectangular-shaped topical delivery system that adheres to the skin. When applied to a painful area such as the upper back, the Lidocaine maintains a wet contact with the skin and anesthetizes the skin nerves. This can create a deeper pain relief that lasts many hours. The patches can be re-applied daily.

Lidoderm has been approved for a post-herpetic neuralgia or persistent pain following shingles attack. An abstract of a recent American Pain Society scientific meeting reported results of functional MRI testing (remember this previously: it "lights up" more in fibromyalgia patients) in a person with post-herpetic neuralgia before and after using Lidoderm patches. The report found reduced brain activity when mechanical stimuli were applied to the painful skin after Lidoderm patch use, meaning the medicine appeared to block pain signals from traveling to the brain so the pain areas couldn't "light up."

I've found Lidoderm patches work well in many of my patients with fibromyalgia, presumably because it desensitizes the nociceptors and reduces some of the allodynia (hypersensitized pain from peripheral stimuli).

Duragesic (Transdermal fentanyl) is a narcotic medicine delivered through the skin from a patch. Two hundred fifty-six patients with chronic non-cancer pain who had been treated with oral opioids were studied with Duragesic patches (*BMJ*, May 2001). The results were better pain relief, less constipation, and an enhanced quality of life when compared to sustained-release oral morphine. The patches actually deliver the medicine transdermally (through the skin) instead of topically (on the skin) and can be helpful to those with fibromyalgia who do not tolerate oral pain medicines. Nausea is one of the most common side effects reported to me by patients.

When applied to a painful area such as the upper back, the Lidocaine maintains a wet contact with the skin and anesthetizes the skin nerves. This can create a deeper pain relief that lasts many hours. The patches can be re-applied daily.

Compound pain creams are individually prescribed mixtures of different medicines made specially by a compounding pharmacist. The medicine is rubbed onto affected areas up to several times a day and can penetrate deeper into the skin to work where oral medicines may not have worked or were not tolerated.

With fibromyalgia I've written hundreds of compound medicine prescriptions over the past few years to help reduce painful symptoms. One cannot bathe in this stuff, so it can't be applied to the whole body! Rather, I think of this approach when selective areas hurt more, or when burning hands or feet are a problem. Common mixtures I've prescribed include a combination of Ibuprofen, Lidocaine and MSM for tennis elbow pain or localized pain, or a mixture of Lidocaine, Gabapentin (Neurontin), and/or Orphenadrine (a muscle relaxant) for painful burning in the hands and feet.

Over-The-Counter Medicines

Many over-the-counter (OTC) medicines are available to all for treating any symptom possible! We used to be bombarded with commercials telling us what OTC products we needed to live better; now we get to see these ads plus ones telling us which prescribed medicine to ask our doctors for.

Although it may seem we have an overwhelming number of choices, there are actually some potentially helpful strategies patients can choose with OTC medicines. The OTC oral pain medicines fall into basically three types of medicine: aspirin, acetaminophen, and NSAIDs (*i.e.*, Ibuprofen, Naprosyn). If there are no reasons to avoid these medicines (sensitivity, allergy, liver problem, stomach ulcer, already on prescribed medicines containing these), they can be tried for pain. If they help, they can be used regularly as long as they are tolerated. Always check with your doctor, though. OTC pain medicines are good pain pre-emptors. If you are planning to do an activity that predictably increases pain, take an OTC pain medicine an hour before you begin the activity as a preemptive "strike" against the potential flare-up.

Another useful category of OTC medicines for fibromyalgia is antacids, especially with our sensitive stomachs, acid reflux, and irritable bowel syndrome. Liquid, dissolvable, and chewable forms of antacids are okay; whatever you prefer. I like to use the OTC forms of Zantac (Ranitidine) or Tagamet (Cimetidine) at night for reflux or upset stomach symptoms.

My first-line recommendation for irritable bowel syndrome is trying a fiber supplement like Metamucil, FiberCon or others. This can help "balance" the two extremes and help keep bowel movements regular and less painful. Diphenhydramine (*e.g.*, Benadryl, Tylenol PM) can help improve sleep and can be used regularly without habituation concerns. I do not recommend taking OTC products to keep you awake, as they contain caffeine which can increase fibromyalgia pain and cause withdrawal headaches.

OTC pain medicines are good pain pre-emptors. If you are planning to do an activity that predictably increases pain, take an OTC pain medicine an hour before you begin the activity as a preemptive "strike" against the potential flare-up.

Numerous OTC topical medicines exist. They include muscle creams that try to decrease pain by creating a "counter-irritant" sensation that is more tolerable than pain (remember Melzak & Wall's gate control theory?). This "substitute sensation" may be heat (*e.g.*, Tiger Balm) or cold (*e.g.*, Biofreeze). Various patches and creams with aspirin, Aloe Vera and other ingredients claim to decrease pain. These appear harmless to experiment with to determine if they work for you.

Supplements are a major OTC industry that I've described in a separate chapter. It's common now to see hybrids of OTC medicines and supplements available in the drug stores and health food stores.

My Basic Strategies

In addition to the variety of medicines available for fibromyalgia treatment, a variety of doctor "strategies" are also available. Doctors who prescribe medicine will usually find, through trial and error, an effective or favorite strategy. There is no single right way to prescribe medicines for fibromyalgia, and more than one strategy may work for different people and different doctors. Over the years, I have discovered basic strategies that seem to work best for me when using prescription medicines.

1. **Educate about expectation with medication.** I tell patients that no medicine will completely cure fibromyalgia or eliminate the symptoms, but it may help improve symptoms and comfort level, hopefully without side effects. Let me give you an example of how educating about medicinal expectation is important.

   Say you came to me with pain, and I prescribed a medication. I tell you to take the medicine to see if it helps your pain. I don't clarify what to expect. You go home, try the medicine and come back. I ask you how the medicine worked, and you say, "It only took away half the pain, I'm still hurting; I need something else."

   Now take the same situation, same exact medicine, but when I give you the medicine I tell you, "This medicine is not going to eliminate all of the pain. It may help reduce your pain, but it will not make the pain disappear. Hopefully, you will find that at least you feel better than you did before, and there will not be any side effects to interfere with the success of the medicine. Give it a try, and let me know how it works." When you come back for the next visit, and I ask you how you did, you will say, "Great! This medicine took away half of my pain. I haven't felt this good in years!" If the patient is educated about what to expect, the medicine can be much more effective.

2. **Try to use the lowest effective dose of medicine** and wean off medicines whenever possible, especially if the patient is at a "stable baseline." Believe it or not, fibromyalgia can stabilize and require less medicine than before. I always try to challenge the fibromyalgia by decreasing the medicine to the lowest effective dose that controls symptoms. Sometimes when decreasing the medicine, we are able to actually stop the medicine altogether, and to our pleasant surprise the symptoms do not return or are tolerable without the medicine. This approach considerably reduces risk of side effects or developing tolerances to the medicines. If the symptoms flare up at a later time, the medicines can be resumed or increased.

3. **Discontinue any medicine that is not working.** Many times patients come to me with a list of a dozen different medicines they are taking, and then report that none of them are helping. Yet they are continuing the medicines! I will instruct the patient to stop or, if needed, wean off the medicine. Sometimes a patient will stop a medicine and the symptoms increase, indicating that the medicine probably was helping. If this occurs, the patient can resume that particular medicine and monitor for improved symptoms. Sometimes medicines help to maintain a stable baseline, and we don't realize how much they are working until we stop them.

   Other times, a medicine had helped in the past, but is no longer effective because the body has developed a tolerance to it, or perhaps a higher dose is needed. I avoid automatically adding any new medicine to the group of medicines that are not working. I often do the "add and subtract" strategy, where I add a new medicine to try but, at the same time, subtract one that does not appear to be working.

4. **Narcotics/opiates can be used sparingly and responsibly for pain control.** There are certainly risks for habituation, dependency, and addiction with the use of narcotic medications. In my experience, most patients are terrified of using narcotics on a regular basis for fear of becoming addicted. If patients use prescription narcotic medications responsibly and as prescribed for pain control, the risk of addiction or other serious side effects is very low. Patients must be instructed on the importance of using narcotics sparingly and responsibly, exactly as prescribed, and agree to strictly adhere to these rules.

   I form a "contract" with each patient before I prescribe narcotic medication. The criteria and terms of this contract include:

   - The medicine is to be taken only as prescribed.
   - No early refills are to be requested.
   - No one else can prescribe any narcotic or opiate medications.
   - No emergency room visits seeking pain medicines for non-acute pain problems are permitted.

   Patients must agree to these terms before I prescribe these medicines, and they understand that failure to abide by all these terms could result in a termination of the doctor-patient relationship. I rarely have problems with my patients misusing narcotic medications. From time to time, there are "red flags" that go up and must be addressed immediately. I have found that the benefits of responsible use of narcotic medications for pain control is much more important than the occasional risk of side effects, but the physician has to monitor these prescriptions closely.

Three things that can happen with narcotics.

The legendary Ohio State football coach, Woody Hayes, loved to run the football at the opponents in a conservative style known as "three yards and a cloud of dust." Woody believed the pass should be used only as an element of surprise. He said "there are three things that can happen when you pass, and two of them ain't good." For those of you whose football expertise ranks up there with my computer expertise, the two "bad" things that can happen when a football is passed are an incompletion and an interception. A completion, of course, is the one good thing that can happen.

> **Prescribing narcotics can be likened to passing a football. I can imagine Woody as a doctor saying, "there are three things that can happen when one takes narcotics, and two of them ain't good."**

Prescribing narcotics can be likened to passing a football. I can imagine Woody as a doctor saying, "there are three things that can happen when one takes narcotics, and two of them ain't good."

The good thing that can happen is that narcotics may work great and reduce pain, improve quality of life, and be well tolerated. The two bad things that can happen are:

- The person is abusing narcotics and is drug-seeking.

- The person is not drug-seeking at first, but eventually becomes dependent on the prescribed narcotic medication. This doesn't mean narcotics should not be prescribed, but a conservative style, indeed a cautious style, is warranted and followed by most physicians when it comes to prescribing narcotic/opiate medicines.

5. **Be flexible and keep it simple.** There are many different strategies, and sometimes we can try all of them and still not have much success. I have my favorites, but I am willing to try different things. I also try to keep it simple, because the more medicines added to the mix, the more the potential for adverse side effects, sensitivity, and interactions among the medicines.

Injection Treatments

Therapeutic injections are a different way to administer medicine for pain management in fibromyalgia. I'll review different types of injections that I've used in treating fibromyalgia. Various types of therapeutic injections include trigger point injections, Botox injections, epidural steroid injections, selective nerve root blocks, facet injections, joint injections and prolotherapy.

Trigger Point Injections

The most common injections used for fibromyalgia are trigger point injections. I recommend that trigger point injections be considered when a few areas, perhaps 1 to 6, are causing most of the patient's severe pain. Trigger point injections are most effective if they are done in the areas where the patient is experiencing the most pain, even though other trigger points may be painful with palpation. The most common muscles I inject are the trapezial, paraspinal and gluteal muscles.

A trigger point injection sends medicine into a painful soft tissue area, usually the muscle. It is a specialized intramuscular injection. I use a local anesthetic (usually Lidocaine) and often a corticosteroid (usually Dexamethasone) which can prolong the effect of the injection.

Painful areas are located and injected with a small diameter needle. Usually the involved area is felt as a tight knot or band. The patient is instructed beforehand on the potential benefits and risks of the procedure. The benefits include significantly reducing the pain and spasm, confirming that the area injected was indeed the source of pain, and hopefully achieving a benefit that lasts for weeks. The risks include a temporary increase in pain, localized bleeding, or a "black and blue" mark and, very rarely, blood vessel or nerve damage, lung puncture, an allergic reaction, or a skin infection. The procedure is carried out in the doctor's office.

For an average trigger point injection, I generally use Lidocaine. I've learned to get the needle in, inject quickly, and get the needle out. I do not "fan" or "pepper" the needle. I find a single stick in-and-out minimizes any needle trauma and helps achieve the quickest and most prolonged benefit from the injection. During the actual injection, a few seconds of increased pain confirms the right location. There may be a muscle twitch associated with the injection. Then, the medicine works quickly to cause a numbing effect. The mechanism of action is a desensitization of the hyperactive muscle area and reduction of the localized spasm. After the injection, I may perform stretching and soft tissue mobilization to decrease pain and relax spasms.

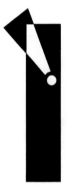

There is no way to determine how long a particular trigger point injection will last in a given person, as it can be anywhere from a few hours to a few months. I've found that the average trigger point injection lasts three to four weeks.

There is no way to determine how long a particular trigger point injection will last in a given person, as it can be anywhere from a few hours to a few months. I've found that the average trigger point injection lasts three to four weeks. Trigger point injections are not a permanent solution. Many times they reduce severe pain and, when they wear off, the pain is not as severe as it was before the shots. Trigger point injections can also help other treatments work more effectively. If injections are helpful, they can be done on a regular basis depending on the patient's needs and physician preferences.

Botox Injections

Botox injections have been used to treat painful tender points. Botox is a purified chemical made from the same botulism compound which causes a potentially fatal food poisoning. When injected into a painful muscle area, Botox causes a disruption of the nerve-muscle junction around the injection site. This releases the muscle spasm by blocking the nerve signals to the muscle area, thereby reducing pain.

Dr. DeAndres, *et al.* recently confirmed the effectiveness of Botox for treating chronic myofascial pain. A 1999 study from Croatia showed Botox helped with tension-type headaches, a common complaint in fibromyalgia. Other studies have supported the use of this specific injected medicine. I previously used Botox injections on a number of people who had tender points that were resistant to usual trigger point injections. About 50% to 60% had improvements lasting several weeks to several months.

Epidural Steroid Injections

Sometimes patients with fibromyalgia find themselves with other painful conditions as well. If a person has disc disease at different levels of the spine (lumbar level most commonly), he or she may have a lot of disc pain. The disc disease could be aggravating the overall fibromyalgia as well. Multi-level disc disease can cause nerve root irritation (pinched nerve) or spinal stenosis.

Epidural steroid injections are injections into the epidural space of the spinal column and are usually done in a series of 3 injections, each one about a month apart. The steroid injection bathes the irritated and inflamed disc and spinal nerve areas and reduces swelling, inflammation and pain. These injections can help for months. Epidural injections are not for fibromyalgia, per se, but can help fibromyalgia pain by reducing the problem from the disc disease.

Selective Nerve Root Blocks

Selective nerve root blocks are injections of medicines (local anesthetic plus steroid) directly onto an inflamed nerve root area (*i.e.*, pinched nerve or radiculopathy). Nerve roots can become inflamed from a herniated disc or a boney spur, and if fibromyalgia is also present, patients will report increased fibromyalgia pain as well.

Remember, fibromyalgia does not cause radiculopathy, but can be aggravated by it. Hopefully, any treatment that decreases radiculopathy pain will decrease fibromyalgia pain as well.

Facet Injections

Facet joints are located along the boney spine and stabilize the spinal column. These joints are of particular interest in the cervical spine when a whiplash injury occurs because they are often damaged. These joints will be discussed further in Section V, Understanding Post-Traumatic Fibromyalgia.

If facet joint pain is felt to be a pain-generating area contributing to fibromyalgia pain, facet injections may be helpful. A mixture of a local anesthetic and steroid is injected into the specific vertebral joints, usually under the guidance of fluoroscopy (using a low intensity X-ray machine that confirms needle placement). If fibromyalgia pain decreases, the abnormal facet joint was indeed a contributing source of the fibromyalgia symptoms.

Joint Injections

Injections into specific painful joints with a mixture of a local anesthetic and a steroid can help with joint pain and inflammation. Often, those with fibromyalgia find themselves with inflamed shoulders, knees, thumbs, and other joints, including the facet joints mentioned above. Remember, fibromyalgia does not cause true joint inflammation even though it causes joint pain. The joint inflammation is from something else: arthritis, trauma, synovitis, bursitis, etc.

Prolotherapy

Prolotherapy is a simple, safe, and effective treatment for numerous painful conditions. The term "prolotherapy" was coined in the 1940s by George S. Hackett, M.D., a Canton, Ohio industrial surgeon who developed and later refined the modern technique. The "prolo" in prolotherapy is short for proliferate because the treatment actually induces growth, or proliferation, of tissue. It is a form of injection therapy directed at weakened ligaments and tendons. Typically, a dextrose (sugar) based anesthetic solution is injected into the injured ligament and tendon areas. These injections stimulate an injury-repair sequence. (Sounds painful ... well it is a little bit ... !) The chemical environment of a fresh injury is recreated in a controlled manner, and this activates the healing cascade.

Studies have shown that ligament and tendon size and strength can increase as much as 35 to 40% in areas treated by these injections. Prolotherapy has been shown to be an effective treatment for chronic low back pain, and usually there is a 75% or greater success rate (less pain, less tenderness) in treatment of other types of chronic musculoskeletal pain, including fibromyalgia.

Prolotherapy has been used successfully in posttraumatic fibromyalgia, particularly neck pain from unresolved whiplash injuries. Sprains and strain injuries that do not heal on their own can go on to develop chronic myofascial pain syndrome/fibromyalgia, and perhaps a major mechanism in this particular pain is persistent weakened ligaments and tendons which "destabilize" a region. Muscles tighten up to try to "stabilize" this region, causing painful spasms. Because prolotherapy actually creates new tissue in the injured structures, it may be considered a more permanent treatment in many instances, and indeed many patients have received long-term benefits (Dr. Vladimir Djuric, 1998).

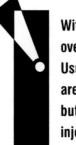

With prolotherapy most patients achieve over 50% improvement in particular areas. Usually a series of proliferate injections are required, anywhere from two to six, but one can usually tell after the first injection if it is going to help.

Prolotherapy has been highly effective in my practice. My associate, Dr. Djuric, has been trained in prolotherapy, and has treated many patients with fibromyalgia. A number of them have gotten permanent improvements with this treatment. The fibromyalgia isn't cured, but certain painful areas settle down and remain in remission. The conditions that have gotten the best results include: persistent spine pain from unresolved whiplash injuries, plantar fasciitis, lateral epicondylitis (tennis elbow pain), knee pain from persistent ligament/tendon strain, and occipital headaches.

With prolotherapy most patients achieve over 50% improvement in particular areas. Usually a series of proliferate injections are required, anywhere from two to six, but one can usually tell after the first injection if it is going to help.

New Medicines

Currently, there is no medicine yet approved for the treatment of fibromyalgia syndrome. There are a number of medicines in the drug pipeline that may be able to help fibromyalgia, however, including one drug that is projected to be the first drug approved for fibromyalgia.

Milnacipran

Milnacipran is forecasted to be the first drug approved specifically for fibromyalgia. It is a dual-acting medicine that inhibits the reuptake of two key neurotransmitters in the human body, Norepinephrine and Serotonin. As we have learned, both of the neurotransmitters are involved with the central modulation and processing of chronic pain and are found to be low in people with fibromyalgia. This drug has already been approved for use as an antidepressant overseas for the past six years (Europe, South America and Asia).

In the United States this drug has been tested for use specifically in the treatment of fibromyalgia. The preliminary results of the Phase II trial indicate that Milnacipran significantly improved pain and fatigue in fibromyalgia patients, as well as causing significant improvement in depressed mood. Cypress Biosciences, which manufactures Milnacipran, has recently launched a Phase III program evaluating the use of Milnacipran as a treatment for fibromyalgia. If the results of this larger Phase III trial continue to be successful, with no untoward side effects or complications, hopefully Milnacipran will soon be available as a prescribed medicine for fibromyalgia.

Duloxetine

Duloxetine (Cymbalta), manufactured by Lilly, is also an antidepressant that acts as a dual-reuptake inhibitor. At the recent annual meeting of the American Psychiatric Association (San Francisco, USA, May 2003), information was presented that a double-blinded placebo-controlled multisite study (United States, Spain, Italy, France) found Duloxetine to be effective in treating depression. It will be submitted for approval as an antidepressant medicine in Europe in the year 2004. We'll need to monitor this medicine as well for possible future availability in the United States to treat fibromyalgia-related symptoms.

Pregabalin

Pregabalin, made by Pfizer, is a gamma-aminobutyric acid (GABA). It is the next generation of Gabapentin (Neurontin) that I discussed earlier in this chapter under "Anticonvulsant Medicines." Pregabalin was shown to improve pain in patients with fibromyalgia syndrome in a double-blinded placebo-controlled study involving 529 patients (data from annual meeting of ACR, October 26, 2002). Pregabalin-treated patients (450 mg/d) showed a statistically significant decrease in pain compared with those receiving placebo. At least 29% of the Pregabalin-treated patients reported at least 50% reduction of pain compared with 13% of the placebo patients.

At the end of 2000, Pfizer was set to file an application with the FDA for the approval of Pregabalin for such conditions as neuropathic pain, anxiety and fibromyalgia. Unfortunately, in February of 2001, there were some reports that mice that were given Pregabalin developed tumors (but the mice's fibromyalgia improved!). The research was reevaluated and, after additional clinical trials, Pregabalin was found to be safe in patients with fibromyalgia and generalized anxiety disorder. This drug may be available soon to treat pain.

Future Medicines

Medicines that are more selective and specific for controlling neurotransmitters, protein factors, enzymes, and even healing factors will probably become available in the future. The ideal medicine would be one that is tolerated, not addictive, effective and free of serious side effects. WePregabalin are looking to our animal friends for help. Powerful pain killers may be developed from natural animal toxins such as snake venom, frog poison, or sea creature chemicals. Drug researchers can modify the molecular structure to remove the toxicity while enhancing the analgesic effect (hopefully, they won't have fibrofog and get those 2 mixed up!). These would be molecular smart bombs.

There is much excitement about conotoxins in biomedicine. These are specialized proteins/toxins made by tropical cone snails that have very specific effects on neurological pathways. Developing drugs from conotoxins to block key neurological pathways could help in the treatment of pain, spasms, inadequate circulation, depression, heart arrhythmias and urinary incontinence, to name a few. We'll watch for conopeptides in the future.

All types of medicine will get better. I expect to see hybrid medicines that perform multiple functions such as replacing deficient substances, boosting certain functions, blocking pain pathways and controlling body responses.

Topical medicines, sublingual (under tongue) medicines, medicine patches, inhalants and injections will be further refined to enhance the delivery of medicines into the bloodstream. Oral medicines that rely on absorption through the stomach may not be the best route for administering certain medicines for those with fibromyalgia. Any medicine that can bypass the stomach, especially in those who have sensitivity or intolerance to oral medicines, may work well.

Prescribed oral medications and therapeutic injections can be considered on an individual basis as part of a multi-disciplinary treatment approach. I use a combination of prescription medicines and injections along with other treatment approaches. We need a lot of weapons to go after this "enemy" of our state of well-being! Hopefully, reinforcement and newer weapons will be arriving soon.

If You Want To Know More

1. Alan L, Hays H, Jensen NK, et al. *Randomised crossover trial of transdermal fentanyl and sustained release oral morphine for treating chronic non-cancer pain.* BMJ 2001; 322: 1154–8.

2. Bennett RM, De Gamo P, Clark SR. *A one year double-blind placebo control study of guaifenesin in fibromyalgia.* Arthritis Rheum 1996; 39: S212.

3. Bennett RM, Kamin M, Karim R, et al. *Tramadol and acetaminophen combination tablets in the treatment of fibromyalgia pain: a double-blind, randomized, placebo-controlled study.* Am J Med 2003; 114: 537–45.

4. Carette S, McCain GA, Bell DA, et al. *Evaluation of amitriptyline in primary fibrositis. A double-blind, placebo-controlled study.* Arthritis Rheum 1986; 29: 655–9.

5. Clark SR, Bennett RM. *Supplemental dextromethorphan in the treatment of fibromyalgia: a double-blind, placebo-controlled study of efficacy and side-effects.* AFSA 2000; 7: 2.

6. De Andres J, Cerda-Olmedo G, Valia JC, et al. *Use of botulinum toxin in the treatment of chronic myofascial pain.* Clin J Pain 2003; 19: 269–75.

7. Djuric V. *Prolotherapy treats pain.* Chronic Pain Solutions 1998; 3: 8–10.

8. Goldenberg DL, Felson DT, Dinerman H. *A randomized controlled trial of amitriptyline and naproxen in the treatment of patients with fibromyalgia.* Arthritis Rheum 1986; 29: 1371–7.

9. Goldenberg D, Mayskiy M, Mossey YC, et al. *A randomized, double-blind crossover trial of fluoxetine and amitriptyline in the treatment of fibromyalgia.* Arthritis Rheum 1996; 39: 1852–9.

10. Hauser R. *The history of prolotherapy.* www.getprolo.com

11. Majar EH. *Treatment of tension-type headache by local injection of botulinum toxin.* Eur J Neurol 1997; 4 (suppl 2): 71–3.

12. Masand P. *Predictors of response to a placebo-controlled, double-blind trial of paroxetine controlled release in fibromyalgia.* Abstract NR36, 157th annual meeting of the American Psychiatric Association, 2004.

13. Nelson KA, Park KM, Robinovitz E, et al. *High-dose oral dextromethorphan versus placebo in painful diabetic neuropathy and post-herpetic neuralgia.* Neurology 1997; 48: 1212–8.

14. Pellegrino MJ. *Inside fibromyalgia.* Columbus OH. Anadem Publishing, 2001.

15. Rao SR. *The neuropharmacology of centrally-acting analgesic medications in fibromyalgia.* Rheum Dis Clin N Am 2002; 28: 235–59.

16. Sosa Y, Balike M, Parrish T, et al. *Chronic post-herpetic neuropathy pain modulation by lidocaine patch: an fMRI-pharmacological study.* Programs and abstracts of 22nd scientific meeting of the American Pain Society, March 2003.

17. St Amand RP. *What your doctor may not tell you about fibromyalgia: the revolutionary treatment that can reverse the disease.* Warner Books, 1999.

Nutritional Approaches In Fibromyalgia

People with fibromyalgia have a number of nutritional deficiencies, so trying to correct these deficiencies through supplements is a logical treatment strategy. All of us require a minimum daily dose of vitamins and minerals to run our bodies' metabolism and key reactions to promote homeostasis. Homeostasis is the body's natural ability to maintain its stable harmony and balance among its hormones, enzymes, muscles and organs to prevent disease or to allow the body to heal itself.

Many people who don't have chronic disease fail to get their minimum daily requirements through their diet. They may not eat the right foods, or foods they eat are deficient in nutrients due to different factors. The food refining process removes many vital nutrients and thus by the time we eat the foods, most of the nutrients may have been stripped away.

Also, the soils are depleted of minerals compared to many years ago so freshly grown foods do not contain the concentration of vital nutrients as needed. For example, studies have shown that about 75% of the population is deficient in magnesium whether or not they are eating a balanced diet. Many diseases affect our ability to eat or absorb nutrients from foods, further depleting necessary vitamins and minerals and exacerbating any deficiencies. The table below demonstrates how nutrients are affected by different drugs.

Nutrients Affected By Different Drugs

Drug	Nutrient Affected
Alcohol	B vitamins, magnesium, vitamin A
Antacids	Calcium, copper, iron, magnesium phosphate, potassium, zinc, protein

Antibiotics	B complex, acidophilus, vitamins C & K
Antifungals	Calcium, magnesium, potassium, sodium
Antivirals	B_{12}, carnitine, copper, zinc
Antihistamines	Vitamin C, melatonin
Beta Blockers	Coenzyme Q_{10} (CoQ_{10})
Cholesterol Lowering	CoQ_{10}, vitamin E
Corticosteroids	Calcium, vitamin D, potassium, selenium, zinc
Diuretics	B complex, CoQ_{10}, potassium, magnesium, zinc
Laxatives	Potassium, vitamins A, D, K, calcium, phosphorus
NSAIDs	B_1, B_5, vitamin C, folic acid, iron
Oral Contraceptives	Folic acid, B vitamins, vitamin C (more if *Candida* develops)
Thyroid Replacement	Iron (indirectly: calcium & magnesium)
Tricyclics	CoQ_{10}, B_2 (major antidepressants also deplete melatonin)
Ulcer Meds	B_{12}, folic acid, vitamin D, zinc, protein

Health Points 2003; 10(4):13. Reprinted with permission from To Your Health.

People with fibromyalgia and other chronic diseases require MORE than minimum daily requirements because their bodies have deficiencies as part of the disease, and extra dosing is needed not only to meet the daily requirements, but to replace and restore the deficiencies. *The Journal of American Medical Association (JAMA)* recently recommended that all adults take a daily multivitamin supplement.

Proper nutrition is important for maintaining health. Medicine has long recognized the importance of nutrition therapy and dietary modifications in diseases such as diabetes, heart disease, osteoporosis, gout, and hypertension. Nutritional strategies can play an important role in the overall treatment of fibromyalgia. In this chapter I'll review supplement and diet strategies.

Supplement Strategies

If our bodies are low in a particular vitamin or mineral, we can't just take any form of this low substance to replace it. If we had an iron deficiency, we wouldn't chew on nails to try to replace the iron. This would be rather silly, plus it could lead to puncture wounds in the mouth!

For supplements to be tolerated and effective, they have to have certain characteristics. The most important one is the bioavailability. Bioavailability is the amount of a nutrient ingested that is absorbed and available to the body for metabolic use. Bioavailability is important because our nutritional intake must be available to various body systems for growth, maintenance of body tissues, and other performance factors. No matter how high the nutrient levels or how well formulated the product, if it is not bioavailable, then it is worthless to the body.

One way to improve bioavailability is to take chelated minerals. When minerals such as zinc, manganese, magnesium and others become surrounded by amino acids, they are bonded into a stable form and this is referred to as chelation. Through chelation, the body is able to transport minerals across the intestinal wall as part of digestion. The body is very efficient at absorbing amino acids, so amino acids can be used to piggyback vital minerals into the body. Otherwise the minerals would not be absorbed without the chelation process.

Another characteristic of a supplement is that it must be well tolerated. This means there should be very few, if any, side effects. Sometimes supplements cause flu-like symptoms, loose stools, nausea, and even rashes. The supplements should be made with very low allergenic materials and of good quality so they are well absorbed and well tolerated.

Over the years I've used a lot of supplements in the treatment of fibromyalgia, and I believe they are effective in many patients. Not all patients benefit but, in general, supplements are safe to try and, if they help, are relatively inexpensive to continue. Today nutritional supplements are one of the most important treatments I recommend for fibromyalgia.

Deficiencies In Fibromyalgia

We discussed some of the deficiencies found in fibromyalgia earlier in Chapter 6. Let's review a number of deficiencies present and how they may affect our fibromyalgia symptoms, and look at specific supplements that may help.

Serotonin Deficiency

Serotonin is an important hormone and neurotransmitter manufactured from the amino acid, tryptophan. Serotonin is important in our food behavior, sleep behavior, neuroendocrine function, mood and energy. The clinical symptoms from low serotonin include depression, fatigue, increased pain and hypoglycemia.

Nutritional supplements to treat low serotonin are:

- 5-HTP. 5-hydroxy L-tryptophan which is a modified amino acid that the body uses to manufacture serotonin. In addition to helping the body produce serotonin, 5-HTP can be an appetite suppressant and a sleep inducer. Typical dosing is 100–300 mg per day. Griffonia seed is a source of natural 5-HTP.

- St. John's Wort. This herbal antidepressant seems to work by raising the serotonin level. Typical dosing is 300 mg up to twice a day.

- SAM-e (pronounced "Sammy"). A natural medicine used in Europe for 25 years to treat mild to moderate depression. It stands for S-Adenosyl-L-methionine and it helps make the body's mood enhancing chemicals. Usual dosing is 200–400 mg twice per day on an empty stomach. Side effects can include upset stomach and headaches.

Magnesium Deficiency

Magnesium is a common deficiency in the general population but even more so in patients with fibromyalgia. Intracellular magnesium is low, which interferes with the muscles' ability to relax and make energy. Magnesium is needed to convert 5-HTP to serotonin.

Magnesium Facts

- 27% of magnesium is stored in muscle tissue.

- Every energy-consuming reaction in life needs magnesium to proceed.

- Less than 1% of body magnesium is in the serum.

- Low magnesium intake results in magnesium depletion from muscles and bones to maintain serum magnesium levels.

Symptoms of low magnesium in fibromyalgia include increased fatigue, increased spasms, and increased pain. Individuals with low magnesium are more prone to injuring their muscles when they exercise, so exercise intolerance or increased pain and spasms after activity is another symptom of low magnesium in fibromyalgia.

Natural supplements to treat low magnesium include products containing magnesium. Magnesium glycinate is the preferred bioavailable form. A magnesium supplement works with the muscles to help them manufacture more energy (ATP molecules). When taken as a supplement, magnesium and its co-factor, malic acid, can enter the muscle cells and improve the muscle energy production.

Studies have shown that this combination reduces pain in fibromyalgia patients and headache patients (Abraham GE and Flechas JD, 1992; Russell IJ, *et al.,* 1995). I have found that 75% of people who use products made by To Your Health, Fibro-Care™ (containing magnesium, malic acid, vitamin B_1, vitamin B_6, vitamin C and manganese) will report improvement with either decreased pain, improved energy, a more stable baseline, or a combination of these. Anywhere from 300–500 mg of extra magnesium supplement a day may be needed. Taking 5-HTP along with magnesium/malic acid will increase your odds of converting 5-HTP to serotonin.

Low Amine ATP Or Energy Deficiency

Biochemical studies show that fibromyalgia patients have low ATP or energy molecules in their muscles due to a deficiency of the compounds that make ATP such as oxygen and magnesium (Abraham GE and Flechas JD, *Journal of Nutritional Medicine,* 1992). Swedish investigators, Drs. Bengtsson and Henrikson, have shown that a lower concentration of oxygen than expected is found in fibromyalgia muscles, which contributes to lower ATP levels. This lower concentration is most probably due to poor metabolism of nutrients and not from true hypoxia (lack of oxygen in body).

A lack of ATP contributes to fatigue, increased pain and increased muscle spasms. Supplements to improve the ATP levels include magnesium and another product called co-enzyme Q_{10} (CoQ_{10}). CoQ_{10} is a vital enzyme in the energy producing pathway of the muscles' energy centers called the mitochondria. Typical CoQ_{10} dosing is 100–300 mg daily. Oxygen therapy is not beneficial and could damage the lungs.

Vitamin B_{12} Deficiency

I have found many people with fibromyalgia have a relatively low B_{12} level. Vitamin B_{12} is important in manufacturing red blood cells (erythropoiesis), improving nerve pathways, improving DNA synthesis and folate metabolism.

Symptoms of low B_{12} include increased fatigue, numbness and tingling, and depressed immune system.

Nutritional supplements for B_{12} include B_{12} lozenges, sublingual B_{12}, or B_{12} injections. B_{12} that is taken in a lozenge or sublingual form is absorbed directly into the blood vessels in the mouth. In many, B_{12} is not absorbed well from the stomach. I frequently prescribe a B_{12} injection protocol in which 1 milligram of B_{12} is injected intramuscularly once a week for 6 weeks or more.

Low Growth Hormone Level

Dr. Bennett (1998) found that people with fibromyalgia have decreased growth hormone levels as measured with IGF-1 (insulin-like growth factor, a derivative of growth hormone). Symptoms of low growth hormone include fatigue, increased fibrofog, decreased metabolism and depressed immune system.

Supplements to increase growth hormone level include colostrum which has growth hormone and immunoglobulins. Bovine (beef) colostrum is taken orally, and is essentially identical to human IGF-1. Bovine colostrum given orally has been found to raise the serum IGF-1 level in humans. I found that over 75% of my patients report improvement in their energy level and concentration abilities when taking colostrum.

Daily growth hormone injections can increase the IGF-1 level and result in improvement. Growth hormone injections are expensive, averaging about $1500/month, and they are not routinely covered by insurance, hence limiting the widespread application for fibromyalgia treatment. Growth hormone is available by sublingual form as well.

Adrenal Hormone Deficiency

The adrenal glands can become dysfunctional in fibromyalgia and cause problems with the immune system and ability to handle stress. Supplements that boost the immune system can be considered. These include colostrum, vitamin C, zinc, echinacea, cinnamon, garlic, and golden seal. Antioxidants are helpful in fighting free radicals, supporting the cellular function, and improving the immune system. Common antioxidants include vitamins A and E, grapeseed extract, and lipoic acid. Licorice root and Eleuthero (previously known as Siberian ginseng) can also help improve adrenal gland function and boost our stress and immune responses.

Supplement Strategies For Treating Specific Symptoms

We discussed treating specific deficiencies in fibromyalgia, and I wanted to address some specific symptoms of fibromyalgia and supplement strategies available. Later chapters will provide more details.

1. **Pain**

   - magnesium and malic acid combinations
   - natural anti-inflammatories such as glucosamine, chondroitin, MSM and flaxseed oil
   - feverfew for headaches
   - guaifenesin is a cough medicine that is reported to have some success in treating patients with fibromyalgia (Dr. R. Paul St. Amand)

2. **Fatigue**

   - magnesium and malic acid combination
   - colostrum
   - co-enzyme Q_{10} (CoQ_{10})
   - vitamin B_{12}
   - ginkgo biloba
   - vinpocetine

3. **Poor Sleep**

   - 5-HTP
   - melatonin
   - valerian root
   - To Your Health Sleep Formula™ (5-HTP, valerian root, lemon balm, passion flower)

4. **Fibrofog**

   - colostrum
   - ginkgo biloba
   - vinpocetine
   - acetyl-L-carnitine
   - phosphatidyl serine

5. **Irritable Bowel Syndrome**

   - fiber supplement
   - acidophilus
   - valerian root
   - peppermint oil (enteric coated)`
   - olive leaf extract

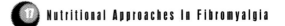

6. **Mild Depression**

- 5-HTP

- St. John's Wort

- SAM-e

- flaxseed oil

Our Daily Needs

We need to make sure we get our basic balanced minerals and vitamins. Supplements are important to replace deficiencies but we mustn't forget that we still have to get all of our daily vitamins and minerals. A good multivitamin such as To Your Health Multi-Gold™ is recommended. Or even better, their product, Foundation Formula™ is a powder formulation that packs a nutritional punch. To meet all of your nutritional needs, you'd have to swallow countless pills. The Foundation Formula™ is a complete vitamin and mineral supplement that you can take for your nutritional needs that replaces 30–40 pills a day at a fraction of the cost.

Food & Drug Administration (FDA)

Many supplements are available to treat fibromyalgia. These over-the-counter (OTC) supplements and health foods are currently not subjected to the same strict FDA regulations as prescription medicine. This does not mean that OTC supplements are not safe to use.

The FDA is a scientific accrediting and regulating agency for prescription medicine. In some instances, the FDA has warned consumers about potential side effects or contamination of health food products that can cause medical complications. For example, there have been FDA warnings about the use of tryptophan because contamination has resulted in a serious blood reaction called eosinophilia. Also, the FDA has warned about using dietary supplements containing both ephedrine and caffeine, as this combination may cause heart attacks, heart arrhythmias, or hepatitis. In December, 2003 the FDA announced a ban on dietary supplements containing ephedra due to health concerns about the product. The FDA does not require products to be approved before they are manufactured but it does regulate vitamins by DSHEA and labeling laws. The National Nutritional Foods Association does encourage members to obtain GMP (good manufacturing practices) which is a stringent certification for manufacturing supplements. For example, I use many products from To Your Health which has its products manufactured in a GMP approved lab.

Many effective nutritional therapies have been used for hundreds and even thousands of years, resulting in a lot of accumulated clinical experience. That is not the same as saying scientific studies have confirmed the success, or that the FDA has approved the use of particular products. We have to remember that not everything we use to treat medical conditions has been studied or approved, and that doesn't mean we shouldn't use it.

We need to be open-minded about nutritional approaches, but we also have to optimize safety and therapeutic efficacy by being responsible and knowledgeable about products that we use. Fibromyalgia patients should work closely with their doctor, nutritionist, pharmacist, or knowledgeable colleagues to learn about a product and make intelligent decisions. You should not try anything unless you know exactly what it contains and your doctor has approved its use.

Be Open-minded

Numerous nutritional products are available, and I work with my patients in an open-minded and responsible manner about trying them. Educate yourself by reading up on various products. Ask your doctor, and basically make these decisions based on your knowledge and expertise and not on the product's good marketing strategy. Try one supplement at a time for one or two months and see if you think the product is helping. If you think it might be helping but you're not sure, try it for another month and reevaluate its effect. Remember to work together with your doctor.

Special Eating Problems Related To Fibromyalgia

Fibromyalgia causes problems with everyday living, so it is not surprising that it would interfere with eating. A variety of conditions can pose unique eating problems.

1. **Pain**
   Pain has a way of making us forget about everything else, including hunger. Pain interferes with eating, cooking, and thinking about preparing food as well. Some people use food as a "reward" for being in pain (I'm in pain so I "deserve" ice cream!).

2. **Fatigue**
   Next to pain, fatigue is the most common symptom of fibromyalgia, and it causes us to not think about eating or cooking at all. Extreme fatigue alters our eating pattern, so we tend to minimize any effort involved in preparing food and enjoying meals. Some people overeat to "try" to get energy.

3. **Depression**
   Depression is common in conditions that cause chronic pain. Part of the depression picture can include undereating, overeating, or eating disorders such as anorexia or bulimia.

4. **Irritable bowel syndrome**
   This common condition causes episodes of constipation, diarrhea, abdominal cramping, pain and bloating. People with irritable bowel syndrome are usually sensitive to foods that are greasy, fatty, or bulky, as well as nuts and raw vegetables. Foods that trigger an attack need to be avoided.

5. **Food sensitivities and allergies**
   People with fibromyalgia have a lot of food intolerances. Practically anything can aggravate our symptoms. I believe if we eliminated all foods that can cause allergies or irritate our symptoms, there would be nothing left to eat!

   If food intolerances are present, the most common foods (sugar, wheat, dairy products, citrus fruits, eggs, and chocolate products) are usually the ones that create problems. Many of us are lactose intolerant, meaning that milk and milk products can cause gastric attacks, gas, cramping, or diarrhea. Others do not tolerate food additives or preservatives such as nitrates and sulfites in processed meats. Also, food smells may be nauseating to our overly sensitive nostrils.

   People with fibromyalgia can be more susceptible to chronic yeast overgrowth infections, especially with diets that are high in refined sugars and fermented foods. This can create additional gastrointestinal symptoms.

If one is sensitive to a particular food, the body may not properly digest this food. This in turn may interfere with the ability to digest and absorb other nutrients and perform other necessary nutritional activities. In other words, the body cannot absorb needed nutrients.

Avoiding foods that cause sensitivities or allergies is certainly the main emphasis in treating this problem. A trial elimination of offending foods may cause noticeable improvement in some fibromyalgia symptoms and pain level; these symptoms may reoccur if the offending foods are reintroduced into the diet. Allergy testing or specific allergy medicines may be necessary as well.

6. **Temporomandibular Joint Dysfunction**
This condition commonly associated with fibromyalgia causes pain in the jaw and can lead to difficulty in opening the mouth and chewing. Chewy foods, sandwiches, and hard foods can pose special difficulties for someone with TMJ dysfunction.

A dental specialist may need to be consulted, and specific treatments could include customized bite splints, crowns and bridges, or other TMJ restorative procedures. People with TMJ dysfunction may notice decreased jaw pain if they avoid hard and lumpy foods, take smaller bites, and chew the food slowly and completely.

7. **Hypoglycemia**
People with fibromyalgia are more prone to developing hypoglycemia, or abnormally low blood sugar. This is probably due to our dysfunctional autonomic nervous system. Hypoglycemia can cause dizziness, lightheadedness, a feeling of passing out, extreme fatigue, and listlessness.

A hypoglycemia attack is usually brought on by eating foods rich in sugar: candy; pastries; cookies; and snack foods. After eating, the sugar gets quickly absorbed into the bloodstream. This rapid increase in blood sugar tells the autonomic nervous system to release insulin. Insulin is a hormone that opens the "sugar gates" in the muscles. Thus insulin allows sugar to leave the blood and go into the muscle cells.

In fibromyalgia, it appears that we are hypersensitive to our insulin effect. The insulin "overshoots," causing too much sugar to be taken out of the bloodstream and put into the muscle, thus leaving too little sugar left in the bloodstream (hypoglycemia).

The brain requires a steady level of glucose in the bloodstream in order to function. If hypoglycemia develops, the brain begins to send signals that it is hungry for more glucose. Carbohydrate craving results and more carbohydrate-rich foods are eaten to satisfy this craving. Within a few hours of eating another snack loaded with sugar, the blood glucose level drops to low again, and the cravings return. Eating another carbohydrate snack repeats this cycle. Adding more carbohydrates simply encourages more hypoglycemia.

I came to realize the effects of hypoglycemia when I found that eating a donut for breakfast would cause me to feel lethargic and irritable within a few hours of this sugar feast. And once I realized that I was having hypoglycemic symptoms from carbohydrate sensitivity, I stopped eating America's favorite breakfast carb and made dietary changes.

One may avoid hypoglycemia by eating meals or snacks that have a higher protein content, eating more natural sugars such as fruits and vegetables, and avoiding refined sugar. I will review a fibromyalgia diet in more detail later.

Weight Gain

A common problem observed in fibromyalgia is weight gain. Many women complain to me that weight gain became a major problem once fibromyalgia established itself. It is not unusual for a person to put on a 25–30 pound weight gain in the first year after fibromyalgia was diagnosed. Various factors are involved in weight gain and include:

1. **Decreased Metabolism**.
   Various hormone changes can slow down the metabolism in fibromyalgia. Studies have shown hormone deficiencies or imbalances (cortisol, thyroid, serotonin, growth hormone) in fibromyalgia. Insulin and other hormones are probably affected as well.

   Dr. Leslie J. Crofford (1998) has described hormonal abnormalities in fibromyalgia and how they interfere with physiologic communication between the brain and the body. Closely linked with hormones is the autonomic nervous system. The autonomic nerves are the small nerves vital in the coordination of the body's hormones, and thus they play a role in the regulation and delivery of nutrients to our cells.

   The hypoglycemic roller-coaster effect is a good example of the combination of hormonal endocrine imbalances and autonomic nervous system dysfunction leading to hypoglycemic symptoms. Overall, neuroendocrine abnormalities in fibromyalgia probably interfere with the body's metabolism (by decreasing it), and part of the treatment involves replacing or supplementing hormones to help improve the body's metabolism.

   A slower body metabolism means fewer calories are burned on a daily basis to "run" the body's machinery. If fewer calories are burned with no change occurring in calories consumed, weight gain will result over time. Also, women in their late 30s and 40s often develop fibromyalgia along the same time as early menopause (decreased estrogen). This can further decrease metabolism and increase the potential for weight gain.

2. **Hypoglycemia.**
   As I mentioned earlier, increased sensitivity to insulin will result in too much glucose being removed from the bloodstream and pushed into the muscle. All this extra glucose pushed into the muscles has nowhere to go as the muscles have very limited ability to store glucose.

   The body is forced to go into a fat-storing mode where it coverts this extra glucose into fatty tissue. Contrary to the popular myth that obesity is a result of eating too much fatty foods, obesity is usually the result of eating too many carbohydrates. A carbohydrate-rich diet causes weight gain by converting the extra glucose into fat and, if fibromyalgia causes more insulin activity and sensitivity, then the weight gain can be even greater.

   Another myth is that most overweight people overeat. Actually, most overweight people do not overeat. They may have a craving for carbs and the carbs are easily converted to fat. Fibromyalgia facilitates this process. A diet modified in protein and lower in carbs may help.

3. **Medicines.**
   Side effects of medicines used to treat fibromyalgia can cause weight gain by decreasing metabolism, altering hormones, causing fluid retention, and increasing appetite. The most common offending medicines are the antidepressants.

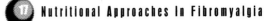

Medicines such as estrogen and prednisone can also contribute to weight gain. If certain medicines are causing weight gain they may need to be stopped or adjusted depending on the individual's medical needs.

4. **Decreased activity due to pain.**
People with fibromyalgia hurt more and are not as active because activity increases pain. Thus, it is difficult to increase the energy expenditure or calorie burning related to exercise and activity. Less calories burned can mean weight gain. Any treatment program in fibromyalgia must include attempts at increasing overall activity level.

Startling Medical Revelation!

Medical experts have found that in order to lose weight, you must burn more calories than you consume!

Diet Strategies For Fibromyalgia

There is no nutritional cure for fibromyalgia at the present time, but we can increase our nutritional awareness as it pertains to fibromyalgia, and make changes gradually and slowly (like we chew our food!). The goals in nutritional therapy for fibromyalgia would be to improve nutrient absorption and entry into the cells, boosting the immune system, eliminating toxins from the body, creating optimal biochemical pathways, minimizing food sensitivity or adverse reactions, maintaining a healthy microorganism balance, improving energy levels, and achieving optimal body weight.

You can control what you eat, so you have the ability to treat your fibromyalgia by dietary modifications. I want you to think about treating and beating fibromyalgia any way you can, and one way you can help is by watching your diet.

Throughout history, the successful "Diet" has been as mythical and elusive as the Holy Grail. Perhaps the Holy Grail is the perfect diet! There are many thousands of diet plans out there and it seems like every few months a new diet "fad" sweeps the country. I've noticed that all diets have some things in common, no matter what the "specifics" are about the particular recommended diet. These common factors include:

- Don't eat between meals (eat less)

- Exercise more (burn off more calories)

- Avoid junk foods (eat less—eat healthier)

- Don't eat at night (since sedentary during evening)

It doesn't take much (a few successful brain synapses!) to realize that following the "common" recommendations will result in eating less and burning more calories which leads to . . . now brace yourself . . . WEIGHT LOSS!

I realize that we don't need to follow any special "diet" to lose weight, because weight loss diets are 90% common sense and 10% medical advice. Sometimes a specific diet strategy makes sense based on the medical condition, and following this specific diet may improve symptoms (such as fatigue) even if weight loss doesn't occur. So for fibromyalgia, let me give you my 10% worth of advice!

A Fibromyalgia Diet

As part of an overall fibromyalgia treatment plan, I try to enhance patients' awareness of dietary possibilities and encourage them to experiment with their diets to see if their fibromyalgia symptoms can improve. Several years ago, I came up with a specific diet to assist patients and give them specific guidelines, and many have found it very helpful.

I have modified the specifics as my patients have given me feedback over the years, but the basic recommendation remains the same: my recommended fibromyalgia diet is higher in protein and lower in carbohydrates than the typical American diet. The diet needs to be balanced so proper vitamins, minerals and nutrients are obtained. Common sense needs to prevail to eat right and make wise food choices.

Traditional Food Pyramid

About 10 years ago we were introduced to the Food Guide Pyramid for recommended dietary guidelines for a healthy diet. The Pyramid emphasized 6 to 11 servings of breads, cereals, rice, and pasta per day, with 2 to 3 servings of meat and sparing use of fats and oils. Over half the daily calories were to be from carbohydrates.

American foods are an easy source of carbohydrates because they are loaded with simple carbohydrates like white flour, white rice and sugars. Added sugars are found in sweets, salad dressings, soft drinks, lunch meats, canned foods, and more.

Americans interpreted the Food Pyramid to say all carbs are good and all fats are bad and we soon became bombarded with all types of fat-free foods that were "good" for us. Americans ate well over half their daily calories in carbs and avoided fats. Those who avoid fats usually end up eating more carbohydrates and too little protein as "low fat" foods are usually high in carbs and low in proteins.

But instead of getting healthier, Americans have been getting fatter and are developing more high blood pressure, diabetes, and coronary artery disease than ever in the past 10 years. What is going wrong?

It turns out that the carbohydrates, always thought to be the foundation of a good diet, may well be harmful. We've learned that too much carbs are bad, but the right kinds of carbs (*e.g.*, fruits, vegetables) are healthy. We've also learned that some fats are good for us (*e.g.*, olive oil, flaxseed oil, fish oil) and need to be part of our diet.

The late Dr. Robert C. Atkins pioneered a different type of diet, a high protein and low carbohydrate diet, over 30 years ago and this has been one of the most widely used diets as well as one of the most criticized diets. Lately, low carb diets are receiving a lot of attention and popularity among dieters and health-conscious consumers alike. Two recent studies published in *The Annals of Internal Medicine* report that low carb diets help people lose weight faster than other diets. Triglyceride and blood-sugar levels improved over time as well.

The editorial accompanying these reports indicated low carb diets can be tried for weight loss but include healthy sources of fat and protein and incorporate regular physical activity. Now, more and more scientists, researchers and dietary professionals are questioning our traditional Food Pyramid.

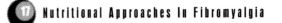

We are changing our thinking pattern to consider a diet that emphasizes good proteins and good fats, and reduces overall carbohydrates.

Rationale

We've discussed some of the basic problems of fibromyalgia, the metabolism changes and the dysfunctional carbohydrate/insulin responses, especially. These problems contribute considerably to many of our most bothersome symptoms, including: aching; fatigue; brain fog; irritability; anxiety; dizziness; carbohydrate craving; irritable bowel syndrome; food intolerance; and food sensitivity. The American "diet" aggravates and perpetuates our fibromyalgia problems. We may have tolerated the higher carb, low fat diet before we got fibromyalgia, but since we got fibromyalgia, this diet no longer works for us and it's probably making us worse.

Because of our slow metabolism, it is difficult for us to eat less and notice a difference. Because of our pain, it is difficult for us to increase our exercise level to burn off more calories. Ideally, we need a diet that improves the efficiency of our calories burned by providing us with the right "quality" of food to enhance our metabolism and calorie-burning abilities.

Foods That Are Okay

1. **Good proteins**

   - Meats, such as lean meats, skinless chicken, turkey and fish. Lean cuts of steaks, sausage and bacon contain higher amounts of saturated fats so they should be kept to a minimum.

   - Eggs. This breakfast staple is a great source of protein; egg whites are healthier.

   - Tofu

   - Soy meat substitutes

   - Dairy products. These include cheese, cream, butter, skim milk, cottage cheese and unsweetened yogurt. Try for low fat dairy products.

   - Legumes. This class includes beans, peas, peanuts, lentils and soybeans.

2. **Good carbohydrates**

   - All vegetables. Vegetables are a source of carbs that are highest in fiber and lowest in sugar. Some vegetables such as corn have more carbs than others.

   - Fresh fruits. Avocado, raspberries and strawberries have the least carbohydrates of fruits. Avoid dried fruits.

3. **Good fats**

   - Plant oils, especially olive oil. Other vegetable oils are acceptable including canola, soy, corn, sunflower and peanut.

   - Fish oils (rich in omega-3)

   - Almonds

   - Avocados

4. Others

- Salad garnishes which include nuts, olives, bacon, grated cheese, mushrooms and other vegetables are allowed.

- Flaxseed oil. A healthy supplement which contains essential fats.

- Artificial sweeteners and sugar-free beverages are allowed in moderation. If you feel you are sensitive to aspartame, avoid products that contain it (NutraSweet) or substitute a different artificial sweetener, such as sucralose (Splenda) or saccharin (Sweet'n Low). Stevia is a sweet supplement alternative to sugar. Xylitol is another one of nature's sweeteners like Stevia that won't raise blood sugar levels and can substitute for sugar.

Foods To Avoid

1. Bad proteins

- Fatty meats. Lunch meat, pork, hamburgers (full of sulfites, nitrates, bad fats, etc.)

2. Bad carbohydrates

- Refined sugars (sweets): These include desserts, candy, cookies, sugared drinks, crackers, baked goods and any good snack foods!

- Breads: White flour can be an especially "bad" carb in fibromyalgia. Even "better" carb breads such as multi-grain breads can interfere with carbohydrate metabolism or impede weight loss. The bread category includes bagels, muffins, waffles, pizza and pancakes. This category also includes cereals.

- Rice: Brown rice is a "better" carb than white rice, but this can interfere with weight loss or carbohydrate metabolism.

- Pasta: Spaghetti, noodles, linguini, and rigatoni. These favorites should be avoided.

- Potatoes: It doesn't matter if they're baked, mashed, smashed, scalloped, sweet and especially if they're fried or chipped, this food category is a major culprit. This category also happens to be a fibromyalgia favorite.

3. Bad fats

- Fatty red meats and organ meats

- Partially hydrogenated oils (trans fats). Includes margarine, lard, vegetable shortening, coconut oil and palm oil.

4. Others

- Alcohol: Alcohol is a source of bad carbs and can cause problems if too much is consumed. I don't have problems with someone consuming a glass of wine a day as a fruit serving because there have been reported health benefits from a daily glass of wine. Obviously, common sense needs to prevail.

- Carbonated beverages: These are a source of bad acids and can aggravate gastric symptoms.

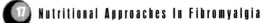

Specific Diet Strategies

1. Think Protein Always

A key with this diet is not to eat any carbohydrate foods by themselves, even if they are considered good carbs. "Orphaned" carbs will increase the risk of hypoglycemia/insulin hypersensitivity in someone with fibromyalgia, so foods that have some protein in them should be consumed every time we eat. Therefore, we shouldn't eat pancakes and syrup for breakfast because it doesn't contain any protein. Insulin is controlled by the balance of protein and carbs each time we eat.

If we want a salad for lunch, we should not just eat plain lettuce and vegetables. We need to have a protein source in our salad as well, such as chicken, tuna, turkey, eggs, cheese and more. We should not eat a plain spaghetti supper. We should have spaghetti and meatballs (made with lean ground chuck meat) or lean sausage. If we crave a snack, we shouldn't eat a sugar cookie. A small bag of cashews would be a better protein-laden choice for a snack. Once you are trained to think about protein every time you put something in your mouth, it becomes easier to stay within the framework of the fibromyalgia diet.

2. Avoid The Rush

Hypoglycemia is often the result of a sudden surge of glucose in our bloodstream after eating a carbohydrate-rich food. The Glycemic Index (GI) of foods is a measure of how fast the carbohydrate triggers the rise in circulating blood sugars. A GI over 70 is high. Examples of food with high GI are:

Rice Crispies GI: 80, corn muffin GI: 95, mashed potatoes GI: 88.

To avoid a carbohydrate surge, take a few bites from proteins first whenever you eat. Even if you are eating good carbs, if you take the first few bites from protein, you can minimize the carbohydrate "rush." Eating proteins first activates the protein digesting enzymes and slows the absorption of carbohydrates. Plus, proteins require hydrochloric acid for proper digestion, carbohydrates don't. If we eat carbohydrates first, hydrochloric acid may not be activated and subsequent proteins eaten may not be properly digested. Foods rich in fiber and fats also slow the absorption of carbohydrates.

3. Eat Until Full

Try to eat at least 3 meals a day and have 1–2 snacks. At meals, eat until you are comfortably full but not stuffed. Some people with fibromyalgia actually do better by eating 5 to 6 smaller meals a day or by eating 3 smaller meals and 2 larger snacks. Those who are bothered by irritable bowel syndrome sometimes can do better by eating smaller portions more frequently. Eat slowly and take your time to chew food well.

4. Weekdays: Behave!

I recommend that the fibromyalgia diet be followed strictly for 5 days each Monday through Friday, and I allow people to splurge a little on the weekends. That is, the diet is 5 days "on" and 2 days not so "on." This allows people to follow the basic rules during the week (more proteins, good carbs, good fats) but also allows the anticipation of favorite foods over the weekend. Anticipation is thus built into the diet, as well as guilt-free enjoyment.

Sample Meal Guide

Breakfast:
- 6 oz. glass of skim milk or juice
- 2 eggs any style

- 2 slices of bacon, Canadian bacon, or 2 links/small sausage patties. Use lean, low fat meats. Consider soy meat substitutes.
- Some days can skip the meat and melt cheese on the egg; some days can skip eggs and eat the meat or melt cheese on the meat.
- One of my favorite breakfast meals is a frittata, made with 2 eggs. A frittata is an Italian omelet with the ingredients (meat, seafood, vegetables, etc.) mixed with the eggs rather than being folded inside. Dozens of variations (go online for recipes!) will keep you from getting bored.

Lunch:
- Chef's salad with ham, turkey, low fat cheese, mixed greens and garnishes.
- Any meat roll-up or mixture of meat, vegetables and lettuce can work for lunch; consider "breadless" sandwiches (is that an oxymoron?)
- Canned tuna salad or salmon packed in water.

Dinner:
- Seasoned chicken; vegetables cooked in olive oil and seasoned; salad garnished with pecans, low fat salad dressing. Be creative with the seasoning.
- Cod with sun-dried tomato marinade with steamed green beans and cherry tomato salad.

Snacks: (1–2 per day)
- Protein and fatty-rich foods are excellent snack foods to satisfy appetite and reduce cravings; consider nuts, sugar-free gelatin dessert with heavy cream, celery with some peanut butter, cherry tomatoes stuffed with low fat cottage cheese.
- Fruit can also be eaten as a snack; mix a cup of your favorite fruit with sugar-free gelatin or heavy cream. Fruit mixed with cottage cheese is also a delicious snack.
- I'm frequently asked if meal replacement bars are acceptable as snacks or even as a meal replacement, especially breakfast. Many people simply do not have the time or energy to cook a breakfast and want a simple solution. Low carb meal replacement bars are okay; some are pretty tasty too (I had to try them out if I was going to talk about them!). Numerous choices of modified protein/low carb bars are available, so try them out if you wish.
- Remember, snack foods should contain protein as required by the fibromyalgia diet.

5. **Mini-Splurges!**
   Weekends (Saturday and Sunday) are your chance to reward yourself for behaving during the week. If you want to start your weekend with Friday's dinner, you can, but your weekend ends after Sunday's lunch and the basic rules are followed again for Sunday dinner. On the weekends, you are allowed to eat your favorite foods again such as pizza, bread, and even desserts. If you splurge too much on weekends, you may feel poorly so you must learn to allow yourself moderate samplings of your favorite missed food but still try to stay within the framework of the diet on weekends.

   A number of my patients have discovered that they can enjoy their favorite foods on the weekend, but still watch their portions or eat their favorite foods within the basic higher protein/lower carb framework and not feel poorly. They appreciate the weekend mini-splurges and they tolerate them. Other patients can balance off feeling somewhat worse on the weekends with the fact that they are eating their favorite foods. Those same people can counteract the negative symptomatology with the positive effects of the weekend (weekends are psychologically a "good" time).

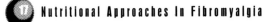

6. **If You Want Less Of You**
   This fibromyalgia diet can help decrease sugar cravings, help rebalance your body's chemistry, especially insulin and blood glucose levels, and can help you shed weight. If slimming down is a goal of yours, on the average you can lose 1–2 pounds every couple of weeks with this diet, based on my patients' experiences. Weight loss is highly individualized, however.

   Record your initial weight and weigh yourself once a week. Keep a log. Also, record how you feel or if you have any problems or questions. You will usually not lose weight for the first 4 days, and when your weekend mini-splurges come along, it is not unusual to stop weight loss for several days or sometimes maybe gain a pound over the weekend. However, patience is needed with the diet for a gradual but steady weight loss over time towards your target weight.

   If you find that you are not losing weight as hoped, it is okay to reduce portions, eliminate snacks, behave on weekends, or be more strict on your carbohydrates and fat. Try not to skip meals to reduce calories because it can lead to low energy and it can be hard on those with adrenal dysfunction. Many of my patients have noted that they lose inches even if they're not losing a lot of weight, and clothes fit them better and they have more energy. This could certainly be considered a successful outcome of the fibromyalgia diet.

7. **Expand Diet, Not Waist**
   Like any other diet, if all is going well, you can add more types of food and still follow the basic rules. For example, if you've gone through several weeks of skipping most carbs and enjoyed your weekend mini-splurges, but want to add more, you may want to add another serving of fruit during the day or add brown rice and whole grain breads, cereals and pastas to your diet on a more regular basis. You can still enjoy improved energy and stable weight or even additional weight loss by adding more to the diet, but each person has to find his or her own balance.

   You want to reach a point where you feel you have better control of your fibromyalgia symptoms through diet, now that you've accomplished a successful lifestyle change where you still follow the basic fibromyalgia diet rules and hopefully enjoy a lifestyle with more energy, more stable weight, and fewer carbohydrate cravings.

8. **If You Must Have It …**
   As long as there are delicious bad carbs and fats out there, we will always be tempted to eat them. The weekend mini-splurges give you that anticipation and craving "release" with this diet, although sometimes we simply cannot wait until the weekend to eat a particular sinful food.

   It certainly is never the intent to feel like you're punishing yourself or feeling guilty when you are following a diet, so I think it's necessary to review some strategies on how you can make some responsible choices even if you are choosing to temporarily go off your diet.

   • **Splurge dessert-style**. If you must eat that donut or that candy bar, it's best to eat it for dessert. That is, do not eat the snack all by itself, but eat it after you've eaten a meal where you've followed the fibromyalgia diet rules. Remember, if you've eaten a "good" meal, you are controlling the rate in which your glucose is being absorbed into the bloodstream. Adding a sugar-rich food item at the end of this meal will add those extra calories but should not give you any sugar surge that disrupts the fibromyalgia biochemistry.

- **Know the dessert proteins.** Dessert proteins include products with egg, cream cheese, cottage cheese, custard, nuts, milk, and cream. Don't be fooled by the protein content, these foods are still very high in sugar. However, if you must have a donut, it is better to have a crème-filled donut with nuts on it than the same-caloried glazed donut. If you must have a candy bar, it is better to eat a bag of chocolate covered peanuts rather than a chocolate bar.

Bread pudding is better than cake. If you have to have a glazed donut all by itself, then I would recommend you drink at least 4 ounces of skim milk BEFORE you eat the donut and another 4 ounces of skim milk while you're eating the donut. Remember, you need to reduce the fast rate of glucose absorption that gets us into trouble.

A couple of dessert foods that have a surprisingly low rate of glucose absorption, *i.e.,* decreased GI, are ice cream and peanut butter. The rich fats and protein in the ice cream can satisfy hunger and cravings while providing sweet and creamy carbs.

Peanut butter contains healthy oils and vitamin E, and a study at the University of Georgia (Dr. Eitenmiller) found that the processing of raw peanuts into peanut butter removed very little of the good vitamin E. Remember, serving size of ice cream is a cup, not a carton, and serving size for peanut butter is 2 tablespoons, not most of the jar! Natural peanut butter is even better because it doesn't have hydrogenated oils which can toxify the liver.

A Few Dessert Recipes

Bread pudding dessert recipe

½ cup raisins	½ teaspoon cinnamon
2 cups bread (use 1–2 days old)	¼ teaspoon salt
2 eggs lightly beaten	½ cup brown sugar
¼ teaspoon salt	2 ¼ cups milk

After mixing eggs and milk, mix with the bread and then combine in baking pan with rest of ingredients. Add 1 cup of water to the ingredients in the pan. For 45 minutes bake at 350 degrees.

Orange cottage delight

8 oz. low fat whipped topping	1 can mandarin oranges or equivalent fresh orange
Orange gelatin (2 boxes, small)	1 ½ lb cottage or ricotta cheese
1 large can of pineapple (crushed) —drain the liquid	

Chill the ingredients combined in bowl. May want to chop the oranges.

continued on next page...

A Few Dessert Recipes

continued from previous page...

A "light" dessert

1 month's supply of sleep modifier

1 month's supply of antidepressant

1 month's supply of nutritional supplements

4 massotherapy treatments

4 biofeedback treatments

12 therapy modalities

12 stretches (mixed)

12 exercise sessions (light variety)

generous helping of fibronomics

Mix sleep modifier, antidepressant, and nutritional supplements together in large bowl. Gently stir in the fibronomics, stretches and biofeedback making sure these get absorbed. Add in the massotherapy, mixing firmly until the lumps are gone. Add the exercises, turning the heat up. Lightly coat this mixture with humor and bake until done.

Serves 1 person for 1 month

- **Make responsible choices**. What about foods craved other than desserts, such as french fries or fast food or fried chicken? If you must, go ahead and break the rules on these foods every once in awhile, but in doing so, try to make responsible choices, *i.e.*, find foods that have higher protein in them or lower carbs to lower the rate of glucose absorption. If you must have a McDonald's hamburger, it would be better to remove the bottom bun and fold the hamburger over to reduce carbs. A number of restaurants and fast food places now offer low carb items that can be tried.

  Craving a baked potato? Eat a loaded baked potato instead because the cheese and bacon bits will slow down the glucose absorption. Gotta have those french fries? I can't think of anything that can redeem this particularly "bad" carb and fat combination, nor would I even suggest a way of modifying this absolutely delicious food!

  I want you to stop and think about everything you put in your mouth and analyze if there's a different way to get the same food but with more favorable biochemistry results. If you do this, you are accomplishing one of your main goals of following a fibromyalgia diet even if you are splurging a little bit now and then.

9. **Other Diet Necessities**

   No diet is complete without mentioning other diet necessities that have nothing to do with the actual foods eaten or avoided. With any fibromyalgia diet, we need to include these necessary recommendations as well.

   - **Drink 6–8, 8 ounce glasses of water per day**. Adequate fluids are needed to run the body's machinery and eliminate waste. Also, people with fibromyalgia are more susceptible to dips in blood pressure which can cause lightheadedness or near-fainting. If too little water is consumed each day, one is likely to have the hypotensive episodes, so make sure you are drinking lots of water. You may substitute sugar-free or artificially-sweetened drinks.

- **Healthy restraints**. Try to avoid consuming nicotine, caffeine and alcohol. These interfere with the body's ability to manufacture energy to carry out efficient biochemical reactions. They act as drugs in our bodies. Most people tell me their fibromyalgia feels better if they are able to quit smoking. Your doctor may be able to prescribe a patch or medicine to help you quit.

  Consider drinking a cup of "real" coffee in the morning and no caffeine after lunch. I've read that chemicals used to remove caffeine from coffee can be hard on your body so watch the decaffeinated coffees too! Common sense needs to prevail when considering whether or not to use these products or how much to consume.

  Also be careful with aspartame (NutraSweet). Artificial sweeteners have been shown to cause a variety of symptoms in some people. These symptoms can include pain, numbness, dizziness, headaches and fatigue. Symptoms are thought to be caused by sensitivity to the aspartame or sensitivity to the by-product of the aspartame breakdown, formaldehyde. Formaldehyde is poisonous in higher concentrations. If you are sensitive to aspartame, avoid products that contain it. Watch your consumption of diet soda as it usually contains both NutraSweet and caffeine. It's actually best to avoid carbonated beverages altogether, or certainly use healthy restraints.

  Don't consume foods that seem to aggravate fibromyalgia symptoms. Consider a trial elimination of certain foods that may exacerbate fibromyalgia symptoms. If you do not notice any improvement after a few weeks, there's probably no relationship between the fibromyalgia symptoms and these foods, so you can reintroduce them. If there are noticeable improvements during the trial elimination, then try reintroducing these foods to challenge your body. If the fibromyalgia symptoms increase, avoid these foods as much as possible. These eliminations/reintroductions/challenge trials can be done with various "suspicious" food categories.

  Many people must avoid gluten in their diet due to allergies. Gluten is a protein in all wheat, rye, barley and oat products. Spelt, a grain from the grass family, is a popular flour substitute that is considered a complex grain for those with gluten sensitivity. I've heard that spelt pasta tastes great!

- **Take nutritional supplements along with the diet**. As discussed earlier, it is important to achieve a balanced diet no matter what type of diet is being followed. Given problems of lost nutrients from food processing, and changes in bioavailability of various nutrients ingested, it is sometimes a problem to get the correct amount of adequate vitamins and minerals even if we follow all the rules of the fibromyalgia diet.

  I feel it's important to take a multivitamin supplement and a good one is Multi-Gold™ made by To Your Health. In addition to a good multivitamin, magnesium and malic acid combinations, colostrum and other supplements may be recommended.

- **A regular activity level**. All diets would say to increase exercise and try to walk more, etc., etc., but let's face it, improving our activity level is a basic goal of treating our fibromyalgia, and I'm working on this aspect with patients through other parts of the treatment program such as physical therapy, reconditioning, and reactivation.

  It's difficult to increase our activity level when we have fibromyalgia, but it is indeed a goal that will also help with optimizing our nutritional and energy level. We try to perform a light conditioning exercise at least 3 times a week (more if able), such as walking at least a mile or some type of similar exercise for 20–30 minutes.

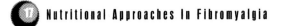

Who Can Benefit?

Everyone's nutritional balance is different, and there are no magical nutritional approaches to cure fibromyalgia. Rather, there are effective nutritional approaches that can be part of its successful treatment. Common sense needs to prevail. If you have a condition that can definitely be treated by nutritional modifications—overweight, irritable bowel syndrome, a yeast infection, lactose intolerance, or an eating disorder such as anorexia or bulimia—prescribed nutritional strategies may be medically required. I frequently work with a dietician and nutritionist to help fibromyalgia people make the changes.

You should notice more energy and less pain, better weight control, and more mental alertness, better sleep, and fewer fluctuations in symptoms. You can control stress better, be less anxious and less depressed. Plus, a good diet for your fibromyalgia will also make you healthier overall. If your fibromyalgia bothers you less, you will feel better about yourself as a result of your nutritional lifestyle changes, and you will have improved your well-being.

Not everyone tolerates this diet. Some people report constipation but this is usually helped by a daily fiber supplement. Other people notice dizziness when attempting to decrease the carbs. If this is a problem, I'll have them increase their fruits as a first attempt to see if this helps. Still others don't report any weight loss.

Sometimes they even feel a lot better, however, and lose inches even if they do not lose weight. Reducing portions may need to be considered if true weight loss is a major goal. If the diet is not tolerated, it can be stopped. As I've mentioned earlier, there are other diets that can be tried and can work for different individuals. I recommend working with your knowledgeable doctor to find the best choices for you.

▶ If You Want To Know More

1. Abraham GE, Flechas JD. *Management of fibromyalgia: rationale for the use of magnesium and malic acid*. J Nutr Med 1992; 3: 49–59.

2. Atkins R. *Dr. Atkins Diet Revolution*. Harper Collins Publishing, 1972.

3. Bengtsson A, Henriksson KG, Jorfeldt L, et al. *Primary fibromyalgia. A clinical and laboratory study of 55 patients*. Scand J Rheumatol 1986; 15: 340–7.

4. Bennett RM, Clark SC, Walczyk J. *A randomized, double-blind, placebo-controlled study of growth hormone in the treatment of fibromyalgia*. Am J Med 1998; 104(3): 227–31.

5. Burton A. *Alternative and complementary therapies*, 218.

6. Crofford LJ, Pillemer SR, Kalogeras KT, et al. *Hypothalamic-pituitary-adrenal axis perturbations in patients with fibromyalgia*. Arthritis Rheum 1994; 37(11):1583–92.

7. Eisinger J, Plantamura A, Ayavou T. *Glycolysis abnormalities in fibromyalgia*. J Am Coll Nutr 1994; 13(2): 144–8.

8. Fairfield KM, Fletcher RH. *Vitamins for chronic disease prevention in adults: scientific review*. JAMA 2002; 287(23): 3116–26.

9. Lister RE. *An open, pilot study to evaluate the potential benefits of coenzyme Q10 combined with Ginkgo biloba extract in fibromyalgia syndrome.* J Int Med Res 2002; 30(2): 195–9.

10. Pellegrino MJ. *Inside fibromyalgia.* Columbus OH: Anadem Publishing, 2001.

11. Pellegrino MJ, Evans AM. *The fibromyalgia chef.* Columbus OH: Anadem Publishing, 1997.

12. Russell IJ, Michalek JE, Flechas JD, et al. *Treatment of fibromyalgia syndrome with Super Malic: a randomized, double-blind, placebo-controlled, crossover pilot study.* J Rheumatol 1995; 22: 953–8.

13. Seelig MS, Rosanoff A. *The magnesium factor*, Avery 2003.

14. Squires M. *What a difference a daily makes.* Health Points. 2003; 8: 16. TyH Publications, Fountain Hills AZ. 1-800-801-1406 (www.e-tyh.com).

15. St. Amand RP, Marek CC. *What your doctor may not tell you about fibromyalgia: the revolutionary treatment that can reverse the disease.* Warner Books, 1999.

16. Stern L, Iqbal P, Seshadri KL, et al. *The effects of low-carbohydrate versus conventional weight loss diets in severely obese adults: one-year follow-up of a randomized trial.* Ann Int Med 2004; 140:778–85.

17. www.usda.gov/cnpp/AHAguidelines

18. Yancy WS, Olsen MK, Guyton, JR, et al. *A low-carbohydrate, ketogenic diet versus a low-fat diet to treat obesity and hyperlipidemia: a randomized, controlled trial.* Ann Int Med 2004; 140: 769–77.

Mentally Managing Fibromyalgia

Fibromyalgia affects your entire body. As a physician, I look at the whole person, not just a bunch of tender points. The body, mind, and soul are all affected by fibromyalgia, and all need to be treated together for healing. We need to consider the mental pain as well as the physical pain; one can't heal without the other.

In the past, fibromyalgia was mistakenly called "psychogenic rheumatism," which suggested that the condition was an imagined one. We know that is not the case, although people can benefit by working on the psychological aspects of this condition. Even if you don't understand at first how fibromyalgia really bothers you, or why therapy may help, you know that having a chronic illness is stressful and has affected your life in many ways:

1. You may have financial stresses because you can't work as much as before and have less money.

2. You may feel you can't give enough to your significant other or your family because of pain and fatigue, and you feel worthless.

3. You may feel cheated and angry because chronic pain wasn't in your life plan.

4. You may be unable to accept fibromyalgia or view yourself as chronically "ill," yet you know you don't feel "healthy."

5. You don't want to reevaluate yourself; you want things to be the way they were before fibromyalgia.

If it is suggested that you work with a mental health professional to help manage your fibromyalgia, that is not the same as saying the pain is "all in your head," or that "you are crazy." Rather, it is a recognition that chronically painful fibromyalgia affects all of you, including your mental outlook. It is okay to get help for *all* of you.

Many people with fibromyalgia develop associated psychological problems. These include decreased self-esteem, depression, anxiety, strained interpersonal relationships and altered coping mechanisms. That is not the same as saying, however, that psychological problems are the cause of fibromyalgia. In fact, studies conclude that depression, stress, and anxiety do NOT cause fibromyalgia, and that people with fibromyalgia have no more psychological problems than other people with chronic medical problems or chronic pain. Nor do past psychiatric diagnoses determine the severity of fibromyalgia (Dr. Lawrence Bradley, 1997).

Chronic physical pain can lead to very real psychological reactions. It is normal to become fearful, frightened, frustrated, angry, anxious, and depressed because of chronic pain. If these feelings lead to decreased self-esteem or depression, psychological therapies need to be considered as part of your overall treatment program. A psychological therapist will not take away your fibromyalgia, but will help you sort things out and support you while you go through the process of accepting your condition. This is not an easy process, but worth the work! A therapist can help you find the "new" you, realistically. Psychological strategies can include a variety of approaches.

1. **Psychotherapy**

   For fibromyalgia, this treatment is designed to evaluate mental aspects of a chronic illness through reeducation, reassurance, and support. Techniques such as psychoanalysis and hypnosis can be employed in psychotherapy. Psychiatrists usually perform this one-on-one intervention aimed at reinforcing your mental strategies, identifying and resolving conflicts, and achieving successful coping strategies. If a person with fibromyalgia is overcome with feelings of depression, anger, or has had negative childhood experiences or traumatic experiences, this technique may need to be considered.

   To give an example, one of my patients reported to me she was feeling more depressed and having suicidal thoughts because of her severe fibromyalgia pain. I referred her to a psychiatrist who was knowledgeable about fibromyalgia. He helped my patient see that she was trying to be a "super woman." Her mother died when the patient was 11 years-old, and the patient, who was the oldest child, always felt she needed to be the "mother" figure for her 3 younger siblings. Later in life, she immersed herself in her "mother" role with her own family, work, and her church. Fibromyalgia came along and prevented this, and caused severe depression. My patient responded to this psychotherapy by realizing what was happening and redefining her role to allow herself to do less and focus on getting her fibromyalgia under control.

2. **Counseling**

   This is professional "guidance" by using information gathered from the patient's history, interviews, and various tests. The counselor gives advice to the individual, couples or a group. A session of counseling is like talking to a friend; you feel comfortable and "safe." This counselor "friend" is an impartial, non-judgmental, but trustworthy professional who will listen to you and offer helpful suggestions. Fibromyalgia creates problems and stresses that not only affect the individual's sense of control or balance, but also can seriously affect the relationships with the significant other, family, and friends. Relationship difficulties, including sexual dysfunction, can occur and may benefit from psychological counseling. I recommend counselors who are knowledgeable in fibromyalgia. Sometimes patients may need some coaxing, but they are usually very pleased with the results.

3. **Pain and stress management**

   This is a more specialized form of counseling which includes cognitive and behavioral therapies. These therapies try to help patients think about themselves and behave in a manner that is "positive" in spite of the chronic pain. Pain management techniques are used to identify problems such as feeling depressed, hopeless, or disabled as a result of chronic pain. The treatment goals are to work on developing successful mental strategies, think more positively, and improve mental and physical outlooks and abilities. These techniques can teach the mind how to relax muscles and decrease pain, stress, and anxiety.

Guided imagery is a popular technique that uses therapist-guided mental images to relieve stress or relax muscles. The therapist may describe a setting and ask the patient to imagine being in this setting and performing imaginary steps to reach goals. For example, one therapist helped patients with burning pain by having them imagine they were using ice to cool it off. The well-known technique of counting sheep jumping over a fence to fall asleep is an example of using guided imagery. Specific programs can be played on cassette tapes to allow patients to practice this technique at home. About 60% of patients do very well with guided imagery.

4. **Biofeedback**

This is a specific technique for pain management in which individuals learn to control their body responses so as to achieve relaxation and pain relief. Numerous bodily functions are automatic, not controlled by our conscious selves. They include heart rate, pulse, digestion, blood pressure, brain waves, and muscle activity. These automatic functions are controlled by the autonomic nervous system. If one can recognize the autonomic nervous system signals, he or she can consciously create favorable autonomic nervous system responses like relaxing muscles or reducing stress.

Biofeedback devices can monitor skin temperature, heart rate, muscle tension, electrical conductivity of the skin and brain wave activity. An individual with fibromyalgia will train with a biofeedback device under the direction of a qualified biofeedback counselor. These devices measure the body's responses to stress or certain brain wave activities, and often give a signal—a noise, beep or visual reading—that the individual can recognize. These responses are automatic at first.

The patient notices these random responses and consciously starts wondering, "What was I doing or thinking that caused this response?" The patient may then appreciate a pattern between what she or he is doing or thinking when the "desired" response occurs. Once the patient identifies this pattern—response relationship, she or he can practice CAUSING the response. The more this learned response is practiced, the better the biofeedback skills become. Thus, the person can learn to consciously achieve relaxation.

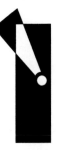

Patients learn to change their attitude and can help make the change from "I can't because of my fibromyalgia," to "I can in spite of my fibromyalgia."

Dr. Stuart Donaldson has been doing research on EEG-driven stimulation as a way of controlling favorable brain waves in the treatment of fibromyalgia. The patient uses biofeedback information to recognize the "good" brain waves on the EEG and tries to consciously "think" good brain waves. The more good brain waves one can think, the less the fibrofog. Any treatment that can give a person feedback can enable the individual to develop skills to control pain, improve concentration, and relax.

Whether it be one-on-one psychological intervention or group therapy, patients can develop better coping mechanisms and improve their outlook with psychological strategies. Psychologists, psychiatrists, counselors, social workers, clergy, and other qualified individuals can assist patients to cope with fibromyalgia and make the necessary lifestyle adjustments. Patients learn to change their attitude and can help make the change from "I can't because of my fibromyalgia," to "I can in spite of my fibromyalgia."

I never hesitate to recommend psychological intervention for someone who may need this help. If you think you may need this help, please make an appointment with someone right away. You may find a professional "good friend" who can help you in ways your other "good friends" can't.

Five REpairs

Physically, fibromyalgia bothers our bodies with pain and other problems. Mentally, it causes depression, mental fatigue, poor concentration, anxiety, fibrofog, and more. The mind can have a powerful healing effect on the body, so we need to keep our minds healthy and use them to help the healing process. Hope is the most important tool in a loaded mental toolbox.

A lot has been written on how to reduce stress, relax, and think positively. If I were to line up every article, book or advertisement on these subjects … well, it makes me stressed, tense, and frustrated to even think about how long it would take!

Mental strategies can reduce the ill effects of stress on our bodies. Notice I said "reduce the effects of stress," not reduce stress itself. Stress is a major factor in fibromyalgia. A catastrophic stress may have caused it, and any stress can certainly aggravate it. Life is stressful, so we can never get rid of stress. I like to say that the last time we were stress-free was when we were in the womb.

We can learn how to reduce stress and minimize its effect on fibromyalgia. Everyone with fibromyalgia can benefit from mental techniques to manage their physical problems. There is no one right way; many ways can work. It takes motivation, practice, and perseverance to learn a new mental management strategy. It is hard!

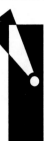

But with encouragement, patients with fibromyalgia are truly impressive in their ability to change their thinking and achieve a positive mental outlook.

Through the years each of us has evolved highly specialized thought processes to view ourselves and our world. For example, we always think of ourselves as young and healthy forever! Then all of a sudden, fibromyalgia comes along. Now these rules and processes are no longer effective. We are then asked to change our lifestyle, not only physically, but mentally. This is not an impossible task, but it involves a willingness to take that first step and to make a commitment to change our lifestyle. It is natural to be scared or even terrified of this process because we are not sure what to expect. But with encouragement, patients with fibromyalgia are truly impressive in their ability to change their thinking and achieve a positive mental outlook.

How can one make mental lifestyle changes? I approach this in a series of small steps that are integrated into a big leap to a successful new mental approach—to change the way you think about life with fibromyalgia. You have to take baby steps before you can jump. I have devised a mental strategy which I call the Five REpairs.

1. REcognize and REdefine

2. REalistic REtraining

3. REliable RElationships

4. RElax and REfresh

5. REspect and REsponsibility

Each pair of "REs" is intimately related and addresses a different aspect of the mental approach to fibromyalgia. The ultimate goal is to be able to integrate all five into a positive mental strategy that works.

1. REcognize and REdefine

Fibromyalgia makes it easy to think negatively. Before we can correct this tendency we need to recognize the ways in which we think negatively.

Here are some examples:

- We over-generalize. One small incident seems like a catastrophe. For example, if we forget something, we think we are getting Alzheimer's disease.

- We anticipate bad things. If someone invites us to a party, the first thing we think of is that the party will cause a flare-up in our pain.

- We blame ourselves for everything. We believe it is our fault that we have fibromyalgia or that we have flare-ups.

- We label ourselves negatively. We think that because we are having a lot of pain, we must be bad or useless people.

- We expect things to get worse. If we talk to someone older than us who has fibromyalgia and is having extreme pain and disability, we expect that we will end up in the same way when we get older.

Continuous negative thinking about ourselves and our situation will ultimately lead to other negative emotions such as anger, frustration, hopelessness, and feelings of guilt and depression.

We also tend to be perfectionists and overachieving individuals, and this can lead to negative consequences when trying to cope with fibromyalgia. Our perfectionist nature can create "negative" traits which include:

- Inability to handle criticism
- Fear of failure
- Fear of rejection
- Feelings of inadequacy
- Anxiety
- Lack of control

By being overachievers, we also risk developing negative behaviors which include:

- Always searching for a fibromyalgia cure
- Doctor shopping for that magical treatment
- Inability to delegate tasks to others
- Feelings of being overwhelmed
- Procrastination
- Impatience
- Extreme guilt when unable to accomplish what we used to be able to do

> **FLAWS (Famous LAst WordS just before a flare-up)**
>
> "No, that's not where it goes. No, you're not doing it right. Here, I'll just do it myself."

Once we've recognized this, we can change our thinking patterns. Fibromyalgia forces us to redefine our physical ability. Since we can no longer do what we used to, we must seek a new physical lifestyle that our fibromyalgia will tolerate. We also have to redefine our thought processes. We must now think of ourselves as persons with chronic pain, and from that perspective, try to imagine how we can feel better about ourselves.

To redefine, we ask ourselves, "What goals do we wish for ourselves?" and "How do we want to see ourselves?" and "What can we do?" A part of redefining our thinking is to redefine what it means to feel good. When we are so focused on feeling bad all the time, it is hard to look for things about ourselves that make us feel good.

You know how a picture can look bad to you at first, but when you move it to a different light it looks better? We must picture ourselves in a more positive light. We were not singled out to have this painful disorder for something we did or did not do, so we must stop blaming ourselves. Redefine ourselves as good, normal people who just happen to have fibromyalgia, and work on believing it. Focus on your strength and expect to live a good quality life in spite of having fibromyalgia.

For our tendency to be perfectionists and overachievers, we should try to redefine those qualities and see the positive. Examples of positive outcomes from our perfectionist tendency include:

- Organization and efficiency
- Industriousness
- Responsibility
- Trustworthiness
- Reliability
- Punctuality

Being overachievers can also have positive consequences:

- Innovative thinking that allows us to create new strategies
- Active participation in our care and decisions regarding fibromyalgia
- Proactive approach by reading everything we can about fibromyalgia and therefore acquiring knowledge
- Flexibility in learning to budget our energy and breaking big tasks into smaller tasks

Ultimately, we need to accept that fibromyalgia is a chronic illness. We need to take inventory of all the thoughts we have and the ways we feel about ourselves because of fibromyalgia. We then sort through this inventory to determine what we want to throw out, modify, or change—what we want to redefine. The next step in the process is realistic retraining.

2. REalistic REtraining

At this step, we ask the question, "How will we change our thinking to accomplish our redefined goals?" With fibromyalgia, it is not realistic to expect to be pain free. However, it is realistic to achieve a low baseline level of pain where we feel we are able to enjoy our lives as fully as possible. Sometimes we may even achieve a remission.

Retraining our thinking is not an easy or quick process. It took us a long time to reach where we are in our thinking process, so it will take time to change our thinking as well. A "quick fix" is not a good strategy since it only captures our initial enthusiasm and motivation as some of the fad diets do. We need a slow but long-lasting lifestyle change that has a higher chance of being successful for a longer duration.

A lot of people have been trained to think in black and white—it is either one way or the other. If we are then forced to start exploring the gray areas, it can create a lot of tension and even confusion in some people. We need to allow ourselves to look into and explore these gray areas. You may be surprised at the new mental strategies you can learn in that territory. Or at least you will be surprised at how many different shades of gray exist!

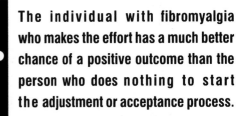

The individual with fibromyalgia who makes the effort has a much better chance of a positive outcome than the person who does nothing to start the adjustment or acceptance process.

The individual with fibromyalgia who makes the effort has a much better chance of a positive outcome than the person who does nothing to start the adjustment or acceptance process. Some of the studies done on fibromyalgia patients over time have found some fascinating comparisons. Individuals who took an aggressive role in seeking strategies to control their fibromyalgia were less bothered by their condition as they aged. Those who took a passive role or were never given the opportunity to become an active participant in the management of the disorder fared much worse.

Set Mental Limits

Like setting physical limits, you need to set mental limits and learn to accept them. You must allow yourself to be forgetful at times without convincing yourself that you have a memory disease. You can be critical of your performance, but don't punish yourself personally and feel that you are worthless or unable to do anything. You can worry about certain activities causing a flare-up, but you have to set a limit on this, too. You can't let it cause you to avoid any type of activity.

Train yourself to change "I shouldn't" to "I'll try." That way, instead of completely avoiding a certain activity, you force yourself to try to find ways of doing it. This is a way of thinking positively, yet still respecting your mental limits. Saying "I'll try" also forces you to think of strategies and mentally rehearse them as a positive and constructive approach to your perceived limitations with fibromyalgia.

If you can train your mind to look for that opening and rehearse a way to get through it, the physical aspect will follow much easier. Here's an example: A minister with fibromyalgia experienced a severe flare-up following the flu. Because of increased pain and fatigue, he is no longer able to perform his hour-long Sunday service that includes a 20-minute sermon. At first he thinks that he shouldn't even try to complete a service because of too much preparation required, the prolonged standing, and the hand gestures that he uses while giving his sermon. His initial thought is to avoid the Sunday service altogether until his flare-up resolves and he is able to perform all of his usual duties.

However, it's uncertain when his flare-up will resolve, and because of the importance of his church involvement, he takes a new approach. He reexamines every motion he makes during his sermon and tries to find ways to participate. His mental plan is to first perform only the sermon, the vital part of the service. He would do this from a seated position, minimizing the hand gestures, and shorten the service from 20 to 10 minutes. From this he envisions being present during the whole service but being seated in a chair. Over the course of several Sundays, he would gradually increase his own participation in the service as he could tolerate it. He mentally rehearses these strategies and constructs his plan, then physically carries it out. He finds out that he is still able to be an active participant in spite of his fibromyalgia flare-up.

The retraining process does not work 100% when you first try it, and a successful behavior is never 100% perfect. Before we learned to walk, we first had to balance, learn to stand, learn to take slow, deliberate and unsteady steps, and practice this pattern until it became easier and automatic. Finally we developed walking skills that became part of our subconscious physical ability. We had to fall down many times before we became proficient at walking and even though we can walk well now, we still fall down occasionally. Our walking skills were achieved by a series of small, successful steps that were inefficient at first but, with practice, gradually became a successful and efficient system. This is how our mental retraining process works.

The retraining process does not work 100% when you first try it, and a successful behavior is never 100% perfect.

Mental retraining strategies can make physical performance easier. But doing physical things can also help us feel better mentally. If we make an effort to physically look good (dressing nicely, keeping our hair neatly styled, basic good grooming), we will feel better about ourselves, and thus receive a mental boost. We must also retrain our thoughts to achieve a proper diet, ideal body weight, and a regular exercise program.

3. REliable RElationships

This REpair step involves others in your life. Relationships mean family, spouses, significant others, friends, and co-workers. Your fibromyalgia affects not only you, but all those around you. Relationships change because of fibromyalgia, oftentimes for the worse. It is your responsibility to make your relationships positive in spite of fibromyalgia.

Even though you are in constant pain, your goal is to treat the ones you care about with compassion and kindness. This isn't easy if you hurt and feel downright mean and miserable. You might find yourself being short tempered and unpleasant with the ones you care about. Then you can feel guilty. You are allowed to feel miserable and be mean and short tempered. You can have these feelings or moods and still be a good person! You simply recognize that these are negative consequences of your chronic pain and you are going to work hard on overcoming them even if you aren't perfect at it.

You may also shut out the family and caring ones because of your pain. Sometimes you shut out the world, and you'll notice the pain more, because the world around you has become so small that there is nothing else in it except you and your pain. Don't shut out your relationships. Keep them in your world, even if fibromyalgia is crowding it.

Many times, families and significant others do not know how to respond to you and your fibromyalgia. If you do not communicate your problems, your family will not be aware of them. They may play a guessing game to figure out how you are feeling at any particular time.

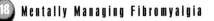

Educate

Some families react to a chronic problem by denying its existence (just as you do sometimes). They think that your fibromyalgia will simply go away someday and you will be back to your "normal" self. You need to educate them about fibromyalgia. Give them literature to read. Let them know the types of things that aggravate your pain, what you are doing to help control your symptoms, and what works for you. Tell them that your fibromyalgia is not a tumor and will not cause deformities or paralysis and that you will not die from it. Hopefully, they will appreciate your teaching attempts.

In relationships, everyone brings his or her own unique perspective. Each person's perspective has been shaped by his or her individual past experiences, traumas, attitudes, limitations, and accomplishments. Everyone has "baggage." Most of our baggage, however, just happens to be from our physical experiences with fibromyalgia. Just as we would not reject someone for something in their past, we would not expect someone else to reject us just because we have fibromyalgia and a "past" associated with this problem. If we give others a chance, they can accept us.

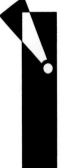

Just as we would not reject someone for something in their past, we would not expect someone else to reject us just because we have fibromyalgia and a "past" associated with this problem. If we give others a chance, they can accept us.

At times you will think that no one is making any attempt to understand your problem, and at times they will think that you are simply using fibromyalgia as an excuse to avoid your responsibilities. A successful family support system recognizes the extremes that occur occasionally, but maintains a stable balance of understanding, acceptance and support that does not falter when these occasional bad times occur. Family life (indeed, any relationship) is difficult even in normal situations. Adding a chronic illness makes everything even more challenging.

Communication

How can individuals work together to form positive and reliable relationships? Open communication with your family and others you trust is important. They also have frustrations, needs and feelings about the fibromyalgia. Share your feelings with them, find out about their feelings, and work together to understand and accept your physical and mental limitations. Work on positively redefining relationships.

It helps if your family reads about fibromyalgia and maybe even attends your support group. When you attend the group, pay particular attention to what spouses and significant others share with the group. They are your best source of information on how healthy people look at and deal with fibromyalgia. Then you can ask your spouse or significant other if they have the same complaints. If so, work to make changes. You will learn to see your illness by others' perspectives. This may open a totally new line of communication.

Have frequent family conferences that function as your own family support group. Find out how everyone is feeling and how family members can help each other out. If you find the problem is too big to handle on your own, you may wish to seek professional help.

An area of concern to many patients with fibromyalgia is sex and intimacy. Chronic pain and illness definitely impact this aspect of relationships. There are particular fears and anxieties about whether individuals will be able to find an accepting life partner or continue to have satisfying and fulfilling relationships once chronic pain and fibromyalgia have intervened. This concern is discussed more in Chapter 39.

Delegate

It is difficult to ask others for help. Feelings of low self-esteem, fear of losing our independence, and concern that we will be bothering this person by asking for help inhibit us. However, if fibromyalgia prevents us from doing things, we must learn to ask for help and delegate responsibility for various tasks to others. Practice on your family first.

Team chores can be performed by different family members with designated tasks. Everyone works together while performing his or her task. You do your part, also, and you can count "supervising" as a chore!

One patient compared this process to a corporation. If you are the CEO of the family, you have the ultimate role of making sure your whole family unit is functioning. However, you can set up your organization so problem solving and simple task completion can be done at different levels. Even though you are overseeing everything, you don't need to be approached directly for every task or problem. With your influence, these tasks are already handled automatically.

It is okay to ask for help from others outside of your family. We need to allow ourselves to approach reliable and trusted individuals to ask for help when we need it. Instead of "bothering" these people, we will probably discover that they will gladly help us.

It is okay to ask for help from others outside of your family. We need to allow ourselves to approach reliable and trusted individuals to ask for help when we need it. Instead of "bothering" these people, we will probably discover that they will gladly help us. Family, friends and co-workers can become trusted people who are willing to help us when we ask. One patient said that whenever she is feeling her lowest, she always calls her most positive friend and can count on her to boost her spirits. We all need to find these positive people who can help pick us up when we are feeling down. We in turn will gladly help these people when asked.

Support Groups

Support groups are an excellent way to form reliable relationships. Sharing with others who know exactly how you feel has incredible power. Many of my patients are active in fibromyalgia support groups, both live and virtual. Other groups can be helpful and therapeutic even if they do not involve fibromyalgia. Card clubs, cooking groups, book clubs, and church groups are other therapeutic groups. Volunteering is an excellent way to stop thinking about our own problems and feel good about helping others deal with theirs.

4. RElax and REfresh

Perhaps one of the most difficult things for people with fibromyalgia to do is to relax. With fibromyalgia we always seem to have tense bodies and minds. One woman described her tense mind as though she is "constantly running a marathon in her brain." We have a more hypersensitive autonomic nervous system, especially the sympathetic nervous system which is responsible for the "fight or flight" response.

The fight or flight response is normally triggered when we are in a threatening situation. Certain hormones, especially adrenaline, are released in large quantities to ready the body's protective mechanism, and we become tense, focused, and primed to either fight or run. It is not often, though, that a tiger jumps out of a bush in a parking lot and starts running after us, nor do we usually find ourselves standing in the middle of a railroad track facing an oncoming train. Yet, thanks to fibromyalgia, we manage to maintain such a continuous state of anxiety and tension.

The relaxation response is the opposite of the fight or flight response. It occurs when natural physiologic mechanisms cause muscles to loosen up, blood flow to improve, heart rate to slow down, and the mind to become calm. Our body's parasympathetic nervous system mediates this response, which is eliminated or distorted when the body is in a constant state of tension and anxiety. Thus, the chances of finding the relaxation response in fibromyalgia are about as good as finding an area on our bodies that does not hurt! If we have lost the ability to subconsciously achieve the relaxation response, we need to consciously retrain our bodies to relax.

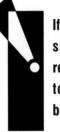

If we have lost the ability to subconsciously achieve the relaxation response, we need to consciously retrain our bodies to relax.

If there ever was something easier said than done, it has to be telling someone with fibromyalgia to relax. It is so difficult to relax that whenever someone tells me to do it, I actually get more tense. Saying the word "relax" elicits a fight or flight response! When trying to teach yourself a relaxation technique, keep in mind that there are literally dozens of techniques, and as I have said before, there is no one way that works best for everyone, but there is probably a way that will work for anyone. For me, I like to read and watch video movies. Whether one is meditating, participating in a sporting event, praying, or performing Tai Chi, a type of relaxation exercise is happening. You too can learn to master the art of relaxation.

Comfortable Environment

The first rule of relaxation is to create a comfortable environment. This means picking a quiet spot and making sure that there is nothing to disturb you. Find a comfortable chair where you can stay in the same position for 20 minutes without increased pain. To get comfortable, wear loose, nonrestrictive clothing, place your body in a neutral position, then close your eyes.

Deep Breathing

The next step in the relaxation response is deep breathing. Once you have reached a comfortable position and told your muscles to relax, you should become aware of how you are breathing, and if you are breathing properly. Your stomach should expand when you breathe in through your nose and contract as you slowly breathe out through your mouth.

Take slow deep breaths through your nose, taking in as much air as your lungs will hold to the count of 3. When exhaling, breathe out slowly through a slightly opened mouth to the count of 6. Placing your hands on your stomach will give you tactile feedback that your stomach is properly moving out and in as it is supposed to with deep breathing. Repeat this cycle for 10 to 15 minutes, then sit quietly for 5 minutes with eyes either open or closed, continuing to think only calm thoughts.

Do not be disappointed if you don't achieve a deep trance or hypnotic state. This rarely happens. Breathing deeply can make you feel dizzy or light-headed at first. Try to stay relaxed as you feel yourself about to pass out! This exercise should be done at least once a day, but can be done several times a day if necessary.

This relaxation exercise can be an important part of your fibromyalgia management, once you practice and master this technique. There are other types of relaxation exercises, many that involve mental imagery. Daydreaming, fantasizing, and recalling pleasant memories are examples of mental imagery that can help you to relax. These techniques can be done while you are performing other activities and with your eyes open. Many people can use mental imagery to induce a form of self-hypnosis which helps achieve successful relaxation.

> **This relaxation exercise can be an important part of your fibromyalgia management, once you practice and master this technique.**

Guided imagery can help. One fibromyalgia patient did a 4-week guided imagery study on volunteers with fibromyalgia. She was completing her training as a counselor and did this project as part of her schooling. She interviewed each participant and made a guided imagery cassette tape that instructed each person what to imagine. The tape was played daily. Nearly all reported better relaxation and improved sleep.

Biofeedback can also help. This technique is taught by trained psychologists or counselors, and involves muscle monitors and skin temperature measuring devices. Depending on the instructors, over half of people have success with relaxation techniques. Success means the ability to learn to relax and carry over this same response into your everyday life.

Ways To Relax

The following are ways people can relax and cope with fibromyalgia.

1. **A regular exercise program.** This is a powerful stimulator of the body's relaxation response. Exercise to relax—sounds like an oxymoron, doesn't it?

2. **Religion and prayer.** Many people are comforted by their beliefs and convictions.

3. **Enjoyable hobbies,** *e.g.,* dancing, reading.

4. **Volunteering to help others.**

5. **A hot bath.** This is a great way to both physically relax the muscles and mentally relax the mind.

6. **Writing.** Keep a daily journal or diary—write a fibromyalgia survivor book!

7. **Music.** A universal stress antidote.

8. **Taking drives** on a rural freeway or country road during the day. (Avoid construction or slow semitrailers in front of you!)

9. **Yoga, Tai Chi, meditation**.

Relaxation is not something that just happens. It is something that you first practice, and in time accomplish. Then you must plan your relaxation response on a daily basis. Set aside time and protect it. This is not the time to take a nap, but an opportunity to manage your fibromyalgia.

Top Ten Fibromyalgia Hazards Found In Church

1. Petrified pine pews and kneelers with scant, if any, padding

2. Speakers too loud for uninterrupted snoozing

3. Burning, perfumed incense entering dry nasal and eye membranes

4. Long, single-file communion lines

5. Single antique ceiling fan that serves as entire church's climate control system

6. 30 inch leg room space for 34 inch legs

7. Noxious mix of smelly cosmetics used liberally by attendees

8. One toilet for 300 parishioners

9. 517 page song books that have fallen under the pew

10. Weekly ritual struggling to remember names of all those familiar faces

5. REspect And REsponsibility

The final step in repairing your mental approach to fibromyalgia is respect and responsibility. Having a painful syndrome is difficult because every day you hurt. I know this from personal and professional experience. We must understand and respect that fibromyalgia indeed does cause lifestyle altering pain, and that we will continue to have pain. Set a goal to achieve a minimal baseline level of pain. Try not to avoid doing something for fear of a flare-up. Rather, do whatever you can in spite of your fibromyalgia and its pain. You remember how you used to be before fibromyalgia, but now it is time to reset your mental thermostat to a level that accommodates some baseline pain.

In spite of doing everything right, we may still experience fibromyalgia flare-ups. However, by controlling what we can, we can reduce their number and frequency.

The issue of control and fibromyalgia comes up frequently. While we have no control over whether or not we have fibromyalgia, we can learn to appreciate and respect the control we do have once we have the condition. We are able to control our posture, our response to stress, our activities, our home program, etc. We focus on respecting what we can control so we can decrease the risk of a fibromyalgia flare-up. In spite of doing everything right, we may still experience fibromyalgia flare-ups. However, by controlling what we can, we can reduce their number and frequency.

Good Pain Vs. Bad Pain

I use the concept of good pain vs. bad pain as part of the control issue related to fibromyalgia. If we have chosen certain activities, we can deal with the consequences of increased pain because it is expected. If we like to wash the car one warm Sunday, then we can do it and accept the increased pain on Monday. After all, we did something we wanted to do. On the other hand, if we choose not to wash the car on Sunday and still wake up Monday with unexpected and severe pain, we consider this bad pain, or pain that we have no control over. It is better to make responsible choices in spite of having fibromyalgia than to use the condition as an excuse to evade responsibility.

Find Balance

You need to seek a balance between detaching yourself from fibromyalgia and integrating it into your everyday lives. Control what you can, learn what you can.

We tend to detach ourselves from our fibromyalgia by trying to ignore it or pretending we don't have it. When the pain level is lower, we may rationalize that there is no need to follow through with our home program since we "don't have a problem." Yet, on the other hand, fibromyalgia goes with us wherever we go. It is always there to remind us that it is part of us. We must respect that part of us. I am an optimist and believe that everyone can eventually find that balance, but he or she has to work very hard at it. The ultimate prize in mental coping is acceptance of fibromyalgia.

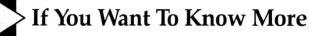

If You Want To Know More

1. Aaron LA, Bradley LA, Alarcon GS, et al. *Perceived physical and emotional trauma as precipitating events in fibromyalgia. Associations with health care seeking and disability status but not pain severity.* Arthritis Rheum 1997; 40: 453–60.

2. Brown BB. *Stress and the art of biofeedback.* Harper & Row 1977.

3. Donaldson S, Gabriel ES, Horst HM. *Fibromyalgia: a retrospective study of 252 consecutive referrals.* Can J Clin Med 1998; 5: 116–25.

4. Pellegrino MJ. *Inside fibromyalgia.* Columbus OH: Anadem Publishing, 2001.

5. Thieme EK, Gromnica-Ihle E, Flor H. *Operant behavioral treatment of fibromyalgia: a controlled study.* Arthritis Rheum 2003; 49: 314–20.

Physical Medicine Program

Top Ten Fibromyalgia Treatments That Did Not Work

1. Hot motor oil bath

2. Surgical excision of tender points

3. Gentle pressure massage by ex-Olympic wrestlers

4. Microwaveable ice pack

5. Daily vegetable soup soaks

6. Drinking daily 8 ounce mixture of wine, fish oil, broccoli juice, dissolved aspirin and holy water

7. Prolonged underwater exercises

8. Acupuncture by ancient Antartican technique

9. Combined electric current and aquatics therapy

10. Hanging upside down by your ankle tendons

A physical medicine program is an important part in the overall treatment of fibromyalgia. A physical medicine program includes such modalities as heat, cold, massage, electric stimulation, or whirlpool. Manual exercises, stretching, strengthening, conditioning, aerobics, and aquatics can also be helpful. Not everyone with fibromyalgia needs a physical medicine program, but most of my patients have benefited from one. Different therapies work better for different persons, and doctors need to determine what is best for that individual.

Different health professionals who might be involved include physical therapists, massotherapists, chiropractors, occupational therapists and exercise physiologists. Any therapy program should be safe, relatively easy to do, affordable, and have a good chance of success. A successful therapy program should be one that patients can learn to carry out as individuals. Chapter 20 will address how to develop an individualized home program. This chapter focuses on initial prescribed therapies that can help get you started. As with any treatment prescription, the patient's therapy response and any changes or modifications should be monitored by a physician familiar with fibromyalgia syndrome.

Let's consider a number of available physical medicine treatments.

Therapeutic Modalities

Therapeutic modalities (physical medicine treatments) include thermal agents and bioelectric therapy. Thermal agents include cryotherapy, or cold therapy, and superficial and deep heat. Cryotherapy is often used for acute soft tissue injuries to decrease edema and spasm. In fibromyalgia, cryotherapy can reduce pain and muscle tightness. Therapeutic heat consists of both superficial heat (hot packs, warm water therapy, and paraffin bath) and deep heat (ultrasound, diathermy, microwave). Superficial and deep heating modalities can help decrease pain and improve flexibility of the soft tissues. About 20 minutes of a thermal application (heat or cold) is the usual treatment time. Sometimes heat and cold are alternated (called a contrast bath). This can help those with neuropathy-type pain.

Heat therapy is more popular with fibromyalgia, particularly moist heat. Cold treatments can be just as effective if the person can tolerate the first 5 minutes of COLD. After the first 5 minutes, numbness and desensitization of the skin allows full tolerance for the remaining 15 minutes of treatment. The deep muscle cooling effect of the cold modality can insulate the tissues and slow the blood flow, neurological signals, and metabolism to give a longer-acting effect than heat. If an exercise program is also being performed, a combination of heat and cold can be used for the best effect. Heat modalities can be used before exercise to assist in the warm-up process, and cold modalities can be used immediately after exercising to help minimize swelling and pain and to assist in the cool-down process.

Bioelectric Therapies

Electric stimulation, sometimes called bioelectric therapy, can also provide relief. Electrical current delivered to the muscles ranges from a mini-electric current that is barely felt, to a stronger electrical current that causes the muscles to contract. Types of bioelectric therapy include transcutaneous electrical nerve stimulation (TENS), functional electric stimulation, interferential therapy, and iontophoresis. Each type works differently; your doctor may prescribe one or more types as part of your program. Drs. Melzack and Wall performed a landmark study in 1965 on the gate control theory of pain (see Chapter 9), and this led to the development of numerous electrical therapy modalities. The mechanisms of the bioelectric modalities include: 1. blocking the pain with "soothing" electrical sensation; 2. facilitating the entry of nutrients into the cells and waste products out of the cells; and 3. biochemical/neurologic reeducation to improve the body's efficiency at a cellular level. Bioelectric modalities are usually well tolerated, and with repeated treatments, the patient can tolerate higher intensities and get even more therapeutic effect, particularly when treating more acute pain and muscle spasms.

Manipulation & Adjustments

Manipulations and adjustments can be performed by trained osteopathic physicians, chiropractic physicians, and manual therapists. These techniques can mobilize joints, improve range of motion and relaxation, and reduce muscle pain, all of which can benefit patients with fibromyalgia. Manipulations are forceful movements of body parts such as the neck to bring about a greater range of motion and relaxation. Adjustments are the application of a sudden and precise force to a specific point in the vertebrae or muscle to properly align the body. The desired outcome of properly aligned vertebrae and muscle is improved circulation and neurologic signals and reduced pain.

Massage Therapy

Massage therapy can decrease pain by relaxing muscles, improving circulation and oxygenation, removing waste buildup in the muscles, increasing muscle flexibility, and reeducating muscles. Various massage techniques include:

1. **Stroking,** which is the gliding of palms and fingers firmly over the muscles in a slow rhythmic motion.

2. **Kneading,** when the muscles are grabbed between fingers and thumb and slightly lifted and squeezed in a slow rhythmic sequence.

3. **Friction massage** penetrates deep into the muscles and uses slow circular motions with the tips of the fingers or thumb.

There are different types of specialized massage. Swedish massage is the traditional massage that involves stroking, kneading and friction massage techniques. Massage therapy is administered by a qualified therapist, and treatments usually last for about 60 minutes. The massage therapist needs to be knowledgeable and experienced in treating fibromyalgia to use the best of many techniques for any given individual situation. This therapy is often combined with other therapies, but my patients love this treatment and consider it one of their favorites.

Self-massage is a simple procedure that patients can be taught. A spouse or significant other can also learn how to perform therapeutic massage. We offer couples massage classes. One criteria for the classes is that the patient with fibromyalgia has to agree to give the significant other a massage every once in a while, too!

Manual Therapy

Some physical therapists specialize in a form of hands-on treatment techniques called manual therapy. Disease processes can cause defects in soft tissues and bones and the body reacts to these changes. In fibromyalgia, neuromuscular defects can lead to muscle spasms, guarding, shifting, abnormal posturing and malalignment which contribute to the pain. A manual therapist has special knowledge of anatomy and physiology and can perform specialized hands-on techniques that try to correct bony alignment, reduce muscle spasms, and enhance the body's normal neuromuscular patterns.

There are a number of manual therapy techniques that can be used in the treatment of fibromyalgia. They include:

1. **Myofascial release.** This technique was developed by physical therapist John Barnes. It is designed to loosen up the fascia (or connective tissue) and allow the muscles to relax and improve blood flow.

2. **Trigger point therapy**. This technique involves sustained pressure applied to pain trigger points/tender points (no needles here!). This sustained pressure helps break up and desensitize the trigger points.

3. **Craniosacral therapy**. This gentle technique was developed mainly by Dr. John Upledger. It enhances the flow of the cerebrospinal fluid which bathes the brain and spinal cord (craniosacral system). This therapy is promoted to reduce stress and enhance the body's natural healing mechanisms, hopefully reducing pain.

4. **Strain/counterstrain**. This technique uses opposing forces on muscles and connective tissue to relieve restrictions and tightness and cause the muscle fibers to lengthen. When properly performed, it will cause relaxation/lengthening of the muscles and improvement in spasms and mobility.

5. **Lymph drainage therapy**. This technique uses light pressure and a hands-on treatment that manually assists lymph to move through its vessels to the main nodes. Lymph is a fluid that leaves the vascular system in the tissues and it contains water, ions, proteins, various cells and blood factors. It has a separate lymphatic drainage system to return the lymph to the blood. This therapy technique helps clear out toxins, reduce swelling and promote a better immune system.

Exercise Therapy

Exercises are beneficial in the long run for everyone and everything! Many people with fibromyalgia reject exercise outright because it's simply too painful. But everyone can find some type of exercise program that is tolerated and helpful, even if it's stretching only. I usually wait until the acute pain begins to subside before introducing exercises, then gradually progress them as tolerated. Patients often experience increased pain after exertion due to a combination of tight muscles and being less aerobically fit overall (Bennett R.M. *et al*, 1989). Fibromyalgia patients who attempt an exercise program often experience an increase in muscle pain which may discourage them from continuing to work on improving their level of fitness. I have found that staying with a prescribed supervised exercise program will gradually coax the patient's muscles to a greater fitness level with more flexibility and functional ability. Different types of exercises include:

1. **Range of motion exercises**. Each joint is moved through its normal range. These exercises help maintain normal joint movements and decrease stiffness.

2. **Stretching and flexibility exercises**. This combines range of motion with a gentle, yet firm, stretching of the muscles and joints. The shoulders, neck, hips, and back muscles tend to be particularly stiff and painful, so they need to have regular stretching and flexibility exercises.

3. **Strengthening exercises**. These increase muscle strength. Isometric exercises (the person tightens the muscle, but does not move the joint) can be helpful if the joints are painful, because it makes the muscle stronger with little joint movement. Isokinetic or isotonic exercises (the muscles tighten using a weight or some type of resistance, and the joints move through the motion) are also effective because they allow for better blood flow and oxygenation. Two popular exercises that combine stretching and strengthening include therabands (long rubber bands) and a Swiss ball (an oversized inflated ball), used in different ways to stretch and strengthen muscles.

   Specialized exercises to strengthen back muscles include McKenzie exercises and Williams flexion exercises. McKenzie exercises are a popular and effective way to strengthen back muscles, particularly the extensor muscles that arch the back. Many of my fibromyalgia patients have learned these exercises from trained therapists and have found them helpful in reducing back pain and improving posture and strength.

4. **Aerobic exercises**. These enhance the condition of the heart and lungs as well as strengthening and conditioning muscles. Common aerobic exercises include walking, biking, jogging, aerobics, and swimming (if the water is close to 90° F).

Aquatic Therapy

This special category of treatment serves several purposes: it can be a modality, provide massage-like benefit, and allow exercises to be done (it doesn't allow safe bioelectric treatments while in the water, though!).

Water therapy is a good modality especially if the water is kept at a comfortable temperature, usually around 90° F. Warm water can be soothing to painful areas of the body, like a comfortable warm bath.

The water can act as a massager as well. The water movement and waves can gently massage muscles and help improve blood flow and reduce tightness and spasms. Those who like the whirlpool can appreciate how water movement can provide therapeutic forces on painful areas.

Aquatic exercises are beneficial even for someone who cannot swim. In water, most of the body weight is buoyed so the gravity stress on the muscles and joints is reduced. Range of motion, flexibility, strengthening, and aerobic exercises can all be done in the pool, and can initially be supervised by a trained professional until individuals feel comfortable with following through on their own. I frequently prescribe water exercises to patients. Those who do well with water aerobics, water jogging, and even swimming say that the achieved benefits carry over well onto the land. Overall, I think aquatic therapy is an excellent treatment choice for those with fibromyalgia if you don't

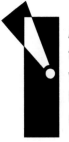

Aquatic exercises are beneficial even for someone who cannot swim. In water, most of the body weight is buoyed so the gravity stress on the muscles and joints is reduced.

mind the routine that's involved with undressing, getting into a bathing suit, getting in and out of the pool, and getting back into clothes (it's very important to remember to dress again after removing the bathing suit!).

A typical prescribed therapy program may start with therapies three times a week for 10 to 12 treatments. The goals of such a program may be to decrease the pain by at least 50% over a month, and to gradually increase tolerance to activity. I want the patient to make progress from the pain management phase to the exercise phase (reactivation and retraining), and ultimately to a successful home program (reintegration phase). Progress is documented in four ways:

1. Pain Analog Scale (patient reports less pain). This scale allows grading of the pain from 0 (no pain) to 10 (worst pain). Many patients rank their pain higher than a 10! This scale is particularly useful and valid for a given individual to note pain before, during, and after treatments to see if the treatments helped (*i.e.*, pain decreases).

2. Tender point examination or "mapping" results (may show fewer painful areas). Objective palpation of soft tissues often reveals less pain and less spasms if the patient is improving.

3. Range of motion (improves). Joint motions can be measured and documented. Less pain usually means less spasm and more flexibility, and the joints move more freely, *e.g.*, neck, shoulders, hips, etc.

4. Functional accomplishments (patient able to do more). Objective rating scales can be used such as Functional Independence measure or Disability Index Scale to document improved function.

Pain Management Phase

This phase is designed to decrease pain and get control over a pain flare-up. It involves education, prescribed medicines and nutritional supplements, and specific physical medicine therapies. I use multiple treatments at the same time because they have a better chance of reducing pain more quickly rather than trying one thing at a time, waiting to see if it works, then trying the next thing if the first treatment didn't help. I want you to feel better FAST! If you should have decreased pain from the different treatments, but can't tell exactly what works, so what?! What a nice problem to have, feeling better but not sure what's working! We can figure out what is helping after you are feeling better. Most people can tell what helps, even if more than one treatment is helping.

Depending on the location of pain and the number of "worse" areas, I may try trigger point injections. Using either a local anesthetic only or a combination of a local anesthetic and cortisone, I may inject from one to six areas at a time. Other types of injections may be necessary including selective joint injections, nerve blocks, epidurals, or prolotherapy.

The first part of my therapy program focuses on pain management. The patient works with me and other team members (therapists, primary care specialists, chiropractor, counselor, and other medical professionals) to decrease the acute pain as much as possible using different therapy or injection strategies. Hopefully, the pain stays settled down. If it does, the patient is ready to begin a progressive exercise program.

Exercise Phase: Reactivation And Retraining

I shift the emphasis from pain management to reactivation and retraining. Now I want patients to increase their physical activity and fitness levels and develop a successful home program. This phase is usually started around the third week of treatment. Pain management modalities are winding down, and there is a progressive increase in stretching and range of motion exercises. Manual therapy/massotherapy is often continued. Pain management therapies may be renewed as needed, and the patient may continue to work with various team members.

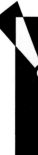

I emphasize postural exercises, stretching, and flexibility exercises of all major muscle groups, and focus on a warm-up period that consists of stretching only.

I emphasize postural exercises (see Chapter 15, Fibronomics), stretching, and flexibility exercises of all major muscle groups, and focus on a warm-up period that consists of stretching only. For some people, stretching may be the only exercise that they can do.

I also try to develop what I call a "light conditioning" program. Such a program can include walking, water aerobics, using an exercise bicycle, or performing low-impact aerobic exercises. This exercise program is introduced and gradually progressed as tolerated with the goal of achieving a stable baseline and developing a successful home program. I instruct patients to do a regular exercise program at least 3 times a week. I emphasize proper posture and body mechanics to minimize strain on the muscles and joints. I always tell patients that it's better to have fit painful muscles than deconditioned painful muscles. In other words, you can improve your function even if the pain doesn't decrease.

Sometimes the progressive stretching and exercise increases pain, even if the acute pain has subsided from the initial therapy program. Manual therapy/massage usually helps, but if this is not controlling the pain, additional pain management techniques can be reintroduced (heat, cold, injections).

Ultimately, becoming knowledgeable about fibromyalgia and learning what works for you will allow you to find a regular program of proper body mechanics, stretching, and exercises that helps.

Home Program: Reintegration Phase

In this phase, the patient is reintegrating into the "real world," armed with knowledge and self-management strategies. Patients use these techniques and lifestyle changes to live their everyday lives, work their jobs, and be themselves in spite of fibromyalgia. Patients will continue their program of medications, nutritional supplements, stretches and exercises, and hopefully will be able to maintain a stable baseline. I do not automatically follow-up with people at this stage unless there is a new problem or a flare-up, but my patients know they are welcome to call me or see me at any time. If there is a new problem or a flare-up, we review together the need for any new treatments or changes in their program.

Regular prescribed treatments may be required. For example, a patient may continue with periodic manual therapies or massage therapies, or have periodic trigger point injections in addition to continuing prescribed or nutritional medicine. The ideal goal, however, is to have the patient be able to control her or his symptoms through a self-responsible and independent home program. The medical professionals are available if needed, and hopefully they will not be needed on a frequent basis.

As part of the home program, the patient may join a support group. I offer a fibromyalgia course that can be taken at any phase of treatment, and it encompasses the overall understanding and management of fibromyalgia. Chris Marschinke, R.N., who co-developed the course with me, teaches the course in my office. The course consists of 6 weekly sessions, 2 ½ hours each week. It includes workbooks, lecture slides, and handouts. A different topic is covered each week and the last week includes a question and answer session with me, and a class graduation ceremony!

This comprehensive Physical Medicine and Rehabilitation approach in the treatment of fibromyalgia can help individuals achieve a realistic stable baseline. A stable baseline is not the same as no pain, rather it is a level where, while there may still be pain, it is not preventing the patient from performing desired activities. The baseline level is different for everyone, but each person can eventually learn what her or his baseline state will be. Actually, we all must learn this; our fibromyalgia doesn't give us much of a choice! At a stable baseline, the spontaneous pain is decreased. We still have painful tender points if poked at, but we can usually get through the day without getting poked!

What Kind Of Results Do I Get?

I do not cure people of their fibromyalgia. Everyone who sees me does not get better. Sometimes people feel worse after they see me! But I try. A lot of factors are involved in determining how people do, including insurance issues, compliance issues, and severity of the fibromyalgia.

There are four categories of fibromyalgia patients that I see in my private office setting. They are:

1. The newly diagnosed fibromyalgia patient with no previous treatment (about 25% of my total fibromyalgia patients).

2. The previously diagnosed fibromyalgia patient who is referred for additional recommendations or follow-up of initial treatment approaches (about 25% of my total fibromyalgia patients).

3. The fibromyalgia patient who is experiencing a flare-up (about 40% of my total fibromyalgia patients).

4. The chronic fibromyalgia patient whose symptoms have been resistant to multiple treatment approaches (about 10% of my total fibromyalgia patients).

Results I Get For Each Category

I monitor the outcomes of treatment programs for my fibromyalgia patients. Certainly, reduced pain is a major goal but sometimes a person can report improvement even if the pain remains the same. That person may be able to be more functional in spite of the pain, or is able to do more activities without increasing the pain. A key way that I monitor outcome is by using a pain outcome chart to determine a patient's pain level over time with treatment.

I reviewed 300 charts of patients treated for fibromyalgia in the first 4 months of 1999. By monitoring the patient's reported pain level over treatment, the following outcome results were noted:

1. In the newly diagnosed fibromyalgia patient (106 patients), 85% achieved 50% or more reduction of their pain level over an average of 10 therapy treatments; 15% achieved less than 50% (and of those, 5% reported less than a 10% reduction of their pain).

2. In the previously diagnosed fibromyalgia patient who was referred for additional treatment (73 patients), 80% achieved a 50% reduction or more of their pain level; 20% achieved a pain reduction of less than 50%.

3. In the fibromyalgia patient experiencing a flare-up requiring treatment (109 patients), 85% returned to their previous stable baseline, and 15% improved but were still higher than their previous stable baseline.

4. In the chronic fibromyalgia patient who has been resistant to multiple previous treatments and who tried a treatment approach under my direction (12 patients), 20% achieved a 50% or greater reduction of their pain level; 80% achieved less than 50% pain reduction (and of those, 15% reported no change at all in their pain level). Newly diagnosed patients seem to get better results, whereas those with chronic "resistant" fibromyalgia respond less favorably.

These results are general guidelines based on an average of 10 treatments. Each patient's treatments are individualized. Some patients may require additional therapies and get additional improvement. Other patients may flare-up shortly after their treatment program and experience a rise in their pain level again. I certainly want everyone to improve, but not everyone does. The goal is to try to help as many people as much as possible.

Here are some examples of patients' pain outcomes as indicated on the pain outcome charts in the following diagrams. Each pain outcome chart demonstrates a different example of a treatment response in fibromyalgia patients. The patient names are fictitious, but the pain outcome charts are derived from real patients. On the chart, the "●'s" represent pain level before treatment and "✖'s" represent treatments represent approximately a 1-month time period.

Diagram 1: Improvement. Sally's pain outcome chart demonstrates an improvement in the overall pain. This is the most common type of pain outcome and shows a consistent response to the treatments and lowering of the pain scores. In this particular example, the pain decreased from 10 out of 10 to 3 out of 10, a 70% improvement.

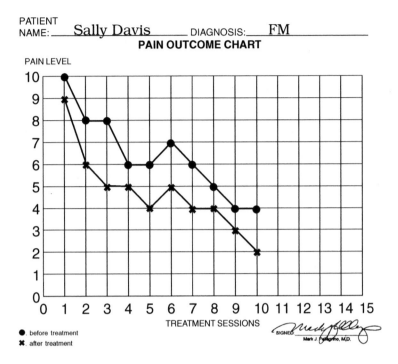

Diagram 2: Resistant Fibromyalgia. Sue's pain outcome chart shows very little response to treatment and a persistent high level of pain that stays around a 10. This is very little improvement in the pain immediately after the treatment.

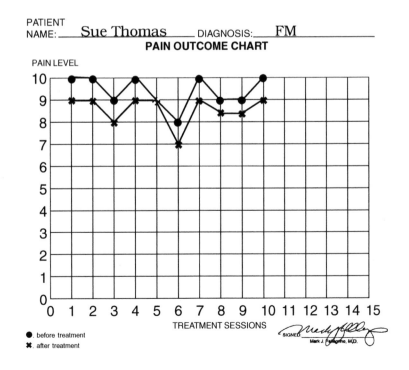

Diagram 3: Unstable Fibromyalgia. Mary's pain outcome chart indicates the pain levels bouncing up and down and variable responses to treatments. This pattern is actually *no pattern* and characterizes unstable fibromyalgia.

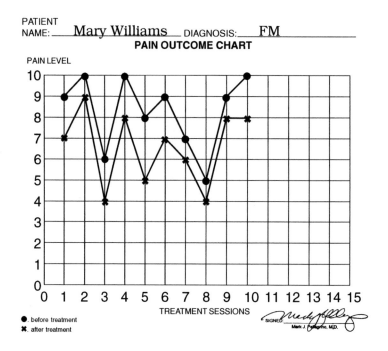

Diagram 4: Flare-up. Jane's pain outcome chart shows an initial good response to therapy with improvement of the pain scores. However, between the fifth and sixth treatments, there is a sharp increase in pain which causes a peak to occur on the graph. In Jane's case, she planted a garden which caused her flare-up. In spite of the flare-up, she continued to improve over time with additional treatments, and in the end her pain decreased from 10 out of 10 during her flare-up to 3 out of 10.

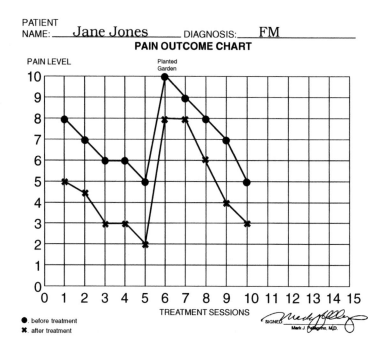

Diagram 5: Stable Baseline. This chart shows that John's pain improved, but around the fifth treatment his improvement stabilized and plateaued, and he remained at a stable baseline even with a few additional treatments. Overall, his pain improved from a 10 to a 4, a 60% improvement.

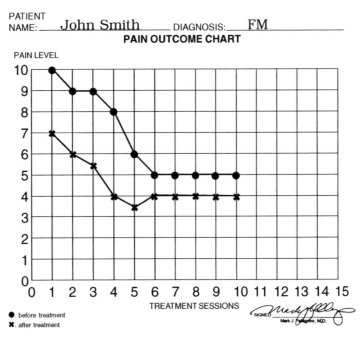

The fibromyalgia patient is a unique individual who has specific problems and needs. There is no generic patient. The physician should approach each patient on an individual basis using the types of strategies I described above. Each patient requires an individualized program, and hopefully everyone will get some improvement.

Personal Profile

by Mark J. Pellegrino, M.D.

In September 1986, nearly two years before I would be diagnosed with fibromyalgia, I wrote an editorial for a newsletter about hearing impairment. As a hearing impaired person, I used to belong to a national hearing impaired organization whose purpose was to educate and support those with hearing impairment (sound like a fibromyalgia support group?). Our local chapter in Columbus, Ohio printed a newsletter and I was the editor for a few years. I recently looked over this particular article again and was amazed how the problems I wrote about hearing impairment could easily be transposed to fibromyalgia. At the time I wrote this article, I didn't know about fibromyalgia but, as you read this, you will probably be able to substitute fibromyalgia for hearing impairment and find the article does not lose any meaning.

The Ostrich Syndrome

When you think about it, everyone has some type of "handicap" whether it be severe or mild, real or imaginary. This list is endless—too heavy, too thin, poor vision, too bald, wears dentures, fatigues easily, too shy, too short, too anxious … and so on. No matter what the shortcoming, each person is forced to deal with it in everyday life.

Until a few years ago, I treated my hearing impairment as a separate part of me. It was some detached disease that always followed me but never really "belonged" to me. My hearing impairment was my weakness. It made me feel inferior, abnormal, stupid, and alone. I was convinced that all my troubles were due to my hearing disorder and if I could just hear normally, even for one day, I would be a "normal" person. I could handle any problem imaginable if I could HEAR.

continued on next page...

Personal Profile

continued from previous page...

I actually felt sorry for myself. I tried to ease my feelings of self-pity by pretending that my impairment did not actually exist. It was separated from me. I could conveniently shift any burden of guilt or any negative feeling onto my detached O'Leary cow. That way, I didn't have to deal with all these "conflicts." (so I thought)

I became an ostrich. The ostrich, when pursued, hides his head in the sand and believes himself to be unseen. I attempted to avoid the uneasiness associated with my hearing impairment by refusing to face it. If any reference was made about my hearing impairment by others, I flinched with painful embarrassment. If the wind blew my hair, I turned quickly to hide my hearing aids. If someone mentioned my nasal speech, I casually managed to evade revealing the true underlying cause. Hide in a hole and everything will magically disappear.

It didn't work, though.

As much as I consciously tried detaching my hearing impairment from the rest of me, I couldn't get away from the reality of the situation: I have a hearing impairment. It is as much a part of me as my right arm is. No matter how hard I tried to avoid them, numerous situations arose daily that reminded me I was hearing impaired. These humiliations battered my ego and created increasing feelings of fear, anxiety, and guilt—the same conflicts I was trying to avoid.

I eventually realized that my biggest problem was not trying to get others to accept me, but to get me to accept myself, hearing impairment and all. I told myself that I was a normal human being and a hearing impairment, like any other "handicap," was simply a part of my life that I had to deal with. There is nothing wrong with having a hearing impairment, and no one is to blame for it either. It is my responsibility to deal with my difficulties, not to avoid them.

I didn't change overnight. Adjusting to an impairment is slow. It is like climbing a ladder; improvement comes a step at a time. Since I have joined this organization and attended the meetings, though, I feel like I've moved up a few rungs. I have met many others with problems similar to mine. We all want to climb the ladder, and by sharing and providing support, we can all climb this ladder together. We are people first, and our hearing loss is a challenge we can learn to cope with.

This organization has helped many people accept themselves for what they really are: GREAT people who just happen to have a hearing impairment. By continuing to grow and provide education and support to hearing impaired people everywhere, undoubtedly the lives of many more people will change.

Many famous people have overcome difficulties to accomplish great things, such as Beethoven and Franklin Delano Roosevelt. We can look up to these individuals for inspiration as we strive to overcome our problems. We can help each other conquer our difficulties.

Together, we can stop acting like an ostrich.

EARnestly yours,
Mark Pellegrino
Editor

"Many men owe the grandeur of their lives to their tremendous difficulties."
—Charles Haddon Spurgeon

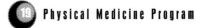

Summary

As complicated as fibromyalgia treatments can be, I still adhere to the philosophy of trying to keep treatments as simple as possible. If medicines aren't helping, they need to be stopped. If they help, use the lowest effective dose. If certain therapies help, teach the patient how to do them on her or his own. Sometimes the best treatment is simply trying to point the patient in the right direction and watching the patient take control of the fibromyalgia!

▶ If You Want To Know More

1. Djuric V. *Prolotherapy treats pain*. Chronic Pain Solutions 1998; 3: 8–10.

2. Manheim CJ. *The myofascial release manual*. Slack Inc., 2001.

3. Pellegrino MJ. *Inside fibromyalgia*. Columbus OH: Anadem Publishing, 2001.

4. Sprott H. *What can rehabilitation interventions achieve in patients with primary fibromyalgia*? Curr Opin Rheum 2003; 15: 345–50.

5. Upledger JE, Vredevoogd JD. *Craniosacral therapy*. Thieme, 2001.

Developing A Home Program

Now that we have reviewed mental strategies and physical medicine treatments, we need to include physical strategies for developing a successful home program. This is a difficult, yet necessary, challenge to help us cope with fibromyalgia. A home program can be time consuming, but it can also reduce the severe pain and keep us at a stable baseline.

Our muscles are painful, tight, and easily fatigued, and when we attempt to exercise them, they often respond by increasing pain. Negative painful experiences may lead to decreased motivation, decreased activity, or exercise phobias. A cycle of increased muscle tightness, spasms, and pain starts again, and we seem to sink deeper and deeper into a painful unconditioned state. We want to accept responsibility for improving our activity level, and we need to choose wisely.

Basic Goals For A Home Exercise Program

- **It is practical.** Buying a 15-piece indoor gym set for which we have to build an additional room isn't practical.

- **It should improve muscle endurance and fitness.** Even if it hurts, it is better to have fit and painful muscles than unconditioned and painful muscles!

- **The program can be easily modified.** If we have a flare-up, we should still be able to do the program, just less of it, or work on other parts of the body that are not painful.

- **The program should help maintain a stable baseline.** This is our prize goal, to reduce pain and keep it stable.

Our home exercise program is our responsibility, and we have to be organized and consistent with it. Various medical professionals can help develop a home program: your doctor, physical therapist, massotherapist, fitness trainer, aquatics instructor, and aerobics instructor. As I have said over and over (and over!), no one program works best for everyone, but everyone should be able to find something that works. Each home program should include the following:

1. Fibronomics

2. Modalities

3. Stretching

4. Massage

5. Light conditioning

1. Fibronomics

Proper postures and fibronomics are the basic building blocks of a home program. There is a proper way of doing everything in our daily lives, whether we are at home, at work, or anyplace else. Once we practice these techniques, they will become automatic and ingrained in our subconscious so we don't have to think about them all the time. These techniques are discussed in Chapter 15.

2. Modalities

Modalities include heat, cold, electric stimulation, and water therapy. They can be applied at home to help relieve pain. Heat is the easiest home modality to apply and usually works the best. Heat can be a recurrent theme throughout the day: a heated mattress pad; an electric blanket; a hot morning shower; a heating pad during the day; heat-producing muscle creams before exercise; hot, jetted Jacuzzi after exercise; and a hot tub in the evening. Since many fibromyalgia patients complain of cold skin and cold extremities, heat is a natural modality to warm the skin, improve the blood flow, relax muscles, and decrease pain.

Some people complain that a jetted Jacuzzi or whirlpool aggravates the tender points due to the direct pressure. Other people describe it as a soothing massage effect. You need to determine if this approach would work for you prior to investing in a jetted Jacuzzi bathtub. A hot tub is a good investment for many people, since it not only allows deep therapeutic heat to relax the muscles, but it is mentally relaxing as well. If that is not feasible, taking a bath in water as hot as can be tolerated and soaking up to the top of your neck for 30 minutes can be an excellent substitute.

Hot showers are a great way to start off your stiff, painful morning. If you have a couple of tender areas that are particularly bothersome, a continuous hot shower stream on these areas can reduce the pain. If you are experiencing a flare-up, you can take extra showers during the day; or soak in the hot tub or a hot bath. You can never overheat your muscles by performing too many heat treatments during the day. Use heat more frequently during flare-ups, and once a stable baseline is achieved again, the usual program can be resumed.

Many people who use electric blankets will still complain of coldness coming from their mattress and sheets. I advise them to use an electric blanket only after having first acquired a heated mattress pad. Heat from below is better for skin and muscles than heat on top because the weight of our bodies pushing down on the heated surface increases the body surface area in contact with the heat, and improves heat conduction to the body. Plus, heat rises, so one wants heat rising from below to meet the body and not rising off the bed.

Some people like cold treatment, especially for muscle spasms. If you can stand the first 5 to 10 minutes of an ice application, then a full 20 to 30-minute treatment may provide considerable pain relief, muscle relaxation, and longer duration than heat. However, very few people can tolerate the cold sensation against skin (including me) and opt instead for heat treatments. If heat is not effective, however, I always advise trying cold treatment, such as an ice pack or ice massage, to see if this

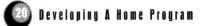

modality is helpful. One patient told me she used a refrigerated gel pack for 10 minutes, then used the ice pack on that "cool" area and the ice pack didn't bother her skin.

Many people have found a TENS unit to be helpful. This is device that emits an electrical buzz that blocks the pain, and can be worn and used for different painful regions of the body. If this particular modality is helpful to an individual, he or she will continue to use it in spite of the hassles that are involved (putting the pads and wires in place, carrying the unit around, adjusting the controls, etc.).

3. Stretching

Stretching is a vital part of a fibromyalgia person's home program, and we need to stretch frequently during the day. Because muscles are so tight, they are more vulnerable to strains, so it is especially important that we counteract this tightness by stretching. I have often been asked if I had to choose one thing to do in a home program, what would I choose; and the answer is: stretching. If you are going to choose stretching, choose to do it regularly and consistently. You should stretch in the morning, stretch during the day, and stretch at night.

How does one begin a stretching program? I like to begin by teaching my patients passive stretching techniques. These do not require any specific equipment and can be done anywhere.

There are some general rules with stretching. Always move slowly and gently without jerking motions, and make sure there is no restrictive clothing or jewelry. Wear comfortable clothing. When you stretch, hold to a slow count of 3 to 10. When you first start, hold for only 3 seconds, and when you become more experienced, gradually increase your ability to hold for the full 10 seconds. Find a feeling of stretch within your comfort zone. Remember to practice deep breathing exercises as part of your stretching.

> I have often been asked if I had to choose one thing to do in a home program, what would I choose; and the answer is: stretching.

Repetitions should be started at a low number and increased. If you have been sedentary for a long period of time, you should begin with a schedule of doing all the stretching exercises, but each one only once, holding each stretch for 3 seconds. Over the first week, progress from stretching once a day to stretching twice a day, each stretch up to 3 seconds of holding. During the second week, progress to stretching twice a day, holding for 5 seconds, and repeating each exercise 3 times.

In each successive week, increase the time held in each stretch by 2 seconds, and the number of repetitions by 2, until you reach a maximum of 10 seconds and 10 repetitions twice a day.

These above guidelines are for a person who has been sedentary for a long while and is just beginning to exercise. Note that I have emphasized slow, gradual stretching over an entire month before even adding any type of conditioning-type exercise. A controlled, gradually increasing stretching program as described should minimize the pain and still allow progressive improvement. Ice after stretching, muscle creams, and over-the-counter antiinflammatory medicines can be used to help smooth over the transition period.

Certainly one can speed up the progression and perform stretching numerous times during the day. I recommend stretching at least twice a day in the training process, and increase as tolerated. I encourage people to always think about stretching as part of their daily routine.

Passive stretching exercises can be done on different body parts: head, neck, trunk, shoulder, upper body, low back, hip, and legs. Dozens of stretching exercises are possible, and all of them can be beneficial if done properly. The following are descriptions and diagrams of these types of passive stretching exercises.

Head and neck forward stretch:

Lie on your back with your knees bent and feet flat. Place hands behind head with fingers on head and thumbs at the bottom of the skull. Gently lift head with hands forward and chin toward chest and go to the comfort zone; hold to a count of from 3 to 10 as tolerated.

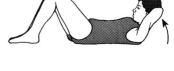

Head and neck lateral stretch:

Place one hand on the opposite side of head below ear, gently pull and turn head so nose points to underarm.

Thoracic or trunk stretches:

Cat back on all fours. Start with hands and knees on floor, head positioned between shoulders. Let back sag, keep head parallel to floor. Lower head with chin to chest, tighten stomach and arch back as high as possible.

Lateral side bends:

These are performed against the wall and are called teapot exercises. Stand so your back and shoulders touch the wall. Cross your arms over your head making sure that your elbows and your head touch the wall, slowly bend your upper body to your right and then to your left, keeping your feet on the floor.

Shoulder girdle and upper body:

Hold a towel overhead with hands at either end of it, and gently pull from side to side. Another exercise is to clasp your hands behind your back and lift your arms upward until you feel a comfortable stretch.

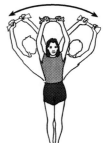
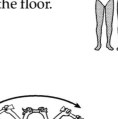
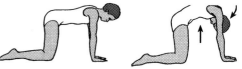
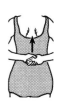
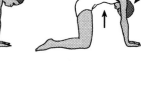
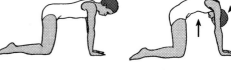

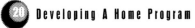

Pectoral stretch:

Stand facing a wall and place both hands on the wall at shoulder height. Turn body away to one side, keeping the shoulders in the same position and keep turning until a stretch is felt in the pectoralis muscle. Lean the body towards the wall to increase the stretch. Repeat the steps for the opposite side.

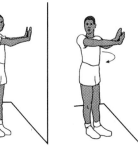
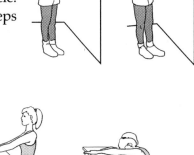

Latissimus dorsi stretch:

Kneel on the floor with elbows and hands placed together on a chair. Slowly move your chest towards the floor and sit back towards your heels until the stretch is felt.

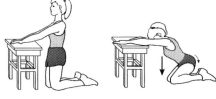

Low back:

Single knee to chest, and then both knees to chest.

Low back and hip:

Lie on back with knees bent and feet flat on the floor. Rotate knees from one side to the other.

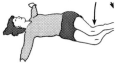

Piriformis stretch:

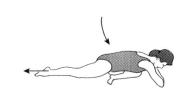
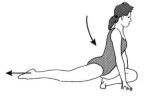

Start on your hands and knees. Place the left foot across your body and directly in front of the right knee. Turn your left knee out slightly to the side. Keep your shoulders and hips square and slide your right leg backwards, gradually sinking down until you feel a stretch in the left buttock/piriformis muscle. Resting on your elbows as you sink down is more comfortable. You should not feel pain in the low back or during this stretch. Reverse technique to stretch the opposite side.

Kneeling hip flexor stretch:

Kneel with the right knee on the floor and the opposite hip and knee flexed to 90 degrees. Maintain an upright trunk and hold onto a chair with the left hand. Position the right leg so the right hip is rotated inward. Place the right hand on the right buttock and flatten the stomach. Contract the right buttock muscle and feel the stretch in the right front thigh. Reverse the process for the other side.

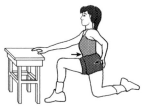

Quadriceps:

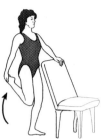

While standing, stabilize yourself with a chair or table. Pull your foot up towards your buttock and keep your hip as straight as possible.

Hamstring stretch:

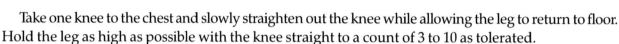

Take one knee to the chest and slowly straighten out the knee while allowing the leg to return to floor. Hold the leg as high as possible with the knee straight to a count of 3 to 10 as tolerated.

Calf-Step stretching:

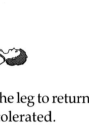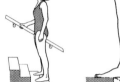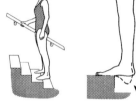

Any step will work, but it is best to use stairs that have a railing for better support. Place the ball of the foot (the padding just before your toes start) on the step, letting your heel sag over the edge of the step and press down until you feel a comfortable stretch.

Bed stretches:

Passive stretching should start in bed before getting up in the morning. Following are suggested bed stretches. These should be done while lying in bed prior to getting up. Stretch and hold each position for 3 seconds.

Arm and leg reach:

Reach your arms up as far as you can with your legs straight out and feet and toes pointed ballet style.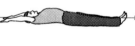

Chin tuck:

Place your arms behind your head and push your head forward so your chin touches your chest.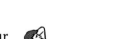

Neck push back:

Look up and back as far as you can, pressing your head into the pillow. Turn your head to the side, pressing your cheek into the pillow. Repeat with the other side.

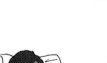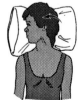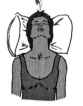

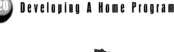

Neck extension with chin press:

Start to tilt your head backward, and at same time try to press your chin into your chest.

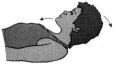

Alternate knee to chest:

While lying on your back, bend your knee to your chest, holding with the arm on the same side. Repeat on the other side. After your stretches are completed, log roll out of bed using proper body mechanics.

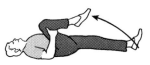

Good Morning!

Stretching in the shower can be especially effective since you can use the warm water. In addition, it helps you start off your morning with stretching at a time when your muscles are usually the tightest.

These pages have given examples of stretches in different situations. One can stretch any part of the body, and I have not demonstrated every possible stretch. An excellent reference book is *Stretching* by Bob Anderson.

Therabands

Exercise using elastic bands (Therabands) can provide dynamic stretching to increase strength and flexibility of our muscles. These are not aerobic exercises, but can be very effective. The rubberized elastic bands come in different colors which represent different strengths or tensions. These bands look flimsy, and one may wonder how they can be effective in an exercise program, but they can provide excellent resistance for the muscles. The harder you pull and stretch them, the more the tension on the muscles. Thicker bands provide more tension.

I have found theraband exercises to be effective for many patients. These exercises require instruction and practice to work best. Sometimes you don't realize how hard you are working with the bands, so you need to be careful not to overdo the first few times you use the bands. Once the exercises are learned, the individual can perform them as part of a self-program.

Here are some examples of basic theraband exercises that can be helpful in stretching and strengthening the upper body and arms especially.

1. Place the theraband behind your head. Your knees should be slightly bent and your back flat. Push your head into the band so that your chin stays parallel with the floor. Push straight back. Don't forget to breathe!

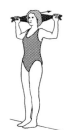

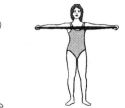

2. Take the theraband in both hands; start with your arms straight out in front and pull them backwards until they touch the wall.

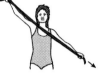

3. Take the theraband in both hands. Start with your arms straight out in front of you diagonally. Pull your arms backwards until they touch the wall.

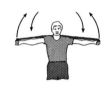

4. Start with your arms overhead holding a theraband. Pull downward until your arms are level with your shoulders. Hold your shoulder blades down as you relax your arms and move them upwards.

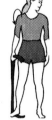

5. Place a theraband under one foot. Turn your head so that your chin is over the opposite shoulder and look down. Grasp the theraband and roll your shoulder up, back and down without bending your wrist.

Practice deep breathing techniques while doing these theraband exercises. Once you are comfortably instructed, begin a regular theraband program ranging from 3 times a week to every day. Like stretching exercises, the theraband should be slowly moved to position and then held to the count of 3 and slowly returned to the starting position. There is resistance from the bands during both the stretch and return. An exercise session can include an increasing number of repetitions up to 10 of each exercise if the individual can tolerate it. I advise my patients to perform therapy and exercises regularly whether or not they are having pain.

One woman with upper back pain found theraband exercises very effective in keeping her pain under control. However, she stopped doing the exercises in January because of various other projects and experienced a flare-up of upper back pain in February. Her flare-up persisted in spite of continuing the other components of her program. Once we realized that she had stopped her theraband exercises, she resumed them and reported that her upper back pain decreased and stabilized again. This is an example of how a particular exercise can be helpful, but it needs to be continued on a regular basis. If the exercises work, do them!

4. Massage

Massages are a wonderful way to decrease pain, relax muscles, improve blood circulation, passively stretch muscles, and overall, let you feel good.

Massotherapy could be done daily if a person had access to this treatment. However, our health care system does not pay for such daily intensive treatment. If massotherapy works for you, try to have it done once or twice a month at least. (If you've won the lottery, have it done weekly!) Family members or significant others can be trained to perform therapeutic massages for you.

Self-massage is a fairly simple procedure that can be learned and performed effectively. Self-massage can be performed anytime, but is often best done in the shower where the hand can glide easily by using soap. Stretching is easily combined with self-massage. One massotherapist who has worked with hundreds of fibromyalgia patients likes to instruct patients to give themselves a hug when taking a morning shower. This provides stretching, self-massage—and starting the day off with a hug! Remember to hug thyself frequently!

Different massager devices are available to purchase. They can be hand-held or devices you sit or lie on that are adjustable to match your comfort level. Many of my patients have some (or all!) of these devices as part of their home program.

5. Light Conditioning

As a general rule, people with fibromyalgia may not tolerate a lot of exercise, but a little bit of exercise is helpful. A light conditioning program means enough exercise to stimulate the cardiovascular system and strengthen the muscles without overworking or exhausting them and causing increased pain. When we resume exercising, our muscles have to go through a "learning curve" again. So expect to be sore at first. Some people with fibromyalgia are exercise intolerant, and any exercise, or even stretching, will aggravate the pain. Most people will be able to find some exercise/stretching program that helps (not hurts!) them. Any increased activity is better than no activity.

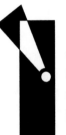

As a general rule, people with fibromyalgia may not tolerate a lot of exercise, but a little bit of exercise is helpful.

Set realistic goals for the body that are well beyond high school! We have to realize what we can reasonably accomplish; for example, a good workout for 30 minutes, 3 times a week. Don't put pressure on yourself to exercise longer and harder in order to feel better. I always tell patients that the amount of time spent exercising is not as important as the actual effort to exercise.

The keys to a successful exercise program are as follows:

1. Emphasize stretching and flexibility exercises of all major muscle groups and focus on a warm-up period that consists of stretching only.

2. Add a low impact, aerobic type program (light conditioning). Such a program can include walking, water aerobics, using an exercise bicycle, or performing a low impact aerobic program.

3. Gradually progress in an exercise program as tolerated. The goal is to achieve improvement and a stable baseline.

4. Continue a regular exercise program at least 3 times a week, even on days when there is increased pain.

5. Follow proper posture and body mechanics to minimize strain of the muscles and joints.

A light conditioning program should not be started until you are comfortable with a regular daily stretching program. For individuals who are more active, a light conditioning program can be started soon after completing a regular instruction program. Perform light conditioning exercises for 20 to 30 minutes at least 3 times a week. As a rule, one should skip every other day to allow the body a chance to rest and recuperate, but this differs according to the individual's abilities and needs. When beginning, it is best to exercise about 10 minutes per session for the first week, and then gradually increase 5 to 10 minutes each week until you reach at least 30 minutes 3 times a week.

Light conditioning does not necessarily entail intensive aerobic activity for 30 minutes. It can involve periods of stretching, strengthening, relaxation, and actual conditioning. This alternating strategy usually works best for fibromyalgia muscles that do not like too much of one thing at any given time. Any conditioning program involves proper warm-up, breathing techniques, good posture, awareness of the body's response, and a cool-down period. Forms of exercise that fall into the category of light conditioning include weights, walking, cycling, stair machines, arm pulleys, aquatics, aerobics, and dancing.

Weight-lifting

Weight-lifting is a category of exercise that emphasizes strengthening, but there are stretching and conditioning components as well, especially if the exercise is repeated a number of times. People with more severe forms of fibromyalgia usually do not tolerate any type of weight-lifting, either free weights or machines. It appears that the continuous resistance on the muscles overstimulates them and increases the pain.

For individuals who have tried weight-lifting and continue to experience increased pain, I usually recommend avoiding weights altogether. These people should use alternative exercises which allow variable resistance on the muscles and are usually tolerated better.

Many people with milder forms of fibromyalgia can develop a very successful weight-lifting program without muscle flare-ups. In these people, the practice should be to use less weight and more repetitions to minimize microscopic tears or strains to the muscles and increase endurance and energy. Free weights and variable resistance weight machines seem to work best. If your fibromyalgia has reached a point where you have difficulty doing any type of exercise, I would not advise a weight-lifting program.

Walking

Walking is a very effective form of light conditioning exercise. Wear soft cushioned comfortable shoes. Rubberized tracks are the best surfaces to walk on as they minimize the impact to your feet and ultimately your back. Walking with a buddy is a great way to motivate and commit yourself to this type of exercise.

When beginning a walking program, you can alternate 5 minutes of brisk walking with 5 minutes of leisurely walking, and repeat this cycle. The goal is to gradually increase your brisk walking to at least 20 to 30 minutes 3 times a week.

Some people do not tolerate walking because of particular pain in the low back, hip, or leg areas. However, others who have predominantly upper body pain may find walking the best way to loosen up these sore muscles. The upper body and arms can get involved with walking, particularly brisk

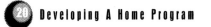

walking with a lot of arm swinging. Increased heart rate and stimulated respiratory drive makes this exercise a beneficial cardiovascular and aerobic activity as well.

I am frequently asked if any certain exercise equipment is helpful in fibromyalgia. I always advise people that anything can be tried, but before making a large purchase, one should try several sessions of exercise on that particular piece of equipment, either at a health spa or at a friend's house. If you like the exercise, tolerate it well, and feel it is helpful, then you can consider purchasing it. Too many of my patients have unused exercise equipment sitting in their basements. Try before you buy!

Here are some considerations for different types of exercise equipment:

Treadmill

Many people prefer to use a treadmill for controlled walking exercise. I thought I would enjoy this type of activity, but after I purchased a treadmill, I found this type of walking to be too artificial. There is something about walking but not seeing things move past me that bothers me. I have a hard time maintaining an exact rhythm as I prefer to be able to vary my pace and I tend to lose my balance every so often. I found that a slight loss of balance on the treadmill could throw me off it entirely! Even though I prefer natural walking, I still encourage people to consider treadmill walking if they are interested, but try it before you purchase the machine. If you like your trial, I know where you can get a cheap treadmill that has hardly been used!

Exercise Cycle

The biggest potential problem with an exercise cycle is malpositioning on the unit. If the seat is too narrow or the handlebars are too far out in front, you could be in a position where you are leaning forward and reaching out with your arms, creating a lot of neck and back strain. A wide, comfortable seat and handlebars that reach out so you can hold them and still be in a comfortably aligned position are necessary. Persons with painful knees may not tolerate stationary bikes at all, although the seat height can be raised to decrease strain and painful movements of the knees. Exercise cycles that allow a reclined position can be very effective for fibromyalgia patients since they minimize the strain on the low back and arms.

Stair Machine (StairMaster)

This equipment emphasizes strengthening the gluteal and leg muscles. Many people with fibromyalgia can only handle this type of machine for a short period of time before cramping increases, especially in the calves. Those with knee pain may find this exercise too aggravating. If you can tolerate and progress with this machine, it is an excellent workout.

Arm Pulley Systems

These systems may be part of a treadmill, stationary bicycle, or other leg exercise apparatus. The main problem with this type of system for people with fibromyalgia is that it puts a lot of strain on the arms, particularly with all the reaching, pulling, and squeezing involved. The arms usually tire very quickly. People who have difficulty reaching out with their arms will usually not tolerate any arm pulley system as part of an exercise program, but some systems, which don't require as much reaching, are well tolerated.

Aquatics

Another popular form of exercise is aquatics. Water exercises provide an opportunity to stretch, strengthen, and condition the body. The water supports the spine and extremities and acts as a brace and massager. Those who have difficulty holding their arms out in front may do so more comfortably as the water buoys the arms. Standing chest high in water will remove much of the gravity in the lower back area, which may dramatically reduce pain.

Numerous aquatic exercise classes are available for people with arthritis and fibromyalgia. Warm water is necessary. Ideally water temperature should be 88 degrees or higher, although many pools keep the temperature for these types of classes around 85 degrees. Various aquatic equipment is available to help work out in the water.

Like other forms of exercise, one needs to first try the water program to determine if it is helpful. Some individuals do not tolerate the cold feeling in the water or the air drafts that cool the skin. Wearing a wet suit or long sleeve shirt in the pool and having lots of dry towels ready as soon as you get out can help avoid the cold.

Others describe the process of changing into a bathing suit, getting into the pool, getting out of the pool, showering, drying the hair, and getting dressed again to be too much of a hassle even though there may be some benefits. However, many people, particularly those who have tried land exercises without success, and who may have particular problems with the low back, pelvic, hips, and leg areas, respond very nicely to an aquatics exercise program. I recommend that these exercises be done first with an aquatics instructor, usually in a class. Choose a pool with warm water and warm, still air around it! Individual programs can be developed if group aquatic exercises are helpful.

Aerobics

Traditional aerobics are not tolerated very well by people with fibromyalgia, since it involves a lot of exercises with the arms out or overhead, prolonged standing, and high bodily impact. Low impact aerobics may be better tolerated. Arm exercises and standing still are difficult for many people. Step aerobics are popular, and some individuals with milder fibromyalgia may do well with these.

Modified aerobics, if tailored to the individual, can provide effective light conditioning. Chair aerobics is an example. The individual sits as much as possible to unload the spine. Activities are done primarily from the chest level and below, avoiding any overhead arm activities. Higher impact movements are modified. For example, walking movements may be simulated by "marching" while seated. Stretching is emphasized and problem areas are moved slowly. Exercises are designed to stretch the tight muscles, usually the chest and quadriceps, while strengthening the weaker muscles, usually the back and hamstrings, and also to achieve a better posture. Therabands are commonly used in chair aerobics.

Dancing

Many of my patients have found dancing to be a great workout that they tolerate well. Jazzercise, line dancing, polka dancing, and good old rock and roll are examples of light conditioning and aerobic exercises that have worked for various people. Some dance to video tapes and others go to public dance floors. Remember to stretch and warm up before turning yourself loose!

Summary

As always, the key to the numerous types of exercise is to actually do something! Professional guidance and supervision are available to help you find the right program for you, but it is your responsibility to do something, and to do it regularly and consistently. You should stretch before and after exercising, and you should stretch just about any other time in between! You may prefer to exercise at home because you can be more independent and flexible in a convenient location. You also don't have to worry about being embarrassed by others watching you, if that is a concern.

On the other hand, working out in a gym or spa allows you to get away on a predictable schedule and be in a social setting. Paying for a membership often motivates a person to follow through regularly, and positive results will increase your confidence and self esteem.

Activating muscles can be painful at first, but it is not harmful. You are not hurting yourself, and you will be able to work through this initial pain. Temporary flare-ups can occur when one is starting an exercise program, but support and supervision from your medical professionals will enable you to overcome any initial difficulties and "get over the hump," so to speak.

Once a successful exercise program is underway, I believe that subsequent flare-ups are very rarely due to the actual exercise program. You may need to modify your exercise program during the flare-up, but it is important that you continue exercising in spite of the flare-up. If you stop using or exercising the other muscles, they will get tighter and will quickly become unconditioned; that is, they will get weaker and have less stamina. It then becomes even harder to reactivate the muscles. Muscles that are flared-up need to be exercised to keep them as flexible and conditioned as possible, even though they hurt more.

Adding extra modalities can also help you return to a stable baseline. Don't stop everything, though. You will be surprised to find you can still follow through with an exercise program even when you have more pain.

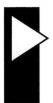 ## If You Want To Know More

1. Anderson B. *Stretching*. Shelter Publications, 1992.
2. Pellegrino MJ. *Inside fibromyalgia*. Columbus OH: Anadem Publishing, 2001.

Alternative Medicine

Alternative, or complementary, medicine has become more and more popular in recent years. This type of medicine has been around for thousands of years, much longer than traditional or conventional medicine. Historically, the United States has embraced the conventional medicine approach, so complementary or alternative medicines have been viewed with skepticism. As patients and the public in general have become more aware of alternative medicine, its popularity has increased.

A study described in the *Journal of the American Medical Association* (Eisenberg DM, *et al*, 1998) found that the total number of visits to alternative medicine practitioners rose by nearly 50% from 1990 to 1997. In 1997, the most popular alternative therapies were vitamins and herbal medicine, massage, energy healing, chiropractic, and homeopathy. In the United States, over 21 billion dollars was spent in 1997 on alternative medicine.

It is not surprising that people with fibromyalgia are interested in alternative medicine approaches. If there is one area in which conventional medicine often fails, it is in the management of conditions causing chronic pain. Conventional medicine emphasizes the diagnosis and pharmacologic treatment of various medical conditions based on scientific research. The main philosophy is to identify the cause of the disease and treat it with medicines or surgeries to eliminate the cause. Conventional medicine is wonderful in curing patients with bacterial infections by treating them with antibiotics, saving persons with diseased organs by transplants, treating diabetes by providing insulin replacement and saving an individual with acute appendicitis by performing an appendectomy. But if someone has chronic pain, does not respond to medications, is not a candidate for a surgical procedure, and has had numerous diagnostic tests that were normal, conventional medicine may be helpless.

Complementary or alternative medicine strategies emphasize the interaction between the body and the mind. The main focus is on maintaining homeostasis, which is the body's natural ability to maintain a stable harmony and balance among its hormones, enzymes, muscles, and organs to prevent disease or to allow the body to heal itself. This type of medicine focuses on the whole individual instead of the individual symptoms, and seeks to optimize homeostasis by promoting healthy lifestyles, appropriate exercise, restful sleep, proper nutrition, and self-responsibility.

Those who endorse complementary medicine will tell you that the body does not end with the skin. Instead, energy fields extend beyond the body that affect one's well being. We can respond to energy therapies. And no, you do not have to be radioactive to emit an energy field, you just have to be alive!

Conventional medicine sets a high research standard for approving certain treatments. Scientific studies are valuable tools in proving effectiveness (or harmlessness) of certain treatments. If a particular drug treatment has been studied and shown to be scientifically effective, this drug may be helpful (and safe) for patients.

Most conditions that doctors treat do not have scientific studies that "prove" a particular treatment is effective. But that does not stop us from treating conditions, nor should it. Medical practitioners need to be open-minded. If we always waited for scientific proof, most diseases that exist today could not be treated.

Sometimes, this scientific standard can be a double-edged sword. Most conditions that doctors treat do not have scientific studies that "prove" a particular treatment is effective. But that does not stop us from treating conditions, nor should it. Medical practitioners need to be open-minded. If we always waited for scientific proof, most diseases that exist today could not be treated. Complementary medicine has long been stereotyped as "failing" to hold up to scientific standards of conventional medicine. An increased number of scientific studies are being published that support the effectiveness of many complementary medicine treatments. Complementary medicine may still need to "catch up" on its scientific credibility, but it already has a long and successful history in clinical applications. Just ask people with fibromyalgia!

Placebo Effect

I remember learning that the placebo effect was "bad." The placebo effect occurred when a person reported improvement in pain (or other symptoms) after being given a sugar pill instead of the actual drug (or other treatment). The placebo effect has to be accounted for in any scientific research study because a placebo response does not measure the effect of the drug or treatment being tested. So as not to mistakenly attribute all of the positive benefits to the drug being tested to a placebo effect, research studies are designed to "cancel out" the placebo effect.

Placebo is derived from the Latin word that means "I will please." It is a positive human response to hopefulness and wanting to get better with a treatment. Even though the person wasn't given an actual research drug, she or he felt measurably better simply because of HOPE. Studies show the placebo effect may happen up to 30% of the time with ANY treatment. This means 3 of 10 people will feel better when given any type of treatment, with no obvious relationship to the actual treatment.

The placebo effect is a powerful physician "tool" that is not limited to a pill. Suggestions that a physician makes can have a dramatic effect on how a patient will respond to a particular treatment. In a study done by Drs. Staats and Hekmat (1998), the role of one's pain threshold in response to suggestion was examined.

Three groups of college students were to place their hands in a tank of ice water. Each group was instructed differently. The first group was told "neutral" things: don't think about anything, just keep your hand in the water until you need to remove it. The second group was told "positive" things: ice water can improve circulation, strengthen the heart, cleanse the skin cells, and other beneficial effects. The third group was told "negative" things: ice water can be dangerous by causing numbness, decrease in blood flow, tissue damage and hypertension. All 3 groups were told to keep their hands immersed until they couldn't tolerate the pain anymore.

Guess what happened? The "positive" group held their hands in longer and reported less anxiety. The "negative" group took their hands out much quicker and reported more anxiety. The "neutral" group was in between the other groups. This study demonstrated how the physician can affect the patient's response to treatment. Reassuring positive words are more likely to increase the therapeutic response—cause a positive placebo response. I have found much better responses to medications in my patients when I explain what to expect and tell them the medicines may help but won't take away all the pain, than if I just gave them the medicines and said, "Take this and let me know if it helps."

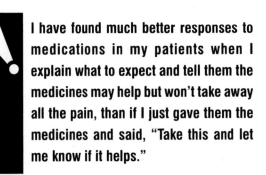

I have found much better responses to medications in my patients when I explain what to expect and tell them the medicines may help but won't take away all the pain, than if I just gave them the medicines and said, "Take this and let me know if it helps."

A number of years ago it dawned on me that the placebo response from hopefulness and one's desire to improve is EXACTLY what we are trying to accomplish in the treatment of chronic pain related to fibromyalgia. We want people to feel better, even if we can't explain how it happened. This approach would seem to be one of the major philosophies of complementary medicine, to improve the well-being of body and mind. With this realization, I've washed out all of the negative connotations I learned about placebos from conventional medicine and have become more open-minded. Now one of my philosophies is: Welcome Placebo! We WANT to achieve a positive placebo response.

My Specialty Blends Both Medicines

My specialty is actually a blend between conventional and alternative medicine strategies. By using a multidisciplinary approach, we blend the best of everything to help fibromyalgia. I was "conventionally" trained at The Ohio State University Medical School, but my training included learning and understanding physical medicine treatments, physical therapy, massage therapy, manipulation therapy, nutritional therapy, biofeedback, and many other areas that are considered "alternative" treatments. I also received training in diagnosis, testing, prescribing medications, and research, which are areas considered "traditional."

Over the years, the line between traditional and alternative medicine blurred. Acupuncture, physical therapy, and nutritional therapies are examples of alternative treatments that have become traditionally accepted. I have already reviewed some alternative treatments in detail (physical therapy, massage, biofeedback, nutritional therapies). I think it is a pointless exercise to try to separate conventional and alternative medicines; we need to recognize that treating chronic pain requires the best of everything.

Many people are frustrated by the lack of improvement with conventional treatments for chronic pain, and if physicians are not open-minded and flexible in their treatment approaches, these people will search elsewhere for relief. A knowledgeable physician treating pain should accept whatever works and not be limited to any particular treatment.

Many doctors specialize in complementary medicine and have undergone years of training to become experts in their field. However, many non-medical people have ventured into alternative medicine treatments with little or no experience, training, or supervision. They promote themselves as so-called "experts" in managing pain. I advise patients to be open-minded, but to check credentials and training and make sure that the practitioner is licensed. If the answers to these licensing and credential questions are too "vague" or "mysterious," stay away from him or her.

This chapter is not meant to be a complete, comprehensive guide to all of the alternative medicine strategies available for chronic pain. There are many good reference books on alternative medicine. A good one is *Alternative Medicine, The Definitive Guide*, compiled by the Burton-Goldberg group. This chapter will highlight some specific approaches I have found useful in the overall treatment of fibromyalgia. Many others, which I have not included here, may be helpful.

Chiropractic Medicine

Chiropractic medicine can be effective in treating back problems, headaches, and other pain disorders including fibromyalgia. Dr. Daniel David Palmer founded the modern chiropractic system in 1895, and today chiropractic medicine is the most popular of alternative medicine fields. Chiropractic treatment can be effective in persons with fibromyalgia since these patients often have pain along the entire spine.

A key philosophy in chiropractic medicine is the holistic approach, with an emphasis on the relationship between the spinal column, the nervous system, and the soft tissues of the body. Proper alignment of the spinal column is necessary to achieve homeostasis and optimal health by allowing unimpeded nerve flow and enhanced neurologic and soft tissue function. In other words, it is believed these treatments enable "clearer" nerve signals to travel through the spine to the brain. If an imbalance, disequilibrium, or misalignment occurs in the vertebrae or soft tissues, nerve pressure can occur. This results in altered signals which eventually lead to impaired nerve function, disease, and pain.

Manipulations are forceful movements of body parts (*e.g.*, pelvis, shoulder) to bring about a greater range of movement and to relax muscles. Adjustments are the application of a sudden and precise force to a persistent point in the vertebra or muscle to properly align the tissue. The desired outcomes of properly aligned vertebrae and muscles are improved balance, better neurologic flow, better circulation and, ultimately, decreased pain and tension.

Many chiropractors use a device called an Activator to perform adjustments. This hand-held device has a spring loaded plunger mechanism which delivers focused pressure energy to a specific body part to achieve proper alignment. A chiropractor is trained in all types of adjustments and can determine which techniques would be most appropriate for a given individual. Chiropractic medicine also deals with preventive, nutritional, strengthening, and fitness measures in helping individuals achieve their highest state of well-being.

I believe the professional relationship and communication between chiropractic and medical physicians will continue to improve, and patients will benefit. I work closely with many chiropractors in my area in treating patients with chronic pain.

Applied Kinesiology

Specific muscles may be overactive causing spasms, or underactive, causing weakness. These muscles can create dysfunction(s) that cause pain and impairment. An applied kinesiologist uses procedures that strengthen weak muscles and relax tense muscles to help return injured or dysfunctional muscles to their normal state. Specific muscles are thought to be related to specific organs, and thus by improving the muscle balance organ function improves. Since patients with fibromyalgia have muscle imbalances because portions of the muscles are overly tense and other portions are weak, applied kinesiology techniques can help. Many chiropractors and manual therapists have learned applied kinesiology skills.

Acupuncture

Acupuncture originated in China thousands of years ago and has been successful in pain relief, particularly as an alternative to conventional pain medications. Acupuncture is based on the theory that energy pathways called meridians are present in the body, and that they link the nervous system with the organs. Multiple acupuncture points within these meridian systems can be stimulated to improve the energy flow. These points are stimulated using special needles, electrical stimulation, or pressure.

Acupuncture stimulates the body's own natural pain killers, endorphins. It also affects neurotransmitters or hormones that transmit nerve impulses in a way that decreases the perception of pain. Many studies have shown the effectiveness of acupuncture as a substitute for surgical anesthesia and the temporary relief of pain.

A growing number of physicians have been trained in acupuncture and are practicing this technique in treating pain disorders. In November 1997, the National Institutes of Health consensus panel on acupuncture issued a statement indicating that pain from musculoskeletal conditions could be successfully treated with acupuncture. Indeed, many patients with fibromyalgia have benefited from acupuncture treatments.

Magnetic Therapy

Magnetic therapy uses magnets to decrease pain by improving energy and blood flow in the body. This treatment has been used successfully for thousands of years. Therapeutic magnets work on the same principle as acupuncture, but without the needle. Magnetic fields surround us, generated by natural mechanisms such as the earth and weather changes. The fields can be man-made, caused by power lines and electrical devices. This theory maintains that these magnetic fields can affect the body's function in both positive and negative ways by influencing the body's metabolism and oxygen availability to cells.

Magnets have two poles, a positive and a negative. It is felt that the positive pole causes negative effects such as decreased metabolic function, especially with prolonged exposure. The negative pole is felt to cause beneficial effects by normalizing the body's metabolic and energy functioning. Magnetic therapy can be used in numerous ways, from magnetic strips applied to parts of the body to magnetic beds, pillows, and shoe inserts.

Some people believe that reduced exposure to the earth's natural geomagnetic fields can lead to a magnetic field deficiency syndrome. People who live in cities, in high rise buildings, or who have minimal contact with the "bare" earth would be at risk for magnetic field deficiency syndrome since asphalt, concrete, bricks, and metal block our exposure to the natural geomagnetic fields. This syndrome causes pain, headaches, insomnia, stiffness, and fatigue (sound like fibromyalgia?). It is felt that magnetic therapy can be used to correct this deficiency and help restore health in some of these people.

Magnetic fields are used in diagnostic testing procedures such as MRI (magnetic resonance imaging), magnetic encephalography and nerve conduction studies to safely and accurately measure structures and electrical activity. Magnetic field diagnostic techniques are already established in mainstream medicine, and therapeutic magnetic therapy is rising in popularity. It is considered a safe treatment, and many qualified health professionals are using magnets in their clinical practices.

Energy Therapy

Energy therapy is a practice of promoting healing by working on the body's energy fields. It is deeply rooted in the ancient practice of laying-on of the hands. If one assumes that human beings have energy fields that extend from their bodies and that energy flows to and from the body, then one can understand how energy therapy may be a helpful modality. Energy therapy can also be called therapeutic touch, although it is not necessary for the energy therapist to physically touch the patient.

Energy therapy has its roots in ancient Chinese medicine that was based on increasing and balancing the flow of Chi, which means "life force." Acupuncture, another ancient treatment, is also based on altering the flow of Chi by identifying and treating specific acupuncture points in the body.

Energy therapists believe that some illnesses are related to blocked or uneven energy. Various stress-related problems such as headaches, irritable bowel syndrome, breathing difficulties and autonomic nervous system dysfunction may be caused by altered energy flow in the body. Energy therapy has been promoted as an effective way of reducing stress and pain and relieving various stress-related symptoms. Accelerated healing and boosting the immune system are the results promoted by energy therapy.

It is believed that energy can be transferred from one person to another, hence an energy practitioner can access an energy field and rebalance or re-pattern the energy of a symptomatic patient. The energy therapist usually accesses the energy field by moving the hands over the body from 2 to 6 inches away. The energy therapist reports that her hands sense cues from the patient's energy field such as a pull, tingling, pulsation or a temperature change. The therapist identifies these specific cues and tries to modulate and rebalance the energy field by moving the hands over the area towards the periphery of the field. Sometimes actual physical touch is needed in combination with non-contact "touch." The average treatment lasts 15 to 20 minutes, and each person responds differently. Patients have reported feeling sensations during the treatment such as tingling or warmth.

The goals of energy therapy are to reduce pain and stress-related symptoms. Certainly any treatment that can help achieve a relaxation response and reduce pain and stress is welcome in the fibromyalgia world.

Homeopathic Therapy

Homeopathic medicine had its origins over 200 years ago with Dr. Samuel Hahnemann. It is a practice that approaches each individual disease as a consequence of an imbalance within the homeostasis. Each individual's condition is unique, and the homeopathic doctor learns as much as possible about the patient and then prescribes natural substances, called remedies, to treat him or her.

Homeopathic remedies are administered by mouth and should have no toxicities or side effects. Homeopathic ingredients are based on the principle that *like cures like*. It is thought that a small diluted dose will stimulate the body to control its symptoms by healing and restoring balance. If the substances were given in larger doses, they would usually cause the symptoms the patient is complaining of, not eliminate them. For example, ipecac is given to induce vomiting after a poison is ingested. However, homeopathic remedies use very diluted doses of ipecac to treat symptoms of nausea and vomiting. Think of remedies as vaccines which are small, harmless doses that stimulate a specific body reaction to actually protect the body against this substance.

If the person is given a homeopathic remedy for inflammation, this should gently stimulate the body to heal the inflammation and return the body to health and harmony, or homeostasis. Homeopathic remedies stimulate the body's own immune and defense system to initiate the healing process. The homeopathic practitioner approaches the individual's unique problems and prescribes individualized medicine based on the person's total symptoms, including physical, emotional and mental.

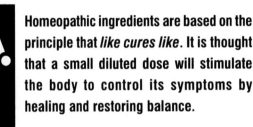

Homeopathic ingredients are based on the principle that *like cures like*. It is thought that a small diluted dose will stimulate the body to control its symptoms by healing and restoring balance.

Conventional medicine has used homeopathic-like therapy. I have already given the example of vaccination to induce a protective immune response against the actual infection. Other examples include using radiation to treat people with cancer (radiation can cause cancer), using Ritalin for hyperactive children (Ritalin is an amphetamine-like drug which causes hyperactivity), and using digoxin for heart conditions (digitalis can actually cause heart abnormalities).

Homeopathic medicine is actually a sophisticated practice in which remedies are prescribed to help the body heal. It is gaining in popularity as more and more people are seeking alternative means for helping pain. A number of my patients have reported substantial benefits in reducing their pain through homeopathic means. If you are considering homeopathic medicine, I recommend you see only a licensed physician who is trained in homeopathic medicine to ensure optimal safety.

Naturopathic Medicine

Naturopathic medicine was founded upon a holistic philosophy that combines various natural treatments with advances in modern medicine. The word naturopathy (naturopathic medicine) was first used in the United States about 100 years ago. But the natural therapies and philosophies on which this alternative medicine is based has been used to treat diseases since ancient times. Hypocrites, a physician who lived over 2400 years ago, is often considered the earliest of naturopathic physicians because he promoted the healing power of nature. Today's naturopathic physicians continue to use nature's therapies, *i.e.*, herbs, foods, water, and tissue manipulation, as the main tools to help the body's own healing power.

Modern American naturopathic physicians are called N.D.s, and they receive training in, and use therapies that include, clinical nutrition, homeopathy, botanical medicine, physical medicine and counseling. The goal of a naturopathic physician is to address the underlying cause of disease and employ therapies that support and promote the body's natural healing process, leading to the highest state of wellness.

In treating a chronic pain problem such as fibromyalgia, naturopathic physicians may use specific individual diets, fasting, nutritional supplements, plant drugs, and small doses of homeopathic medicine to try to reduce pain and spasms and improve the body's immune system. Various physical medicine treatments such as manipulation, exercise, massage, water therapy, and electric therapy can also be utilized to try to reduce pain and spasms. Some naturopathic physicians are trained in the fundamentals of Oriental medicine, including acupuncture, acupressure and Chinese herbal medicine to promote improvement in fibromyalgia. Counseling and stress management are also important components of naturopathic treatments in individuals with chronic pain and stress problems such as fibromyalgia.

Relaxation

As we discussed in Chapter 18, stress, worry, and negative emotions can cause your well-being to deteriorate. Specifically, it can affect your immune system, cause depression and increase chronic pain. Relaxation is a type of alternative treatment that can help decrease stress-related symptoms of fibromyalgia.

A number of structured programs that combine mental and physical aspects of relaxation can help individuals with fibromyalgia learn to relax and incorporate regular (prescribed) relaxation into their lifestyles. Different types of relaxation techniques are available and you need to determine which one is right for you. Let's review some techniques again.

Biofeedback
Biofeedback is one method of learning how to achieve relaxation by controlling your body's responses and reactions to stress. Specific monitoring equipment provides biofeedback information from the body such as heart rate, blood pressure, brain activity or muscle tension. We can learn to identify this feedback information and achieve a change in the body's reaction, such as reducing heart rate, reducing blood pressure, and decreasing muscle tension. A biofeedback professional is required to train the individual on biofeedback devices.

Guided imagery
This technique uses pleasant or relaxing images to try to calm the mind and relax the body. Visualizing a soothing image and doing deep breathing exercises can help achieve a state of relaxation. This method is relatively easy to learn and various tapes can help with the sounds and visual imaging.

Meditation
This popular technique to achieve physical and mental relaxation can be done literally hundreds of ways. The meditative state is one in which there is a deep centering and focusing upon the core of one's being. The goal is to quiet the mind, emotions and body. The meditative state can be achieved through a structured daily routine or sometimes can be done in an unstructured manner, such as "being alone" in the middle of an activity. Various teachers of meditative arts are available, and some techniques can be learned through books or on-line tutorials.

All religions incorporate some form of meditation-like prayer or chanting into their traditions. Scientists have found churchgoers who pray often live longer than others. Meditation reduces blood pressure, improves neurotransmitter activity in the brain, reduces stress and anxiety, and improves overall health. Religion is a private matter, but I encourage fibromyalgia patients to allow their beliefs, faiths, and prayers to help them feel better.

Progressive muscle relaxation

Progressive muscle relaxation is a method developed in the 1930's in which muscle groups are tightened and then relaxed in succession. This method is based upon the concept that mental relaxation is a natural consequence of physical relaxation. This can be practiced 10–20 minutes a day and no special skills or conditioning are involved.

Martial arts (Quigong, Tai chi)

The martial art Quigong is an ancient Chinese healthcare system that combines physical training such as isometrics, isotonics and aerobic conditioning with Eastern philosophy and relaxation techniques. Quigong has been used for hundreds of years in China for the treatment of various medical conditions and learning this art involves a lot of time, commitment and patience. Instruction from a Quigong master or learning in a group setting is recommended.

Tai chi is another Chinese martial art that has been termed a "meditation in motion." It is characterized by soft flowing movements that stress precision and force. Like Quigong, this method has been around for many years, and it requires a lot of patience, determination and instruction to learn properly. If one is considering trying martial arts techniques for relaxation, first check with your doctor before beginning training since motion, force, and physical exertion are required.

Yoga

Yoga is an ancient Indian form of exercise that has been around for thousands of years. The goal of yoga is to restore balance and harmony to the body and emotions through various postural and breathing exercises. Yoga actually means joining or union in Sanskrit and has been called the "search for the soul" and the "union between the individual and the divine."

Yoga helps improve flexibility and relaxation. There are different forms of yoga, including those that are less strenuous for individuals who may have chronic pain or fibromyalgia.

A systematic review of published studies on complementary medicines in fibromyalgia was done by Dr. L. C. Hordcraft, *et al.* recently. A standardized evaluation of the different results published was used to determine the quality of the studies, the effect of the studies, and the effectiveness of the alternative treatment approaches.

The review determined that acupuncture, nutritional supplements, magnesium, SAM-e, and massage therapy had the best evidence for effectiveness with fibromyalgia. Less effective, but still with positive results, included biofeedback and relaxation. Magnetic therapy, homeopathic therapy and dietary modifications had positive results from studies that had some scientific flaws in their research design. Finally, chiropractic cure did not have well designed studies or positive results for fibromyalgia, according to the review and authors.

You are encouraged to be open-minded when it comes to complementary/alternative medicine strategies. Numerous treatments are available and many people have benefited from them. Like any other treatments, there can be side effects from, or lack of response to, complementary treatments, so you need to work with qualified, knowledgeable health professionals. Choose your care wisely and responsibly, and hopefully you will find many ways to control your fibromyalgia!

If You Want To Know More

1. Bennett RM, Clark SR, Campbell S, et al. *Low levels of somatomedin C in patients with the fibromyalgia syndrome. A possible link between sleep and muscle pain.* Arthritis Rheum 1992; 35: 1113–6.

2. Bennett RM, Cook DM, Clark SR, et al. *Hypothalamic-pituitary-insulin-like growth factor-1 axis dysfunction in patients with fibromyalgia.* J Rheumatol 1997; 24: 1384–9.

3. Bennett RM, Clark SR, Walczyk J, et al. *A randomized double-blind placebo-controlled study of growth hormone therapy in the treatment of fibromyalgia.* Am J Med 1998; 104: 227–31.

4. Eisenberg DM, Davis RB, Ettner SL, et al. *Trends in alternative medicine use in the United States, 1990–1997; results of a follow-up national survey.* JAMA 1998; 280: 1569–75.

5. Hershoff A. *Homeopathy for musculoskeletal healing.* North Atlantic Books, 1997.

6. Holdcraft LC, Assefi N, Buchwald D. *Complementary and alternative medicine in fibromyalgia and related syndromes.* Best Pract Res Clin Rheumatol 2003; 17: 667–83.

7. Kalb C. *Faith and healing.* Newsweek Nov 10, 2003; 44–56.

8. Lenarz M. *The chiropractic way: how chiropractic care can stop your pain and help you regain your health without drugs or surgery.* Mosby, 2003.

9. Lister RE. *An open pilot study to evaluate the potential benefits of co-enzyme Q10 combined with ginkgo biloba extract in fibromyalgia syndrome.* J Int Med Res 2002; 30: 195–9.

10. Pellegrino MJ. *Inside fibromyalgia.* Columbus OH: Anadem Publishing, 2001.

11. Pizzorno JE, Murray MT. *Textbook of natural medicine.* 2nd ed. Churchill Livingstone, 1999.

12. Russell IJ, Michalek JE, et al. *Treatment of fibromyalgia syndrome with Super Malic: a randomized, double-blind, placebo controlled crossover pilot study.* J Rheumatol 1995; 22: 953–8.

13. Staats P, Hekmat H, Staats A. *Suggestion/placebo effects on pain: negative as well as positive.* J Pain Symptom Manage 1998; 15: 235–43.

SECTION IV—TREATMENT OF SPECIFIC FIBROMY- ALGIA RELATED PROBLEMS

This section addresses those "other" problems in fibromyalgia. We've reviewed the treatment of fibromyalgia's biggest problem—PAIN—and have regarded fibromyalgia so far as a monster that rears its ugly pain-head at us. We haven't forgotten that other fibromyalgia-related problems also require their own separate treatments. Fibromyalgia is actually a multi-headed monster (remember Hydra from Greek mythology). Sure, pain is its biggest and ugliest head, but we can attack the other heads as well to try to control the beast. Hopefully you'll learn some "beast-busters" here (and be like Hercules … remember, he slayed Hydra!?)

Getting A Good Night's Sleep

Top Ten Complaints About Sleeping In The Same Bed With A Fibromyalgia Patient

1. Every night: Same old, same old

2. Continuous tossing and turning causes motion sickness

3. Restless legs activate security system motion detectors

4. Racing thoughts create annoying draft

5. Acts too dopey from all of the night medicines

6. Too many pillows impair breathing

7. Nocturnal myoclonic injuries

8. Prays too loudly for stage IV sleep

9. Noisy, hissing electric blanket

10. Cold feet cause frostbite

Most of us with fibromyalgia complain about our sleep, whether it is difficulty falling asleep, frequently waking at night, or both. We have a defect in our ability to get into a good deep sleep. It is during deep sleep that our body repairs itself, makes vital proteins, and replenishes our energy supply. Thus, we need to devise some strategies to ensure the best and most restful sleep so our bodies can "rebuild" us at night.

In 1975, Dr. Moldofsky proposed the term "non-restorative sleep syndrome" as a name for fibromyalgia. When he studied 10 patients with the diagnosis of fibromyalgia, he found that seven had an abnormality in the Stage 4 delta sleep (the deep sleep stage). There was an intrusion of alpha rhythms into Stage 4 delta sleep, and this alpha-delta sleep pattern at first was thought to be diagnostic and possibly the cause of fibromyalgia. However, this finding is not unique to fibromyalgia. It can be found in other conditions that cause chronic pain.

Five stages of sleep have been defined. When a person is relaxed but still awake, alpha waves are present on an EEG. As the person begins to fall asleep, the alpha waves disappear (Stage 1). In Stage 2 sleep, bursts of sleep spindle waves occur. Stage 3 is the beginning of deep sleep, and Stage 4 is deep sleep where delta waves predominate on the EEG. The last stage (Stage 5) is called REM sleep, or rapid eye movement stage where most dreaming occurs. Fibromyalgia people dream most about trying to get into Stage 4 sleep and staying there!

Pre-Sleep Routine

The first step in sleeping better is preparing to sleep better. Fibromyalgia doesn't like change, so a consistent sleep schedule, going to bed and getting up at the same times, is helpful. If you want extra sleep, it is better to go to bed earlier than to sleep late. What you do prior to going to bed is important to your sleep routine.

You have to unwind and cleanse the mind before lying down to sleep. Taking all of your problems to bed with you only heightens anxiety and makes it difficult to relax your mind. Allow yourself to get as much accomplished as you can in the evening, but reach a "limit" where you allow yourself to say, "I've done as much as I can on this for now, and I'll address it further tomorrow." By reaching this limit, you can close the book for the night and plan to open the book the next day. Do something relaxing before going to bed: listen to music, read a book, watch a TV program, or take a hot bath. Writing a list of things to do the next day and then "clearing the mind" is helpful to me and enables me to close the day. Practice some of the relaxation techniques that you have learned. Avoid caffeine in the evening.

People who work during the night and sleep during the day have even more difficulty getting restful sleep. Our bodies prefer to sleep at night. The pre-sleep routine needs to be followed if you work the evening shift, and it is especially important to allow your mind to unwind when you get home from work.

Sleep Medicines

Many medications are used to treat sleep disorders. Some of these medicines can be habit forming, but if they are used as prescribed and used judiciously, very rarely do I find any problems with side effects. The logic is that fibromyalgia is a chronic condition associated with a chronic sleep disorder; therefore, one is expected to sleep poorly most of the time. Given this, I believe an individual is justified in taking a nightly medicine to improve sleep as long as the beneficial effects far outweigh the potential risks.

I advise my patients to try to use sleeping medicines on an as-needed basis, perhaps during a flare-up or a persistent period of poor sleep.

I advise my patients to try to use sleeping medicines on an as-needed basis, perhaps during a flare-up or a persistent period of poor sleep. I also "rotate" different medicines (prescribed or natural) for sleep. One medicine may be used during the week, and a different one used on weekends. This enables the beneficial effects of improved sleep, but also allows the body a periodic wash-out effect, and decreases the chance of developing a tolerance to, or side effects from, the medicines. Weekends are not the time to try to "catch up" on your sleep; you need to stay in a consistent pattern all week.

An ideal prescribed sleep modifier would be one taken at bedtime that starts working when you have "naturally" reached deep sleep, and acts to continue deep sleep for several more hours. Instead of waking up at 4:00 AM , you wake up at 7:00 AM and feel refreshed. The medicine shouldn't cause any morning sedation, confusion, or hangover effects. I prescribe a number of sleep modifiers, including Sonata, Ambien, Restoril and others.

Many recommended natural sleep modifiers are available over-the-counter. They include melatonin, valerian root, 5-HTP, St. John's Wort, Passion Flower, and Kava Kava. To Your Health (Fountain Hills, Arizona) markets a product called Sleep Formula™ (a combination of 5-HTP, Valerian, Lemon Balm and Passion Flower), which I frequently recommend as a non-drug way to increase serotonin and improve sleep. Some people do well with over-the-counter medicines that contain Diphenhydramine (Benadryl). Others can get headaches, morning hangovers, or increased fatigue when taking Benadryl at night. I always advise that you work with a knowledgeable medical professional when considering natural sleep modifiers. Natural medicines can sometimes interact with prescribed medicines or have side effects that can cause problems. You want to sleep well, not for all eternity!

The Bed

I'm frequently asked what type of bed is best. Should a water bed be considered or a mattress? I personally have found the most comfortable bed to be one that has a good firm mattress with a soft "pillow top" pad. This type of mattress provides good support for the spine, but also provides some cushion effect on sore skin. Many people report that water beds are hard to get in and out of and do not support the spine as well, so they are not as comfortable. If your mattress is soft and you sink into it, or if you find that you are more comfortable sleeping on the floor instead of on your bed, you need to consider investing in a firm new mattress. Some patients benefit from an egg crate pad on top of the mattress, others have had success with purchasing a form-fitting mattress. Some patients like to use magnetic mattress pads and say their pain is decreased and energy level improved. Consider a one week trial with a magnetic mattress before you purchase one to be sure it helps first.

The Pillow(s)

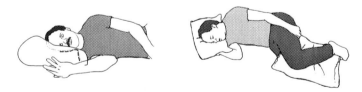

You probably have seen hundreds of pillows offered to improve your sleep. I prefer the old-fashioned, lightly packed feather pillow that I can mold and fluff to fit. Your goals for proper head position during the night include:

1. The pillow should be soft and comfortable.

2. Your head and neck should be supported in a natural position. The pillow shouldn't be too thick or fluffy as to push your neck upward, or so flimsy that your head sinks down too much, but just right so that your head is in the neutral position, centered between your shoulders when you are lying on your side.

3. Your pillow should adjust to your changing positions during the night. A pitfall of customized, fabricated pillows is that they work great for one position only. In reality we shift into many positions during the night.

Your pillow should be shaped so that it allows your head to be in the neutral position and properly centered, yet it should have a fullness to support the neck gap between your head and shoulders when you are lying down (on your side or your back). This "neck gap" support is important to enable the neck muscles to relax during the night by having some support. If you change positions, you naturally adjust your pillow. A customized pillow can be moved as needed. I've had many patients tell me that the water/gel pillows are comfortable for them. A specialized head pillow containing biologic magnets have been helpful to a number of people.

Body pillows can be added. Some people do well with the very long body pillow that intertwines the head, neck, arms, and hip areas. Others prefer to have a separate head pillow and arm and leg pillows. Other people have gotten lost under a pile of pillows in their bed!

When lying on the side, a pillow should be placed between the knees to properly align the hips and pelvis. Use a small thin pillow that separates the knees only a few inches. This reduces the stress on the hips and sacroiliac areas and increases comfort. If a thicker pillow that separates the knees too far (more than a few inches) is used, there may be too much stress placed on the hip and sacroiliac joints.

Many patients have discovered that an extra long pillow, not a body pillow, will help with the head and neck positioning and arm cushioning and support. I prefer the extra long pillow to position my head and neck, and also to cushion my arms. You may need to experiment with different pillows and be creative. If you are not comfortable with a particular pillow, no matter how highly recommended it comes, get rid of it and find another one. Likewise, if you find a perfect pillow, take it with you wherever you go and guard it with your life!

Other Sleep Necessities

Other sleep necessities in terms of equipment include a bed sheet and a blanket. If you are bothered by hot flashes when you first lay down at night, use the sheet only, but have the blanket ready to cover yourself in the middle of the night when you start to feel the other extremes of your autonomic nerves kicking in, the cold limbs. An electric mattress pad or an electric blanket, when used properly, can help keep you warm. Many people have done well with a magnetic mattress pad but others, including me, find that it makes them too hot and causes uncomfortable night sweats, particularly in the neck and upper back areas.

A clock is optional since we all have excellent internal alarm clocks, and we simply will ourselves to get up at a certain time. However, to keep us company while we are clock-watching during the night, it is not a bad idea to have a clock with nice big numbers so we can easily see how long it is that we are not sleeping! To minimize the cold chills, keep limbs covered with long sleeves and long-legged clothing, and wear cotton socks to bed. The tubular athletic socks work well when it comes to keeping your feet warm. The higher the socks, the warmer the legs!

Keep the room temperature comfortable, about 72 degrees. During winter, be sure to keep warm; you may have to turn the thermostat up during the night. You can always turn it back down in the morning after you are up and about. NEVER sleep with an open window or be in the path of direct drafts from vents. Central air conditioning is okay, and is preferred by those who do worse with temperature fluctuations, but avoid the direct cool air drafts. Air drafts are synonymous with muscle spasms!

Body Position

What is the best sleeping position with fibromyalgia? I believe it is lying on the side in a modified fetal position. To assume this position, you lie on your side with your knees bent up, tilt your head forward, and place your arms to your side, bent at the elbows. The hands and wrists need to be in the neutral positions, though, because the fetal positions of these joints (fingers curled and wrists bent down) are usually painful. So sleep like a baby but keep your wrists and hands neutral.

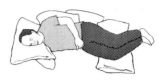

If you haven't been sleeping in this position, it can take about a week to become accustomed to this new position. Once you make the change, your body will adapt to this new position and automatically make the adjustments while you are asleep.

Sleeping on the stomach usually hurts. In this position, your stomach sinks into the bed and arches the back, which puts strain on the back during the night. Likewise, sleeping on the back causes your shoulders and buttocks to arch your back and form a "bridge" which can increase pain. Bending the knees can help relieve some of the low back pressure when lying on your back. In the stomach or low back positions, the muscles in the neck and back are working hard instead of relaxing even though you may be sleeping.

The head and neck should maintain neutral position. Once you are in the final sleeping position, the head and neck should be aligned properly with the shoulder. In this position, individual neck muscles are not strained. Make sure the pillow does not allow the head to sink too far into the bed or be pushed too far away from the bed once your comfortable position is assumed so as not to cause unnatural positioning of the head and neck.

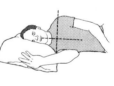

Another position that can be comfortable is lying mostly on the back but tilting to the side with a pillow under both knees. This pillow under the knees prevents the legs from straightening out and thus arching the back. Remember your fibronomics.

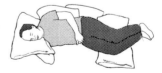

The arms and legs also need to be positioned as part of the overall proper sleep posture. Your arms are not pillows, so avoid lying on them or resting your head on your hands. This puts pressures on the muscles and nerves and will often cause you to wake at night with a numb arm. Avoid stretching your arms over your head also. If you are lying on your side, the arm closest to the bed can be tucked under the pillow. Be careful to keep your elbow out in front of you so you are not lying directly on the elbow. The other arm can be draped over the pillow, if you have a longer pillow, which prevents the arm from resting on your body.

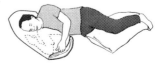

The legs seem to do best in a bent position, with the knees separated by a pillow as mentioned above. If the knees are on top of each other, the hardness of both knees can often cause pain, and the pillow between the knees helps this problem. The ankles can be overlapped so they are not directly on each other, or if you are using a pillow between your knees that reaches down to the ankles, cushion the ankles with this pillow. If you are lying on your back, keep the knees bent. Remember, it takes some time to train yourself to become comfortable in these new body positions; then your subconscious will take over and put you into these positions during the night.

Getting Back To Sleep

Invariably, for one reason or another, we awaken during the night. Our goals are to decrease the number of times we wake at night and to increase the speed at which we can fall back to sleep. If you are on prescription sleep medicines, it is usually easier to fall back to sleep quickly. If you wake up, don't make a big deal about it; just tell yourself you will quickly fall back asleep. If you need to use the bathroom, have a night light in the bathroom. Some studies have shown that a red light minimizes eye glare and "irritation" at night, so try a red night light. The key is to not turn on a bright 150 watt light, 12 inches from your eyes! Make sure there is enough lighting so you can see and don't fall over something.

If you get back in bed but find yourself unable to fall asleep again, repeat your relaxation strategies, or try a mental rehearsing strategy. That is, think about something that might involve numbers and calculations and try to do mental math. You know, boring stuff that hopefully will signal your body to get so bored that it just falls back asleep. Some prescribed sleeping medicines can be repeated in the middle of the night from time to time. Your doctor may allow you to take an extra dose of sleep modifier if everything else fails.

Hopefully, you can develop good sleep habits and go through the various sleep stages. Ultimately, you can experience good Stage 4 sleep!

Managing Fatigue

Chronic fatigue syndrome (CFS) is a condition that is very similar to fibromyalgia. In fact, many medical professionals believe that the two are actually the same condition. CFS may be a subset of a broader fibromyalgia syndrome. Table 1 lists the 1994 International Research case definition of CFS.

Table 1: 1994 International Research Case Definition Of Chronic Fatigue Syndrome

CFS is a syndrome characterized by fatigue that is :

- Medically unexplained
- Of new onset
- Of at least six months' duration
- Not the result of ongoing exertion
- Not substantially relieved by rest
- Causes a substantial reduction in previous levels of occupational, educational, social, or personal activities

In addition, there must be four or more of the following symptoms:

- Impaired memory or concentration
- Sore throat
- Tender neck (cervical) or armpit (axillary) lymph nodes
- Muscle pain (myalgia)
- Headaches of a new type, pattern, or severity
- Unrefreshing sleep
- Post-exertional malaise (lasting more than 24 hours)
- Multi-joint pain (arthralgia without swelling or redness)

Conditions that would exclude a diagnosis of CFS include other medical disorders known to cause fatigue, major depressive illness, medications that cause fatigue as a side effect, and alcohol or substance abuse. Fukuda, *et al*. The chronic fatigue syndrome: a comprehensive approach to its definition and study, *Ann Intern Med* 1994; 121: 953-959.

In the fibromyalgia spectrum I've described (see Chapter 11), I would put chronic fatigue syndrome in subset 6: fibromyalgia with a particular associated condition. The particular associated condition is chronic fatigue syndrome.

In CFS support groups and fibromyalgia support groups I have attended, both pain and fatigue are frequent topics of discussion. A person with CFS who sees me usually has other associated conditions, including sleep disorder, headache, muscle pain, joint pain, difficulty concentrating, and neurologic symptoms. Not surprisingly, the exam usually reveals typical painful tender points. Overall, I treat patients with CFS pretty much the same way I treat patients with fibromyalgia, especially if those with chronic fatigue syndrome are having a lot of pain.

I think one person describing her fatigue said it best. She said her eyelids felt like cement weights and she felt like she was wearing cement shoes. Fatigue can be an overwhelming problem in fibromyalgia, and unfortunately, many people get the double curse, both severe pain and severe fatigue. Why do patients with fibromyalgia (and CFS) have such a problem with fatigue? There are multiple factors involved. These factors include:

1. **Non-restorative sleep disorder**. As we reviewed in the last chapter, restoration that should be occurring during the deep stage of sleep is not happening. Manufacture of proteins, replenishment of energy stores, and repair of tissues are incomplete. Poor sleep leads to increased fatigue.

2. **Deconditioned muscles**. Deconditioned muscles in fibromyalgia have lost their ability to make the body's energy molecules called ATP (adenosine triphosphate). This energy molecule is stored in our tissues, particularly muscles, and is used as fuel to enable the body to perform all of its functions, including muscle contractions. The less ATP around, the less energy available, and once the stored supplies are used up, fatigue occurs. If this process occurs quickly, one may feel a sudden, unpredictable energy crash. In fibromyalgia, our chronically low ATP contributes to chronic fatigue.

3. **Constant pain**. The body's process of monitoring pain, recording pain, and expressing pain is energy consuming and involves nerves, neurotransmitters, and other enzymes and hormones. The patient in constant pain will use up more energy and have less stored energy than normal.

4. **Decreased oxygen use by the muscles**. Studies have shown that muscles with fibromyalgia do not use oxygen as well as normal muscles. This may reflect a problem with the muscle mitochondria, the small organelles that use oxygen and manufacture ATP. A biochemical problem may prevent the available oxygen from being used efficiently and adequately to create ATP.

5. **Associated clinical depression**. Depression is seen in nearly half of patients with fibromyalgia and can cause extreme mental fatigue.

6. **Associated chronic conditions** such as arthritis, hypothyroidism, or other disease. People with fibromyalgia may have other conditions that consume a lot of energy and contribute to excessive fatigue.

7. **Cognitive factors**. Fibromyalgia causes difficulty with concentration and attention, increased anxiety, increased sensitivity to depression, and absentmindedness. This is our fibrofog which I will review in the next chapter.

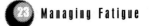

8. **Dysfunctional autonomic nervous system**. We are more prone to anxiety and panic attacks, Raynaud's phenomenon, fast heart rate (especially in response to stress), rashes on the skin (especially in response to touch), throat tightness, irritable bowel syndrome, irritable bladder and other symptoms that are all consequences of an over-sensitized autonomic nervous system. Fatigue can also be a consequence of our dysfunctional autonomic nerves. I will review the autonomic nerve dysfunctions in more detail in Chapter 26.

9. **Visual overload**. I use this term to describe the overwhelming information our eyes receive and have difficulty interpreting, as I reviewed in Chapter 4. We try to spot a particular object but are confronted with a variety of shapes, sizes, colors, and lines in different directions that literally overwhelm our visual senses and at times cause a feeling of dizziness, light-headedness and increased anxiety. I believe this contributes to fatigue by demanding so much energy to sort out this information.

10. **Decreased respiratory endurance**. Many patients with fibromyalgia complain about their shortness of breath with short bursts of activity such as climbing steps, running or walking swiftly. They may actually have difficulty catching their breath. This respiratory complaint may be from sudden exercise-induced fatigue of the respiratory muscles that disrupts the breathing rhythm. The complaint seems to be independent of whether or not the person is out of condition or living a sedentary lifestyle. Since an efficient breathing process is necessary to deliver oxygen to the bloodstream, any problem in this area will certainly create potential for fatigue.

11. **Constant muscle movements**. People with fibromyalgia are frequently shifting their bodies to find more comfortable positions. Habitual movements such as tapping fingers on the table, tapping or bouncing the feet on the ground, frequent crossing of the legs, and kicking out a leg are probably subconscious movements to relieve muscle stress, keep the blood flowing, and readjust the muscles and posture to try to decrease the pain. However, the side effect of these movement patterns is increased energy consumption.

12. **Hormonal problems**. Decreased supply of hormones or inefficient use of available hormones may factor into fatigue. Low growth hormone and low thyroid levels are common in fibromyalgia and can decrease energy metabolism and hence increase fatigue. Altered stress mechanisms in our bodies will increase energy consumption and interfere with efficient use of energy, hence fatigue is worsened. Other hormones that can cause fatigue when in short supply are estrogen and serotonin.

13. **Hypoglycemia/insulin hypersensitivity**. In Chapter 17, I discussed the role of hypoglycemia and insulin hypersensitivity in causing fatigue. Our brains require a steady dose of glucose and if our nutritional dysfunctions lead to hypoglycemia, our brains will react by signaling: "You'll feel lousy until I get more glucose!"

14. **Low magnesium**. As I reviewed in Chapter 17, magnesium levels in the cells are low in most fibromyalgia patients. Magnesium is a key mineral in the formation of ATP/energy molecules in the muscles. Low magnesium means low ATP, which means more fatigue.

15. **Candidiasis**. *Candida albicans* is a yeast normally found in healthy intestines. In fibromyalgia, *Candida* can overgrow in the intestines and become "unfriendly." This can lead to systemic symptoms including fatigue. Chapter 25 discusses this problem in more detail.

Fatigue creates problems in our daily activities, regardless of the cause or causes. A major negative effect of fatigue is increased pain which in turn consumes more energy and causes further fatigue—

a self-perpetuating cycle of pain and fatigue. Fatigue interferes with our ability and motivation to socialize, carry out daily routine chores, and perform our jobs properly.

When one is fatigued, it is difficult to converse or communicate, thus interfering with our relationships. Muscles become more deconditioned and we experience decreased overall cardiovascular fitness. We may develop feelings of depression and overall decreased well-being. Even if we have no energy, we still tend to feel stressed and, like the pain, the additional stress consumes more energy and further increases our fatigue. Fibrofog further aggravates fatigue (see next chapter).

Treating Fatigue

There are many strategies for treating fatigue. Fatigue will probably never be completely eliminated, but many things can be done to control its consequences and minimize its impact on everyday life. Your doctor may first want to investigate for underlying diseases such as hypothyroidism, sleep disorders, anemia, and connective tissue disease, which involve different treatment approaches. If there are no significant underlying diseases present, the fatigue may be attributed to the fibromyalgia syndrome (or chronic fatigue syndrome).

Some specific labs that I frequently order in fibromyalgia patients with significant fatigue include:

- Complete blood count (to evaluate for anemia or blood disorders)
- Sedimentation rate (to evaluate for any underlying inflammation)
- T4, TSH levels (to evaluate for any thyroid abnormalities)
- Insulin-like growth factor 1 level (to measure for growth hormone deficiencies)
- Magnesium RBC level (to measure for any intracellular magnesium deficiency)

If labs are in the normal range but low/normal, I may interpret these to be "abnormal" for an individual patient. That is, the patient's level is still too low for what the patient needs even though the level may be within the normal range.

What steps can be taken to minimize the potential debilitating effects of fatigue? Below is a list of strategies that I have found helpful:

1. **Develop good sleep habits**. Quality sleep is necessary for the body to manufacture energy. Develop a good sleep routine.

2. **Avoid long daytime naps**. Although fatigue may be compelling at times, it is best to try to avoid taking naps since this alters the body's sleep rhythm. Naps are often non-refreshing and time-consuming. Upon awakening, many people feel even less energetic and have more difficulty getting going again. They may even have a period of increased confusion and mental fogginess.

In some people, however, a strategic nap (less than one hour) accomplishes its goal by refreshing and restoring the individual for more successful completion of the remainder of the day. As long as the primary nighttime sleep is not disturbed any more than usual, these naps are not to be discouraged. However, it is my experience (and sleep studies show) that most people who try to overcome fatigue with a nap actually do not accomplish

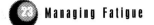

the refreshing and restoring mood that they are seeking, and the evening sleep pattern is disrupted.

3. **Proper nutrition.** I reviewed a dietary strategy in Chapter 17. A higher protein/lower carbohydrate diet has helped many people improve their energy. Diets too rich in fat can put the body into a lazy mode, but if you reduce your fats at the expense of getting too little protein, you may have more fatigue, so find your balance.

4. **Medications (natural and prescription).** The dozens of natural supplements advertised to increase energy are successful for some people. However, many energy products contain the stimulants caffeine or ephedrine, which can have long-term adverse effects on the body and can be dangerous if taken together. Before trying any natural energy product, I recommend first consulting with your doctor.

   I recommend a Magnesium and Malic Acid combination (especially Fibro-Care™ from To Your Health) and Colostrum as the top two supplements to try to improve energy levels. Magnesium and Malic Acid combinations work by increasing energy formed in the muscle. Colostrum promotes improved metabolism and energy by increasing growth hormone levels.

   If the B_{12} level is low/normal, I may recommend vitamin B_{12} in either lozenge, sublingual or injection form. B_{12} pills may not absorb well from the stomach, whereas the other forms of B_{12} are absorbed differently (lozenges and sublingual forms are absorbed into the blood from the capillaries in the mouth and underneath the tongue, and injection B_{12} is absorbed into the bloodstream from the muscle).

   If the thyroid is low or low/normal, I may prescribe Armour Thyroid in the morning. Co-enzyme Q_{10} (CoQ_{10}) is another supplement that can help increase ATP/energy levels in the muscles.

   Prescribed medicines that increase serotonin levels can help improve energy as well. These include the selective-serotonin reuptake inhibitors (SSRI's) such as Prozac, Zoloft, Paxil, Celexa, Lexapro and Effexor.

   Wellbutrin is a different type of antidepressant that is reported to increase the norepinephrine level instead of the serotonin level. Norepinephrine is important in improving our focusing, concentration and energy levels.

   5-HTP is a natural nutritional building block for serotonin which can help improve sleep and mood and decrease pain, all which can help fatigue. St. John's Wort and SAM-e are other natural herbal antidepressants that can help increase serotonin levels. If underlying depression is a problem, your physician may opt to prescribe an antidepressant medication because improving the depression will usually improve the fatigue as well.

   Certain prescription medicines known as central nervous system stimulants can be prescribed by your doctor in cases of extreme fatigue causing debilitating functional problems. These medicines are similar to the ones used for children with attention deficit disorders. They include Ritalin, Cylert and Provigil.

5. **Follow proper fibronomics.** Maintaining proper body posture at home and at work will not only conserve energy, but decrease pain.

6. **Plan scheduled activities, especially in the evening.** The late afternoon and early evening are often the most difficult times for persons with fatigue. After supper can be an especially

difficult time, especially if the person sits down to relax or lies down to read the paper. "Crashing" and inability to do any useful activity for the rest of the evening may occur.

My advice is to routinely plan some activity, especially for after supper, that includes running errands, getting outside, visiting people, or just staying up on your feet. You will be surprised to learn how frequently a second wind will come. Many people have a natural rhythm that causes low energy in the late afternoon and early evening, but then the mood and energy level swings back up again. If you are a night owl, you tend to feel better and more energetic around 9 PM and may have a few good hours where you feel alert and can accomplish a lot. Recognize your own biorhythm and take advantage of it to plan your best work around your high points and to try to stimulate yourself through the low points by involving yourself in an activity.

7. **Divide your task into smaller projects** instead of one big one. Do a little at a time and do more at your best time. For example, yard work can be divided into specific chores for different nights of the week. You may mow the front lawn one night, the back another, and trim on a third night, instead of doing all three in one day. If we are moving and decide to do our own packing, it is much easier to pack a box per day for the six weeks prior to the actual moving date, than to try to do all the packing in one or two days before the actual move. This type of self-discipline is also needed when vacationing and decorating for the holidays. (Actually, self discipline could help a lot of things!)

8. **Perform regular exercise and relaxation.** Exercise increases endurance, cardiovascular conditioning, and a sense of well being. In fact, regular exercise is the best way to improve the ATP/energy manufacturing within our muscles. Relaxation decreases stress and reduces pain. A 30-minute brisk walk after supper provides exercise and mental relaxation and counteracts the low biorhythm point at the same time. One does not have to sit perfectly still to physically and mentally relax; in fact, this often increases fatigue and the tendency to sleep. Remember to relax, not nap.

9. **Make a daily schedule** and check off things as you accomplish them. Allow plenty of time to complete the task. By keeping a structured list, you have a better chance of motivating yourself to reach daily goals.

10. **Delegate chores to others**. One of the best energy-saving techniques known is to have someone else use his or her energy to do your task! While delegating responsibilities is difficult for many people, there are others who will gladly perform certain chores for you. It is best to be as independent as possible, but it is better to allow someone else to help if it means you will have energy for a longer portion of your day.

Hopefully, some of these weapons can help you combat fatigue. Remember that fatigue, like pain, is a "relative" problem (no, I don't mean cousin Vito!). The problem is always there, but you try to achieve a lower, more functional state that, relative to the previous level, is considered a successful, manageable level.

Fibrofog

Top Ten Ways To Know Your Brain Is Affected By Fibromyalgia

1. You confuse your right arm with your left leg.

2. You discover 14 different routes home from work, when in actuality there are only two.

3. You avoid salad bars because too many decisions are involved.

4. Pre-schoolers challenge you to chess games.

5. The national weather forecast issues a fog warning in your brain.

6. You get distracted by clouds while driving.

7. People seem more interested in talking to your pets than to you.

8. You write yourself daily reminders that read "don't forget to breathe, eat, and sleep today."

9. You consistently lose memory games played with your two-year-old son.

10. You've made mistakes on your last 50 checks written.

Hello fibromyalgia sufferers! Have you forgotten your best friend's name recently? Did you try to call your older son "Sadie" (and your dog's ears perked up)? Do you frequently mispll words? Have you stopped in mid-sentence to figure out which side is right and which is left? Do you dread being asked directions, or wonder how to properly tell people you've forgotten what you were going to say? Have you read this paragraph three times and it still doesn't make any sense?

If you've answered yes to any of these questions, then you are probably suffering from fibrofog. Fibrofog is a potent by-product of fibromyalgia, capable of quickly rendering intelligent, articulate individuals into bumbling zombies.

But now there's an amazing new product that's destined to end the fog forever. That's right, one product, once a day and you'll never forget again. Hard to believe? Well listen to what Matt has to say about it:

"Hello my name is Matt. I used to, you know, like, stumble my words all the time okay? I would, umm, like, not know my girlfriend's name and I'd call her Sandy, but her name is really Cindy okay? And she'd get mad at me and call me names and make me feel, like, what's the word? Like I'm sad or bummed out, okay? But now I'm doing better because … DEPRESSED! That's the word I was looking for. Now I'm not depressed, okay? This product makes my mind like clearer, more in focus. Now I think my thoughts better, you know, and I am happier, okay? You should try this stuff, okay?"

"You can have this amazing product today. Just call 1-555-I-FORGET and we'll send you what you need. This product is only available through us. Your doctor doesn't even know about this wonderful product made from our top secret formula containing our patented double-ionized magnetized water molecules. Call now. Don't forget. Write down the number so you won't forget."

Perhaps the most frustrating complaint I hear from patients with fibromyalgia is the fibrofog. Unlike the pain and fatigue which are usually constant nuisances, this problem causes unpredictable difficulties with our thinking. The unpredictability is the very reason it's most frustrating. You never know when it will strike.

Fibrofog, as you may recall from Section I (or may have forgotten already!) is the cognitive dysfunction brought on by fibromyalgia. Its symptoms include:

- Forgetfulness
- Absentmindedness
- Concentration problems
- Confusion
- Disorientation (get lost easily)
- Difficulty finding or saying words
- Short-term memory loss
- Difficulty understanding what you've read
- Difficulty calculating simple math problems
- Mixing up words
- Right-left confusion
- Poor ability to give directions

Additional cognitive symptoms with more emotional components include:

- Depression
- Irritability
- Anxiety
- Panic attacks

Fibrofog is not a dementia or early Alzheimer's. We demonstrate normal learning and memory although we process information more slowly because of our fibromyalgia.

Causes

Multiple factors are probably involved in causing symptoms of fibrofog. On a hormonal level, we have lower than normal concentrations of serotonin and norepinephrine in our brains. Serotonin is important for controlling pain in our central nervous system and relaxing our brain. Norepinephrine is responsible for focusing our thoughts and helping us concentrate. A low level of these 2 hormones will increase fibrofog symptoms.

Our brain's attention centers are overwhelmed with signals which may contribute to neurological causes of fibrofog. At the attention centers, sensory signals arrive and are relayed to different areas including centers for emotion, motor reactions, and memory. If the attention and relay centers are continuously bombarded by pain signals, the centers may be "overwhelmed" and signals get processed more slowly, or blocked, or even lost altogether. This can result in symptoms such as word-finding difficulties, inability to remember something, or delayed recall.

Pain and fatigue demand attention from our brain. Our brains continuously monitor these extra "doses" of symptoms in fibromyalgia. This engages so much of our brain's attention that very little attention "space" is available to allow us to process, retain and recall "routine" information.

Analogy: The Cluttered Hallway

In order to explain fibrofog to my patients, I have come up with the "cluttered hallway" analogy. Picture your brain as the upstairs of a house. In this house, the upstairs bedrooms are neat, organized, and behind closed doors. The common hallway leading to each bedroom is cluttered with laundry baskets, piles of clothing, boxes, shoes, toys, and furniture. One has to navigate the clutter in order to access a bedroom, causing some delay in reaching the door.

The person trying to get into the bedroom is like the nerve signal trying to access a memory trace. The person (nerve signal) climbs the steps (spinal cord) up to the second floor (brain) and is standing in the common hallway (attention center). The egress to the bedroom door (memory) is slowed by all the clutter (neurochemical changes from fibromyalgia). Sometimes it seems to take forever to get to a door, and at other times the person can't remove all the clutter to open the door in a timely manner. This leads to either delayed processing, or inability to read the intended thought or memory.

Once one gets to the bedroom door and opens it, the room (memory) is in good order and can be accessed freely. In fibromyalgia, the bedrooms are neat. In dementia, the bedrooms would be in a disarray. The bottom line is: keep your bedroom clean and let's work together on clearing the hallway.

Another Analogy: Cable Access vs. Dial-Up

To those of you who are computer literate, a simple fibrofog analogy is like having dial-up internet service on your computer instead of cable access. If you have internet service through your phone line, you often experience nuisance delays, or even get "kicked off" before you can get online. Once online, the computer's memory and web pages are in order, but you may experience long delays to access them. Sometimes the delays are so long that you get "timed out." Signals trying to get through the phone line to retrieve web pages are like signals trying to get through our attention center to retrieve memories. Why don't normal people without fibromyalgia have these delays? Because they have cable connections for their computer and their signals travel quickly without delay.

Doctors with fibromyalgia who try to write about fibrofog analogies often make things more complicated and confuse themselves in the midst of their writing, or whatever it was they were trying to do.

Handling Fibrofog

There are a number of strategies to try to treat fibrofog. We can try to take advantage of every strategy available to keep our minds less befuddled.

Write Things Down

Write notes frequently and organize the notes. When I write material for my book, I go through a routine where I jot down ideas and notes on pieces of paper and collect these papers. Then I start to organize these notes in an outline format. I think of details and let my thought processes evolve over days and weeks, while continuing to write notes and organize these notes. From there on I can write my first version of the chapter, revising and categorizing along the way.

If one writes down notes and plans his or her days, or writes down names of people met or key pieces of information for an upcoming meeting or visit, the writing preparation serves two purposes. First, the writing actually reinforces what you are trying to remember. When you write something down you are delivering information via a different pathway to the brain and make it easier to remember by just "thinking it." Second, when you write something down, you can allow your mind to relax and not worry about forgetting it because you can simply refer to your written notes.

Consistent Routine

You need to consciously train yourself to follow a routine and strive for consistency. I always try to follow a specific routine. For example, my car keys can only be in three places: my pocket, on top of my desk, or on the kitchen counter. When I come home from work, I've trained myself to put them in those places. If I throw the keys on the bed, for example, I must consciously tell myself to stop everything and take the keys to the proper location. I used to think "I'll remember where they are," but a few seconds later that memory was completely gone and later on I would spend many minutes searching for my keys.

You can train yourself to follow a consistent routine with practically everything you do, from the time you go to bed to the time you get up: the order in which you approach your morning routine; the locations where you've placed all your necessary items; the day planner that you check off as you complete different tasks and so forth. Once you have trained yourself, it will become automatic for you. Plus, the routine will save you a lot of time and frustration. In this case, the best desired strategy is "same-old, same-old."

Relaxation

Because we have difficulty with our attention spans and our ability to recall information, we are more prone to increased mental stress, which further contributes to mental fatigue.

Achieving a relaxation response helps to counteract episodes of fibrofog. So practice your relaxation strategies that you've learned. Make this routine part of your day. Many times we think our best thoughts and remember the most when we are relaxing, lying down, and trying to get to sleep.

Medicines

A number of prescribed medicines can be considered to help counteract the symptoms of fibrofog. Selective serotonin reuptake inhibitors (*e.g.*, Prozac, Zoloft, Lexapro, Paxil) can work by helping to increase the serotonin level in the brain and facilitate neurobiological connections between the attention center and other brain centers. Medicines that include norepinephrine (*e.g.*, Wellbutrin) can help as well. Medicines in the central nervous system stimulant category (*e.g.*, Cylert, Ritalin, Provigil) may also help by improving our brain alertness and attention. Any medicine strategy that helps reduce pain and improve energy level can help the fibrofog by reducing all the overwhelming signals that bombard the attention center and clutter the hallways.

Prescribed medicines can also interfere with memory, so they need to be evaluated and adjusted if they are aggravating fibrofog. Examples of medicine categories that can affect memory include selective serotonin reuptake inhibitors, tricyclic antidepressants, muscle relaxants, beta blockers, anti-anxiety medicines, anti-seizure medicines, and other medicines that have been used in the treatment of fibromyalgia. Any medicine that causes sedation or fatigue has potential to aggravate fibromyalgia as well.

Supplements

Some of the supplements that can be used to try to improve fibrofog include 5-HTP, colostrum, ginkgo biloba and vinpocetine. The 5-HTP works by providing a substrate for the body to build more serotonin. Colostrum works by increasing growth hormone level which enhances brain activity. Another supplement that can improve fatigue and fibrofog is ginkgo biloba. This supplement is thought to work by enhancing short and long-term memory by improving recall and retention, improving systemic blood flow, and facilitating nerve signals. A pilot study published in 2002 found that 64% reported improvement when taking a combination of ginkgo biloba and CoQ_{10} for fibromyalgia. Vinpocetine is a specific supplement that is felt to improve blood flow to the brain. Increased brain blood flow can boost glucose and oxygen use and improve fibrofog symptoms; dosing is 10–30 mg a day.

Don't Be Too Hard On Yourself

We try to do the best we can with forgetfulness and fibrofog symptoms. Some people can do well with memory association tricks such as trying to associate a person's name with a familiar object. I think the most reliable way is to write things down and knowing where to look for this written information. You reinforce the memory by writing it down, and you can relax your mind better because you know where to look for this information when you need it. You give yourself "permission" to forget.

Even though we may strive for a routine and may be successful at it, we will still forget things. We should not get mad at ourselves when this happens and try to simply work around what we're forgetting. Simply recognize that fibrofog is part of your fibromyalgia and if you forget something, it's really not your fault.

Sometimes I can't remember a particular medical word for a particular physical exam finding. When this happens, I'm not too hard on myself for not remembering the word and I compensate by trying to describe the abnormal finding. For example, I might not remember the term "Spurling's Sign" so I will say the person has radicular paresthesia when the head was fully rotated, laterally flexed, and extended, and a downward compression was applied to the top of the head. I guess it would have been a lot easier simply to say the patient had a positive Spurling Sign!

Dr. P's Memory Diary

by Mark J. Pellegrino, M.D.

Just to show you that this happens all the time, I've decided to keep a memory diary for one day in April 1999. I have summarized my memory diary for the day as follows:

In the morning I was using a red pen to make some corrections. I set the red pen down, made a copy of my changes and could not find the red pen to resume my work. Eventually I found it on the shelf by the copy machine.

I wrote the wrong date 5 times on various prescriptions and notes throughout the day. This occurred in spite of wearing a watch with the date on it.

I told a particular patient, "Nice to meet you," even though I had met the patient before. After I examined the patient and was finishing up, I said again, "Nice meeting you," and caught myself and said "again!"

I wrote down that a patient was a mall carrier instead of mail carrier. I spelled pain, p-a-i-n-e, and wrote that spasms were caused by waltzing instead of spasms caused by walking. Instead of writing "dry eyes and numb face," I wrote "dumb face." I have no clue why I wrote these things, and please don't ask me to psychoanalyze myself!

After seeing patients, I got ready for track practice (I am a coach). I set my keys down, got dressed and forgot where my keys were. And I'm always bragging that I don't lose my keys. I was out of my ordinary routine, however, and misplaced the keys and had to find them.

Later in the evening I realized I didn't have an important paper with notes on it. I had worked on it earlier in the evening and thought it was on my desk, but no, it wasn't. I spent 30 minutes (yes, I did!) looking through my briefcase, my car, my desk, and various piles of paper in the office. I couldn't find the paper, so I assumed I had left it at the sports facility. I went to bed and one minute after I laid down, I thought maybe I had mixed the piece of paper up with my bills, so I got up and checked the basket with the bills in it and there was the paper! How's that for a typical day!

We must realize that a typical day with our fibromyalgia may include betrayal by our brains. Our brains befuddle us, seemingly capable of only random acts of cognizance. We must recognize that we are capable of overcoming the fibrofog by following strategies that minimize the fog and by taking advantage of the times when the fog is temporarily lifted. Hopefully we can find clearer pathways through the clutter.

▶ If You Want To Know More

Ley BM. *Vinpocetine, boost your brain power with periwinkle extract*. BL Publications, 2000.

Candidiasis

What would you say if I told you we had millions of Mr. Hydes living in our bodies, each waiting for the opportune time to turn into Dr. Jekyll? Would you think I'm nuts or would you think I'm an expert!? ("He's losing it," says a reader from Michigan.) We all have little round whitish organisms in our body known as *Candida albicans* that can lose their innocence and become rather vicious creatures that attack our fibromyalgia bodies and make us feel worse.

Candida albicans is fungus or yeast that normally thrives in the mouth, gastrointestinal tract, vagina, and skin. In healthy individuals this yeast is helpful in digestion and vitamin production, and it is harmless because it is kept in check by beneficial bacteria and other yeast such as *Lactobacillus acidophilus* that occupies the same space.

When the balance of intestinal bacteria and yeast is altered, or your immune system becomes compromised, the *Candida* can overgrow, transforming from a benign yeast into an aggressive fungus that releases numerous toxins and can cause many symptoms. When fungal growth exceeds the body's ability to control it, the friendly *Candida* becomes unfriendly and causes a yeast infection.

Causes

Various causes of Candidiasis (*Candida* infection) include:

- Chronic illnesses or stress, *i.e.*, diabetic patients, hospitalized patients, and cancer patients all have low resistance to infection.

- Antibiotic use. This destroys normal bacteria and *Lactobacillus acidophilus*, but spares the *Candida*.

- Birth control pills. The estrogen favors *Candida* multiplication.

- Cortisone medicine

- Immunosuppressive drugs

- Pregnancy. Hormonal changes favor increased *Candida* growth.

- Diets high in sugar and carbohydrates. *Candida* loves glucose!

- Thyroid medicines. Increases *Candida* risk.

- Warm moist areas. Tight nylons, wet diapers, people who work as dish washers; all this can lead to *Candida* dermatitis.

- Alcohol. Another food for the *Candida*.

Those with fibromyalgia often have multiple risk factors, particularly the altered immune system, the chronic stress, and the carbohydrate sensitivity. Throw in the woman (I don't mean actually throw her!) who is on birth control pills, thyroid medicine, and recently took a course of antibiotics for bronchitis, and you have a recipe for "Candisaster!"

When *Candida albicans* transforms into an invasive fungal state, it produces rhizoids which are long root-like structures. Rhizoids can penetrate the intestinal walls and leave microscopic holes that allow toxins, undigested food particles, bacteria and yeast to enter the blood stream. This "invasion" leads to many symptoms.

Candidiasis Symptoms

- Bloating
- Irritable bowel syndrome (IBS)
- Chronic heartburn
- Oral thrush (white spots on the mouth and tongue)
- Vaginal yeast infection
- Skin rashes
- Skin itching
- Vulvar pain and itching
- Rectal itching
- Fatigue
- Irritability
- Fibrofog
- Food cravings (especially carbohydrates)
- Malnutrition (poor nutrient absorption)
- Food allergies
- Depression
- Bad breath

As you can see there is much overlap of Candidiasis symptoms with fibromyalgia symptoms. These two conditions "feed" into each other where the fibromyalgia makes one have more problems with the Candidiasis and the Candidiasis causes symptoms that can aggravate the fibromyalgia.

If I suspect Candidiasis, I will treat it separately from the fibromyalgia because this often leads to much improvement of fibromyalgia symptoms as well as correcting the *Candida* problem.

Testing for *Candida*

A simple home test for Candidiasis can be performed. Dr. Kelly Hannigan described a test you can take (*Health Points* 8 (2) 2003). Before you go to sleep at night set a clear glass of water next to your bed. When you wake up in the morning (before you clear your throat, swallow or speak), deposit your saliva into the glass of water. If within 30 minutes your saliva sinks to the bottom or there are strands of saliva running down into the water or the water turns cloudy you probably have an abundance of yeast in your body.

Lab testing can be done for a definitive diagnosis of Candidiasis. Saliva, stool and blood samples can all be tested to look for specific immunoglobulin antibodies against *Candida*. These tests are not routinely covered by insurance companies so the patient has to pay for these tests, which are usually several hundred dollars.

Since intestinal Candidiasis is so common and easily identified with careful history of symptoms, and since treatments are low-risk and well-tolerated, I will usually treat Candidiasis based on the clinical exam (history and physical) and not always order a specific yeast test.

Candidiasis Treatment

The strategies for treating Candidiasis are focused on rebalancing the intestinal bacteria and yeast. *Candida* that has overgrown needs to be killed and suppressed. The "good" yeast and bacteria needs to be replenished, and the gastrointestinal tract needs to be rebalanced. Here are some strategies used to rebalance the intestinal tract.

Antiyeast Products

Prescribed medicines to treat *Candida* include Nystatin (Mycostatin) and Fluconazole (Diflucan). Nystatin is available in tablet and liquid form. The liquid form is used to treat oral thrush ("swish and swallow.") The tablet forms are used for intestinal Candidiasis and they are usually well tolerated, although some people have some nausea or diarrhea with them. Patients may need to be on this medicine for several months and some of them need to be on maintenance dose for long-term *Candida* management. Nystatin kills off *Candida*, but does not harm the Lactobacillus or bacteria.

Fluconazole is another antifungal medicine that is given to treat Candidiasis. Sometimes one tablet or two tablets only are used to treat a vaginal yeast infection. However, a vaginal yeast infection or recurring vaginal yeast infections in women are a sign of more widespread Candidiasis; the vaginal yeast infection is actually the "tip of the iceberg." In treating intestinal or more widespread Candidiasis, Diflucan may need to be used for weeks instead of days.

Natural antiyeast treatments include herbal products such as enteric coated oregano extract and olive leaf extract (Oleuropein).

Olive leaf extract has the ability to attack *Candida* and other potential harmful microorganisms while sparing the helpful ones. To treat *Candida*, two capsules every eight hours on an empty stomach are recommended. Olive leaf extract can be used in conjunction with the prescribed antibiotic, or can be used as a first line anti-*Candida* treatment.

Herxheimer's Reaction

Herxheimer's reaction can occur when the *Candida* die off. A sudden die-off of *Candida* can release a lot of toxins and the result may be aggravation of symptoms. Whereas this is not necessarily a bad thing, this type of reaction can cause significant discomfort so we usually back off on the medicine to a lower dose to avoid a rapid die-off and to allow a slower and steadier die-off of *Candida*.

To minimize Herxheimer's reaction when taking Nystatin I have patients start with one Nystatin tablet on the first day and then increase by one tablet a day until the desired dose of six tablets a day is being taken. A slow die-off of the *Candida* is preferred as it allows the gastrointestinal tract to better rebalance and not create sudden acute changes that a rapid die-off can cause. Plus a slower die-off allows the friendly yeast and bacteria to gradually fill the spaces and help rebuild the intestines.

Friendly Replenishers

Lactobacillus acidophilus and the good bacteria are called probiotics. These "friendly" yeast and bacteria help with digestion and vitamin production, and when *Candida* has died off, these friendly probiotics are necessary to help rebuild the gastrointestinal flora by filling the spaces where *Candida* used to be and restoring proper balance.

> These "friendly" yeast and bacteria help with digestion and vitamin production, and when *Candida* has died off, these friendly probiotics are necessary to help rebuild the gastrointestinal flora by filling in the spaces where *Candida* used to be and restoring proper balance.

An *acidophilus* supplement is recommended to help replenish the flora. Fructooligosaccharides (FOS) are the food source for healthy bacteria. Any good nutrient (FOS) for the probiotics (*acidophilus* and other friendly bacteria) is called prebiotic. I like to use a product by To Your Health called *Acidophilus ES*, which is a prebiotic and probiotic blend that helps counteract *Candida* buildup and maintain healthy intestinal flora. Acidophilus supplements have done an excellent job of treating irritable bowel syndrome, which reinforces the theory that a lot of irritable bowel flare-up can be related to Candidiasis. I usually have patients continue the acidophilus on an ongoing basis, especially when fibromyalgia increases their risk of Candidiasis.

Dietary Strategies

The *Candida* thrive on high sugar concentrations, so a basic diet strategy is cutting back the number of carbs. Fermented foods such as soy sauce, vinegar, pickles, cheese and yogurt have high sugar concentrations that feed yeast so these should be avoided. The fibromyalgia diet that I described in Chapter 17 is also a good antiyeast diet.

In addition to watching the carbohydrates, you should make sure to get enough fiber in your diet because that will help eliminate toxins and unwanted yeast in the bowel. Many people can learn to control *Candida* yeast overgrowth simply by modifying the diet. Often a combination of yeast antibiotic and friendly replenishers is also necessary along with dietary changes.

Avoid Aggravating Factors

If possible, avoid drugs, chemicals and foods that can trigger the *Candida* and its symptoms. Since alcohol can aggravate *Candida*, it should be avoided or used in moderation. Obviously it is not practical to stop thyroid medicine, hormone medicines or other necessary prescribed medicines.

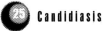

Likewise, if you develop a bacterial infection, you may require an antibiotic. If you must take an antibiotic for a bacterial infection, you might want to also take Nystatin or a natural yeast antibiotic to counteract the potential for *Candida* overgrowth while on the antibiotic. Any prescription medication that you have identified as a cause of Candidiasis should be reviewed with your doctor to see if it can be reduced or changed.

If you have Candidiasis, you can successfully transform the *Candida* back to Mr. Hyde where he can live peacefully in the normal flora neighborhood. (located on Large Intestine Avenue and Skin Street, between Oral Road and Vaginal Way!)

Those Dysfunctional Autonomics

Top Ten Signs That Your Autonomic Nerves Have Gone Astray

1. You have anxiety attacks while napping.

2. Clam fishermen gather around and stare at your hands.

3. Your sweat freezes.

4. When you get embarrassed, neighbors plan impromptu cookout and barbecue hot dogs on your face.

5. The pounding in your head drowns out the loud music.

6. When taking a leisurely stroll, you uncontrollably scream out "I can't stand it anymore!"

7. Puncture wounds from the hair standing up on your arms.

8. Skin rashes begin to form messages like "I hurt all over."

9. Entomologists request permission to study "whatever is crawling under your skin."

10. Your teeth begin to sweat.

Our autonomics have gone astray in fibromyalgia. In addition to causing pain and fatigue, the dysfunctional and hypersensitive autonomic nerves can cause a number of distinct conditions which are part of fibromyalgia but may require separate treatment approaches to try to calm them down. In this chapter, I will address six such conditions that are the result of those dysfunctional autonomics: irritable bowel syndrome, irritable bladder, depression, anxiety disorder and panic attacks, migraine headaches, and near-syncope.

Irritable Bowel Syndrome (IBS)

IBS is seen in the majority of patients with fibromyalgia syndrome and can cause cramping, bloating, gas pains, diarrhea and constipation due to dysfunctional autonomic nerves. Shortly after a meal, cramping and diarrhea may result. If the bowel is stretched from gas or constipation, there can be increased pain. There is no actual damage to the bowel, but the syndrome produces distressing symptoms. In addition to the cramping pain and diarrhea alternating with constipation, other symptoms can include swollen or bloated abdomen, mucus in the stool, or a feeling that you have not emptied your bowels completely after a bowel movement.

Certain foods can trigger IBS symptoms, including nut products, chocolate, caffeine, carbonated drinks, fatty foods and alcohol. Women with IBS will tend to have more symptoms during their menstrual period. And, intestinal Candidiasis can aggravate IBS. Different tests may be ordered to investigate IBS. Tests that can be done include: lab tests to evaluate liver and pancreas; abdominal ultrasound to evaluate gallbladder and liver; and barium enema to lower gastrointestinal tract or endoscopy to look inside the bowel to check for problems.

Usually these tests are normal with IBS, as the problem with IBS is not a structural problem but more of a functional problem with the autonomic nerves. There is no cure for IBS, but if it becomes a problem of its own, different things can be done to relieve symptoms. Treatments include:

Avoid Foods That Make IBS Worse

Specific foods may be identified as causing IBS flare-ups. French fries, ice cream, chocolate, alcohol, soda and caffeine are examples of foods that can make IBS worse. Some foods tend to make IBS better, such as foods that contain fiber. Fiber is found in whole grain breads, cereal, fruits, beans, vegetables and bran. If you are adding fiber to your diet, add a little at a time to let your body get used to it. Too much fiber all at once may aggravate IBS symptoms.

Alter Your Eating Style

Large meals can trigger IBS symptoms. Try eating four or five small meals a day or if you have your usual three meals, eat less at each meal.

Medications

The following medicines can be prescribed to help IBS symptoms. They include:

- **Fiber supplements:** Examples include Metamucil, Citrucel, Flax seed.
- **Laxatives:** These can help treat constipation. Examples include Senokot and Ex-Lax.
- **Antispasmodics:** This type of medicine helps slow contractions of the bowel and can help decrease cramping, pain and diarrhea. Examples include Bentyl, Levbid, Levsin.
- **Antidepressants:** This class of medicine including tricyclics and serotonin reuptake inhibitors can help reduce pain and cramping.

Reduce Stress

Stress doesn't cause IBS but once we have it, stress can aggravate the symptoms. Whatever techniques you are using for your fibromyalgia, you can use these stress relieving techniques for IBS as well.

Irritable Bladder

Irritable bladder is a sister of IBS. Sometimes it is called Interstitial Cystitis. The symptoms of irritable bladder include an urgent need to urinate frequently day and night, feelings of pressure, pain and tenderness around the bladder and pelvis, and decreased bladder capacity. Irritable bladder can also cause painful sexual intercourse in women especially, and in men there can be discomfort or pain in the penis. In most women symptoms can worsen around the menstrual cycle as with IBS.

Your doctor may need to rule out other conditions before considering a diagnosis of irritable bladder. A urinalysis and urine culture are frequently done to identify if any urinary tract infection is present. In men, prostate secretions may be cultured to rule out prostatitis. Cystoscopy is a test where a doctor uses a special instrument to look inside the bladder. Any suspicious tissue noted in the bladder or urethra may be biopsied to rule out cancer.

Treatments for Irritable Bladder Include:

Medications to reduce urgency. Specific prescribed medicines to reduce bladder spasms and urgency include: Imipramine (Tofranil), a tricyclic antidepressant; Ditropan; Detrol; and Urimax.

Bladder distension. Some patients may benefit from bladder distension, a procedure which increases the bladder capacity. The bladder, after distention, decreases the number of pain signals transmitted so symptoms lessen. In women, urethral dilation may also be effective.

Biofeedback. Women can learn to strengthen pelvic muscles to better control the bladder and increase blood flow to the bladder through biofeedback techniques. These techniques can be effective in treating severe irritable bladder symptoms.

As part of a biofeedback program, bladder training can be done. Basically the patient is taught to void at designated times and to use relaxation techniques and distraction to help keep on a voiding schedule. Gradually the patient tries to lengthen the time between the scheduled voids and hopefully the end result is to decrease the number of voids during the day and night.

Depression

Depression is seen in over half the people with fibromyalgia, and it can be serious and disabling. Low serotonin is found in those with depression, just as low serotonin is found in fibromyalgia, so it's no surprise that depression and fibromyalgia are often seen together. Sometimes the depression requires its own separate treatment in addition to treating fibromyalgia.

Being depressed is a normal reaction to life's stresses, but sometimes the depressed feelings take on a more sustained nature and lead to clinical depression that requires treatment. Symptoms of depression include:

- Sadness
- Fatigue and loss of energy
- Feelings of hopelessness or worthlessness
- Lack of enjoyment from things that were once pleasurable
- Difficulty concentrating and making decisions

- Increased need for sleep or difficulty sleeping
- Decreased sex drive and sexual problems
- A change of appetite causing weight loss or weight gain
- Thoughts of death or suicide and even suicide attempts

If I suspect depression I will usually refer the patient to a depression specialist (psychiatrist) for treatment. The most common treatment for depression includes a combination of antidepressant medicines and psychotherapy. Psychotherapy is performed by a licensed mental health professional to focus on understanding and identifying the problems that are contributing to depression and how to regain a sense of control and happiness.

Medicines commonly prescribed for depression include tricyclic antidepressants and selective serotonin reuptake inhibitors, or a combination of medicines. For severe clinical depression, I do not think that the natural antidepressants (5-HTP, St. Johns Wort, SAM-e) are strong enough or potent enough to work. In milder forms of depression these natural supplements may work. I think the prescribed medicines need to be considered for the more severe forms of depression, and a psychiatrist should review those with more severe clinical depression.

Anxiety Disorder & Panic Attacks

Everyone experiences anxiety throughout the day, but those with an anxiety disorder have much more than normal anxiety. Plus, the anxiety is chronic and unprovoked, and persons who have this are always in fear of impending disaster and worry excessively about health, money, work and family. Since fibromyalgia causes dysfunctional autonomic nerves, it's not surprising that the chronic anxiety symptoms are present.

People with generalized anxiety have a difficult time relaxing and have trouble falling asleep or their fibromyalgia-related sleep disorders are aggravated. Physical symptoms can develop including tremors, twitching, increased spasms, headache, irritability, sweating, hot flashes, lightheadedness, dizziness and shortness of breath. Sometimes people feel nauseated. They may feel like they have a hard time swallowing or feel a lump in their throat.

People with panic disorder experience frequent and unprovoked panic attacks that involve a lot of anxiety symptoms such as:

- Rapid heart beat
- Chest pains
- Fear of dying
- Flushes and chills
- Dizziness and lightheadedness
- Tingling, numbness
- Difficulty breathing

Many patients with fibromyalgia have anxiety disorders and panic disorders that blend together to cause significantly bothersome symptoms. These may require separate treatments in addition to the fibromyalgia treatments.

Treatments include psychotherapy and medications. Part of the psychotherapy and behavioral approaches include anxiety-reducing techniques involving breathing exercises, relaxation strategies, refocusing strategies and other measures.

Prescription medicines can help, and two categories of medicines that are used to treat anxiety and panic disorders are antidepressants (tricyclic antidepressants and selective serotonin reuptake inhibitors) and benzodiazepines (*e.g.*, Ativan, Xanax, Klonopin, and Valium).

Near-Syncope

People with fibromyalgia often have problems maintaining blood pressure in an upright position. Near-syncope is the result of the dysfunctional autonomic nerves that cause fluctuations in our blood pressure, especially when we go from a sitting to a standing position. People with near-syncope and fibromyalgia do not have loss of consciousness (true syncope), but we get a lightheaded feeling as if we are about to faint but we don't actually faint. We have unsteadiness, a feeling of weakness or fuzziness without loss of consciousness. This is often synonymous with orthostatic hypotension or orthostatic intolerance. With orthostatic hypotension or intolerance, the blood pressure drops when we change positions because we with fibromyalgia tend to overshoot and undershoot nerve responses to the blood vessels when we change positions. Thus, we are more at risk for fluctuations in our blood pressure, particularly a drop in our blood pressure, when we change positions.

Increased stress and certain medications including muscle relaxants, antidepressants and migraine medicines make us more at risk (on top of the risk we have with fibromyalgia).

Evaluation of near-syncope can include checking blood pressure and pulse in the standing and lying down positions and examining the heart. An EKG, cardiac stress test, and tilt table testing may need to be considered.

The tilt table test is one of the ways to confirm orthostatic hypotension and document dysfunctional autonomic nerves as the cause of near-syncope in fibromyalgia. This testing was described in detail in Chapter 6 and can indicate neurally-mediated hypotension.

Treatment of near-syncope includes the following:

1. **Drink extra fluids.** Many times we are subclinically dehydrated, meaning we haven't been drinking enough fluids each day. If we do not have enough blood volume we are more at risk for a drop in our blood pressure and thus more at risk for near-syncope. I recommend 64 ounces of water per day.

2. **Increase salt intake.** Sodium helps maintain our blood pressure and thus helps prevent decreased blood pressure in near-syncope. Many people are so concerned about salt intake because they think it is bad that many times they don't take enough salt. Too much of anything can be bad including too much salt but if we are bothered by near-syncope it is recommended that we be more liberal with our salt because extra salt will help keep our blood volume up and decrease the risk of hypotension or near-syncope. A trial of 2–6 grams of extra salt a day may help.

3. **Prescribed special diuretic.** Florinef (fludrocortisone) can be prescribed in severe cases of near-syncope. This is a salt-retaining diuretic that acts to increase blood volume and hold up our blood pressure.

4. **Beta blockers such as Metoprolol.** It may seem like a paradox to treat someone with low blood pressure with a blood pressure medicine. Beta blockers block beta nerve signals from the autonomic nerves. If someone has hypertension, blocking the beta nerves can help reduce blood pressure. However, these beta nerves are thought to play a major role in causing the low blood pressure in near-syncope, so blocking these beta nerves with a beta blocker can help reduce near-syncope episodes by stabilizing the blood pressure.

5. **Compression garments.** Tight-fitting leg garments or stockings (*e.g.* thigh-high TED hose, or Jobst stockings) can help minimize orthostatic blood pressure changes by decreasing the amount of "pooled" blood in the legs. Gravity forces tend to pull the blood into the legs more when standing, increasing the risk of an orthostatic drop in blood pressure. The stockings "press" the blood from the legs and keeps it in the body's trunk, the main blood "pool," to help maintain the blood pressure.

6. **Posture change strategies.** Often times it is the sudden change from sitting to standing that triggers the autonomic-mediated drop in blood pressure (near-syncope). A treatment strategy is to eliminate any sudden changes in posture. This means gradually changing positions. For example, when first getting out of bed in the morning, one should sit in bed for 15–30 seconds first, then swing the legs over the edge of the bed and sit there for 15–30 seconds, then plant the feet on the floor and stand up slowly but stay next to the bed for 15–30 seconds, then start walking. This gradual step-wise process can help eliminate near-syncopal episodes.

Migraine Headaches

Migraine headaches are a common disorder in those with fibromyalgia. Many migraine sufferers have typical warning symptoms (auras) before the headache begins. Typical auras can last for a few minutes and include:

- Bright spots or blurring in the vision
- Increasing neck pain radiating up the back of the head
- A feeling of increased anxiety or pressure
- A tingling or numbness feeling

Migraine Headaches

Migraine headaches are usually one-sided and may switch sides from one attack to the other. The type of pain is described as throbbing and pulsating and can last from a few hours to up to several days. Twenty percent of people with migraine headaches report visual symptoms such as double vision or blurred vision which may be part of an aura or part of the actual migraine headache. Women outnumber men 3:1.

Tension headaches usually arise in the back of the neck and radiate to the forehead and temples. There may be a band-like pressure or pain over the head. The type of pain is usually described as a steady dull ache that can last all day. There is usually no aura, nausea, sensitivity to light or sensitivity to sound reported with tension headaches. These types of headaches may be chronic or episodic and can lead to migraine headaches. Women outnumber men 5:4

Reference: National Headache Foundation, Headache Diagnosis and Management Guidelines, 1999.

Migraine headaches are caused by autonomic nerves causing excessive dilation of blood vessels in the head. The pain is not coming from the brain; rather, the pain arises from blood vessels, muscles and meninges (membranes that cover the brain) that are stretched, tensed or hypersensitized, causing the nerves to signal more pain.

Many people with fibromyalgia have different types of headaches, including migraine headaches, tension headaches and sinus headaches. If the headaches are severe enough, there may be a diagnostic work-up that includes a head CT scan, brain MRI, or an EEG to evaluate for any other types of pathology. Typically all these tests are normal for migraine headaches.

A number of factors trigger migraine headaches, including:

- Foods such as cheese, chocolate and other food. People with food allergies can have frequent migraines as well

- Alcohol, especially red wine

- MSG (monosodium glutamate). This is a common ingredient in Chinese food

- Withdrawal from caffeine or other drugs which constrict blood vessels.

- Emotional changes and stressors

- Hormonal changes

- Increased fatigue

- Side effects from certain medications. It is common to have rebound headaches when taking pain medicines and migraine medicines, especially Ergotamine. Certain serotonin reuptake inhibitor medicines can also cause headaches as a side effect.

My Treatment Strategies For Migraine Headaches

Most fibromyalgia patients with migraine headaches actually have mixed type headaches. That is, they may have both migraine headaches and tension type headaches. The headaches are cervicogenic (arise from the neck). Painful neck muscles, ligaments and facet joints, common in fibromyalgia, can lead to tension headaches which "spill- over" into migraine headaches. I want to treat all components of the headache, *i.e.*, treat the tension headache, but also try to treat the source of the headache—the neck.

1. **Dietary modifications.** If certain foods trigger migraine headaches, or food allergies exist, it's best to avoid these foods altogether. Foods such as chocolate, beer, wine and cheese should be avoided if they are identified as migraine precipitators.

2. **Decrease the pain.** The patient who enters my office with a severe headache needs something that can provide immediate pain relief. Pain medicines (narcotic medications), central acting medications (such as Ultracet or Ultram, muscle relaxers, migraine medicines) can all be used. I don't give patients every single medicine at once! The strategy is to decrease the headache that is present NOW.

   Injection strategies are helpful for acute headaches whether they be migraine or tension headaches. Trigger point injections to the upper cervical paraspinal muscles or suboccipital areas can help relieve migraine headaches. Trigger point injections to other neck muscles and trapezial muscles can help relieve neck and trapezial tender point areas that can be triggering the headaches. Another type of injection called occipital blocks can be given to anesthetize the occipital nerve, a major contributing nerve to migraine headaches. The headache can disappear or decrease in intensity considerably following injections.

3. **Decrease the frequency of migraine headaches.** This strategy is a preventive one: reduce the frequency of migraine headaches or decrease the opportunity for migraine headaches to evolve from tension headaches. Several categories of medicines can be used including beta blockers, antidepressant medicines (tricyclic antidepressants and selective serotonin reuptake inhibitors), anti-seizure medicines such as Neurontin, Depakote and Keppra, as well as anti-spasticity medicines including Zanaflex.

The patient keeps a headache diary to determine if overall headaches have decreased over time. It is not realistic to completely eliminate headaches, but if someone who suffers from a couple of migraine headaches every week can reduce the frequency of migraine headaches to one or two a month, this would be reported as a substantial improvement.

4. **Rescue medications.** These medicines are designed to stop a headache that break through your preventive defenses. It's great if you can reduce the number of headaches that occur, but if a headache does break through, it's really great to have a medicine that stops it in its tracks. The same medicines used in stopping the headaches described in #2 above can be used as rescue medicines. The most common one used would be the migraine medications such as Midrin, Imitrex, Maxalt, Axert, Amerge and Zomig. I have had success with using Feverfew, 5-HTP and magnesium as natural products in patients who prefer to avoid prescription medicines or switch them around as necessary.

5. **Physical medicine treatment.** Trying to reduce the neck pain and spasms as part of the fibromyalgia will help in reducing the headaches. A therapy program can include modalities such as ultrasound, electric stimulation, specific hands-on manual therapy and instruction on stretches and exercises.

Just as everyone requires an individual approach to treating fibromyalgia, everyone also requires a unique treatment for his or her headaches. A combination of different strategies will usually work, and I try to help each patient find that right combination. I try to be Dr. Locksmith!

Those Unique Pains

Not all symptoms are related to fibromyalgia, believe it or not! This chapter addresses other conditions that cause painful symptoms and may be coexisting with fibromyalgia. People with fibromyalgia can have other conditions that cause chronic pain, and the challenge is to identify and treat all problems that cause pain and not automatically blame everything on fibromyalgia.

Dr. Vlad Djuric is a colleague of mine who has extensive knowledge and experience in diagnosing and treating these unique painful conditions other than fibromyalgia. Over the years we have worked together on many patients to try to get the best outcomes possible, and we have learned a lot from each other and from our patients. I asked Dr. Djuric to write a chapter on various painful conditions that we often see either as part of fibromyalgia or in addition to fibromyalgia. I hope you find this chapter helpful and can learn from Dr. Djuric as I have.

Vladimir Djuric, M.D.

- Board Certified Physiatrist

- Fellowship trained in non-surgical spinal interventions

- Specialist in spinal injections and prolotherapy

- Private practice Ohio Rehab Center, Canton, Ohio

  www.OhioRehab.com

Those Unique Pains, by Vladimir Djuric, M.D.

The diagnosis of fibromyalgia does not preclude the coexistence of other joint and spinal problems. It is important to identify underlying conditions which may also be causing pain. Treatment could lead to a substantial reduction of regional pain; pain which may in fact be perpetuating more diffuse fibromyalgia symptoms.

Introduction

These relatively common conditions can frequently be overlooked by treating physicians for a number of reasons. First and foremost, many patients exhibit signs and symptoms which mimic those of fibromyalgia. Joint and spinal dysfunction, for example, are often accompanied by an increase in adjacent muscle tone or spasm. If movement is painful, this protective reflex is our body's attempt to restrict motion of the painful joint or "motion segment." Over time, chronically tense muscles develop trigger points, similar to those found in fibromyalgia.

Second, because of the subtle physical findings and lack of diagnostic tests to confirm these unique diagnoses, recognizing such conditions can be difficult. Therefore, a high level of suspicion and thorough evaluation is needed if such conditions are to be identified.

Another reason these conditions may be missed is that most physicians are usually not trained in musculoskeletal medicine and therefore may not have learned the diagnostic skills necessary to identify mechanical joint dysfunction. Pain which is actually due to joint dysfunction may be attributed to being of soft tissue etiology instead.

Whiplash, defined as trauma causing cervical musculoligamental sprain or strain (due to hyperflexion/hyperextension) is probably the single most common cause of traumatically-induced fibromyalgia.

In this chapter we will discuss many common and several uncommon conditions seen in our practice, either in isolation or in conjunction with fibromyalgia. Trauma, prolonged postural abnormalities, and repetitive occupational stresses are responsible for a majority of these conditions. Since the same treatment principles apply for all the conditions described, treatment strategies will be covered at the end of the chapter. Unique interventions will be covered as well.

Whiplash, defined as trauma causing cervical musculoligamental sprain or strain (due to hyperflexion/hyperextension) is probably the single most common cause of traumatically-induced fibromyalgia. It also accounts for a majority of non-fibromyalgia related headaches, neck, shoulder and back pain that we see in our practice. In most cases underlying spinal dysfunctions caused by the trauma are responsible for a majority of the symptoms.

Repetitive activities, particularly those requiring holding one's arms suspended in front of the body for prolonged intervals, places strain on joints, ligaments, and muscles. Over time, such activities result in wear and tear (repetitive microtrauma), leading to joint, ligament, and muscular pain. Muscles that are being used frequently will grow stronger while those that get very little use will weaken. Because joints aren't being put through their full range, motion is lost. Muscles tighten and become shorter.

Under such circumstances chronic muscle imbalances and joint restrictions develop. This combination of joint and muscle pain, muscle shortening, and reduced joint mobility will ultimately lead to a deterioration of posture. The body assumes a position of comfort, or more accurately, the position of least discomfort. In doing so, the head drops down and shoulders migrate forward, placing chronic strain on supportive soft tissues. This "protective" posture is typically assumed by someone already in pain or about to experience pain. Such postural changes become deeply imbedded in a relatively short period of time, making their correction all the more difficult.

Cervical Dysfunction

Although the majority of neck sprain/strain injuries heal on their own, a significant number go on to become sources of chronic pain. This pain can range from a mild discomfort, only aggravated with heavy exertional activity, to severe, unremitting and incapacitating pain. Prognosis after common whiplash is typically quite good with nearly 75% of individuals recovering completely within 6 months. Unfortunately for those individuals that do not recover, persistent neck pain, headaches, shoulder pain and a variety of other symptoms may linger indefinitely. In 10% the symptoms are severe, intruding on everyday activities. Four percent are unable to return to their previous occupation due to the severity of pain and functional compromise. The reason for this ongoing pain can frequently be traced back to injury of ligaments and tendons, tissues that have a poor healing capacity, have a poor blood supply, and have an abundance of painful nerve endings. This structural combination predisposes these tissues to chronic pain generation.

Over the past decade our understanding of the pathophysiology of whiplash has improved a great deal. Extensive research has identified cervical zygapophyseal joints (facets) as the most common cause of neck and shoulder pain after whiplash. Small tears in the intervertebral disc wall have also been implicated in causing persistent pain after trauma. Other injured structures include the vertebral bodies, ligaments, fascia, and muscles. Injury to the cervical sympathetic nervous system can result in a form of reflex sympathetic dystrophy known as Barré-Lieou syndrome, which will be reviewed later.

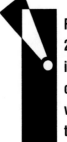

Researchers have discovered that over 20% of individuals sustaining neck injuries went on to develop symptoms consistent with fibromyalgia, making whiplash one of the most common traumatic causes of this condition.

What may start as a very localized pain can spread to adjacent areas and even extend to the other side of the body. This "regionalization" of symptoms may be due to the development of compensatory posture and movement patterns in an unsuccessful adaptation made by the body in an effort to minimize pain, similar to a limp due to a painful hip, knee, or ankle. Sleep disturbances, difficulty with concentration, depression, and anxiety are other common complications of whiplash. In most cases these symptoms can be directly attributed to unremitting pain. Researchers have discovered that over 20% of individuals sustaining neck injuries went on to develop symptoms consistent with fibromyalgia, making whiplash one of the most common traumatic causes of this condition.

Interestingly, speed of impact correlates poorly with pain after whiplash. Possibly the single most important factor predictive of chronic pain after such trauma is head position at time of impact. A rotated or inclined head predisposes to more severe injury. Shorter time before onset of initial symptoms, higher initial pain rating, the presence of pre-traumatic headaches, and cervical degenerative joint disease are all predictive of more severe and persistent symptoms. As in fibromyalgia, an increase in generalized muscle pain and increased sensory sensitivity can occur soon after whiplash injury. Such changes are also associated with poor recovery.

Table: Predictors of Chronic Pain after a Whiplash Injury

• Head rotated or inclined at impact	• Prior headaches
• Immediate pain	• Prior cervical arthritis
• Initial high level of pain	• Prior fibromyalgia

Barré-Lieou Syndrome

Thought to be due to a dysfunction of the cervical sympathetic nervous system, Barré-Lieou syndrome is characterized by any combination of the following: headaches, facial, neck, dental, and ear pain, dizziness, ringing in the ears, nausea and vomiting, visual blurring, impaired balance, sinus congestion, tearing, and salivation. A variety of other symptoms such as facial swelling, facial numbness, hoarseness, muscle weakness, fatigue, shoulder pain, dysesthesias involving the upper limbs, and swelling and stiffness of the fingers may also be present. Jean Alexandre Barré, M.D., a French neurologist and Yong-Choen Lieou, a Chinese physician, each described the condition independently in 1925 and 1928, respectively.

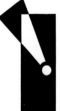

Because of stretching and/or tearing of the cervical stabilizing ligaments, whiplash can have a destabilizing effect on the cervical spine.

The sympathetic and parasympathetic nervous systems together make up the autonomic nervous system (ANS). In general, the ANS is responsible for the subconscious monitoring and control of bodily functions such as heart rate, blood circulation, blood pressure, body temperature, gut motility, etc.

Function of the cervical sympathetic chain, which rests just in front of the cervical vertebral transverse process, can be adversely affected by injury to the cervical spine. Such injuries most commonly occur in whiplash-type trauma. Because of stretching and/or tearing of the cervical stabilizing ligaments, whiplash can have a destabilizing effect on the cervical spine. Chronic instability probably leads to irritation of the sympathetic chain, ultimately resulting in ongoing sympathetic dysfunction. This could explain the multitude of head, neck, and upper extremity symptoms that develop after neck trauma.

Rib Dysfunction

One group of structures that has received very little attention in the allopathic (M.D.) medical literature, but appears to be a major source of pain and altered sensation involving the upper back, shoulder blades and upper extremities are the ribs. Causes of rib dysfunction are numerous, paralleling those of neck pain (*e.g.*, whiplash/trauma, repetitive activities, altered posture, etc.). Very little force is necessary to provoke a rib subluxation (a minor dislocation). Sometimes, just a quick turn of the head or awkward positioning during sleep will lead to shifting of a rib head. This places strain on the rib's joint capsule and stabilizing ligaments which causes increased tension of overlying muscles. Chronic muscle tension can eventually become a source of additional pain.

Most commonly pain is localized to the back of the shoulder, between the shoulder blades, or the upper back. Symptoms can be provoked with deep breathing. The pain can be sharp and stabbing or dull and aching in character, occasionally radiating around the side and into the front of the chest. When the first and second ribs are involved, arm pain, numbness, and tingling can also be elicited. This sensation can extend as far as the hand. Although the entire arm and hand can be affected in this manner, the ring and little finger (C8-Tl nerve root or ulnar nerve territory) are most commonly involved. Rib and thoracic dysfunction can increase muscle tension in the neck, ultimately resulting in headaches.

Many practitioners classify this phenomenon as Thoracic Outlet Syndrome, a condition marked by compression of the neurovascular bundle in the neck/shoulder area. Various etiologies of this compression have been proposed and some drastic treatment measures have been recommended. Treatments range from stretching and postural correction to surgical rib resection. In our experience, rib dysfunction of this nature responds well to standard non-surgical therapy directed at correcting the dysfunction.

T4 Syndrome

Another little-recognized condition which can be responsible for a variety of complaints involving the middle back and arms is T4 syndrome. Common complaints include arm discomfort and paresthesias (abnormal sensations) that do not follow any specific nerve territory. Because of hand numbness and tingling, the condition is frequently mistaken for carpal tunnel syndrome. However, a work-up usually fails to reveal any significant nerve entrapment.

The underlying cause of this syndrome is hypomobility (too little movement) involving the upper to mid thoracic spine. The worst area is usually between the second and sixth thoracic vertebrae (T2 and T6), most commonly at T4. Typically, vertebral rotation accompanied by elevation of the associated rib places tension against the nervous structures in the area. If the thoracic spine is too stiff (hypomobile) in an area, more force is transmitted to the nerve structures when one twists (rotates the spine) and reaches (elevates the ribs). Although the exact mechanism producing these symptoms is unknown, sympathetic nervous system involvement is theorized to be largely responsible for the unusual clinical presentation.

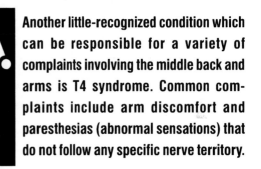

Another little-recognized condition which can be responsible for a variety of complaints involving the middle back and arms is T4 syndrome. Common complaints include arm discomfort and paresthesias (abnormal sensations) that do not follow any specific nerve territory.

The condition responds well to mobilization techniques. Occasionally, thoracic para spinal blocks may be necessary to desensitize the affected area, particularly if tissue hypersensitivity prevents effective mobilization.

Thoracolumbar Junction Syndrome (Maigne's Syndrome)

Spinal dysfunctions occur most frequently at junctional levels. Junctions are transitional zones in the vertebral column where motion preference and degree of mobility change dramatically from one level to the next. The vertebra change in size as you descend down the spinal column. More importantly, orientation of the small joints in back of the vertebra (zygapophyseal or facet joints) changes as well. Facet joint orientation dictates motion preference. Other factors such as intervertebral disc height dictate degree of movement.

The cervical spinal segments are designed to move well in multiple directions, having the greatest degree of motion in flexion and extension. Because of the stiffening effect of the rib cage, the thoracic spine has very little intersegmental (between the vertebrae) motion. However, facet orientation dictates that rotation is preferred over all other movements. The lumbar spine, with its large thick discs, is capable of substantial intersegmental movement and does best with flexion and extension. By comparison, side bending and rotation are quite limited.

The cervicothoracic, thoracolumbar, and lumbosacral junctions are the areas where problems are encountered most commonly. Transitioning from one type of motion to another is a complex mechanical phenomenon. Because of biomechanical weaknesses of the human spinal column, which are attributed to upright posture and walking on two legs, spinal dysfunctions tend to develop, particularly at these transitional levels.

A French osteopath, Robert Maigne, diagnosed the condition at the thoracolumbar (T-L) junction which now bears his name. Features of thoracolumbar junction or "Maigne's syndrome," include pain and deep tenderness at the posterior iliac crest (see diagram), usually one side only, thickening and hypersensitivity of the skin and underlying tissues in the same vicinity, and tenderness with palpation of the spinous processes and facet joints at the T-L junction. What's interesting about Maigne's syndrome is that the more prominent symptoms are quite distant (typically some 6 to 8 inches) from the actual site of pathology. This occurs because the thoracolumbar facet joints and skin at the iliac crests share the same nerves. Such dual innervation frequently leads to a phenomenon known as "referred pain."

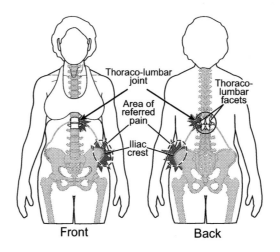

Lumbar Spine

In the past century there has been extensive deliberation over the specific causes of low back pain. Imaging studies such as x-rays, CT scans, and MRIs help shed light on underlying structural abnormalities. Whether or not these abnormalities are responsible or even partially contributing to the symptoms is many times uncertain. In large part, the focus of both imaging and electrodiagnostic studies (EMG's) is the intervertebral discs and their effect on the adjacent spinal nerves.

A herniated disc can either press against a spinal nerve directly or inflame it by leaking inflammatory substrates. Clinically, this results in sciatica-type symptoms, *i.e.*, pain extending from the hip or buttock into the leg, sometimes as far as the foot. In addition to pain, symptoms such as numbness, tingling, and weakness are also frequently present. Treatment for a simple disc herniation is relatively straightforward. Standard conservative measures including medications, physical therapy, and epidural steroid injections typically lead to an eventual resolution of symptoms. In instances where such measures fail or if there is danger of permanent neurologic loss, surgical intervention is usually successful.

Primary back and buttock pain (as opposed to buttock and leg pain—the most common symptoms with lumbar disc herniation) is an altogether different phenomenon. In this pain problem, nervous system pathology is usually not present. Until recently this type of pain was classified as "non-specific low back pain" in the medical literature. This term suggests that determining the exact cause of back pain was difficult, impossible, or inconsequential. Simply put, our understanding of the more complicated presentations of back pain remains inadequate. Furthermore, even though our understanding of the problem may be quite thorough, treatment options may be very limited.

Intervertebral Discs

Lumbar degenerative disc disease is a common condition and considered to be painless and part of the normal aging process. We depart from normality when these degenerative discs cause pain. Treatment options for painful degenerative disc disease are limited. For those failing to respond to standard conservative care, invasive treatments such as intradiscal electrothermal annuloplasty (IDET) and surgical fusion are sometimes considered. In most instances, even though these high tech procedures may be available, the patient is not a candidate; the criteria are very stringent.

In order to determine whether IDET is an option, lumbar discography is the diagnostic test of choice. Discography can determine if degeneration (determined by disc height loss) and painful discs are present and help clarify the potential benefit of IDET. Treatment of multiple discs and more advanced stages of disc degeneration decreases IDET's success rate. Long term studies of IDET are ongoing and so the ultimate benefit of this procedure remains to be determined.

As with IDET, surgical lumbar fusion and a variety of other surgical interventions directed at the intervertebral discs have also been studied extensively. Their usefulness in the treatment of chronic back pain remains controversial. Such procedures permanently change the anatomy of the spine, decreasing the amount of available motion. Mechanics altered in this fashion can lead to problems involving adjacent motion segments in the levels above and below the level of surgery. Such problems may not surface until several years after the procedure and may lead to more surgery.

In our practice we have seen many patients who undergo such procedures, only to later discover that it has not changed their pain. Other times they will experience a recurrence of their symptoms several years and sometimes even months following the surgery. The lesson to be learned is that surgery for back pain is the very last resort. An exhaustive search for other treatment options needs to be done. Several opinions should be obtained prior to making a decision.

Facet Joints

Facet (zygapophyseal) joints are another potential source of chronic low back pain. These small joints located in the back of the spinal canal help guide segmental motion and to a lesser extent, assist in weightbearing. Especially with spinal arthritis, spondylolisthesis (slipped vertebra), and trauma these structures can become sources of pain. Again, treatment choices are limited. Steroid injections into the joints may provide substantial relief but the benefits are often temporary and repeated injections are contraindicated. Neurolysis, procedures involving chemical or thermal destruction of the nerve supplying pain fibers to the joint, has been of limited success in the lumbar spine. Occasionally, lumbar fusion may be considered as a last resort, but is usually not advocated.

Sacroiliac Joint

Despite its prevalence, sacroiliac joint dysfunction (SIJD) is vastly under-recognized and often misdiagnosed. Although it may be present in as many as 40% of individuals who experience back, buttock and leg pain, it is frequently overlooked as the cause of these common symptoms. Many clinicians familiar with SIJD feel it holds the distinction of being the single most common cause of chronic or recurrent back pain.

There are many different ways in which SIJD can manifest itself. In some cases the symptoms develop gradually without an obvious cause. More frequently, trauma involving the SIJ leads to injury of the SIJ ligaments. Because of its very complex mechanics, restoring normal function can be extremely challenging and in some cases virtually impossible.

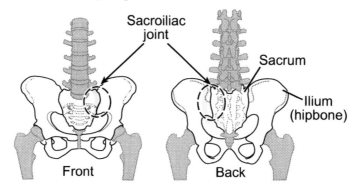

The SIJ is a transitional structure; it can be thought of as either the bottom of the spine or the top of the leg since it really functions as both. The joint is not very large, especially considering the forces which cross it. Its stability is due to a combination of factors: irregular joint surfaces, the wedge-like shape of the sacrum, and most importantly, the ligaments which hold it all together. These ligaments, considered the strongest in the body, function like cables of a suspension bridge. In order for the joint to function properly each cable needs to provide a certain degree of tension and support; each plays a role in bridging the spine to the leg, thus facilitating a fluid gait and normal body mechanics. When the ligaments are stretched or torn, either as a result of single trauma or because of repetitive impact loading, joint motion is compromised and joint dysfunction results.

Some of the most powerful muscles in the body surround the SIJ but these muscles influence SIJ motion only indirectly. However, the effect of the SIJ on these muscles can be profound. The piriformis, iliopsoas, gluteals, lumbar paraspinals, quadratus lumborum, tensor fascia lata, and hamstrings can all be affected to various degrees. With SIJD these muscles can become tense or spastic, and are not able to perform effectively. This can lead to an abnormal gait, spinal dysfunction, hip bursitis and leg pain.

The most common symptoms with SIJD are pain in the buttock, hip and/or low back. Groin, thigh and leg pain can also be present. Burning, numbness, and tingling in the same distribution are also common.

The most common symptoms with SIJD are pain in the buttock, hip and/or low back. Groin, thigh and leg pain can also be present. Burning, numbness, and tingling in the same distribution are also common. SIJD is sometimes mistaken for sciatica pain or a lumbar herniated disc. A sense of joint looseness or instability may be present on exam. This looseness can lead to joint subluxation and locking. Patients frequently comment that their hip or back "is out." Inability to find a comfortable position and activity intolerance are common complaints. Bowel and bladder irritability, sexual dysfunction, and a host of other symptoms can also result.

Treatment

As mentioned at the beginning of this chapter, in order to properly treat the conditions discussed, they must first be identified. Treatment approaches are remarkably similar, regardless of the condition being treated. Factors that need to be considered and properly addressed include altered joint mechanics or dysfunction, muscle tone, muscle strength, regional imbalances, and ligament weakness.

Manual therapy serves to realign and re-educate the body. Various mobilizations help to realign the spine and pelvis. When possible, self mobilization techniques can be taught to enable patients to

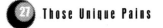

restore alignment on their own or with the help of a partner. Instruction in body mechanics and activity modification help to avoid reaggravation of the condition.

It is important to restore proper function and coordination of movement with specific exercises. Tight and shortened muscles inhibit progress by perpetuating joint dysfunction. Such situations call for a focused stretching program. Stretching serves to restore muscles to their proper length. It also improves joint mobility. If, on the other hand, hypermobility (too loose) is the problem, then muscles need to be trained to re-establish control of movement through a combination of strengthening and coordination exercises.

Injection Therapy

When persistent pain stemming from tense muscles or irritated ligaments limits progress, injection therapy can facilitate a more rapid response to treatment. Trigger point injections, dry needling, and acupuncture are useful adjuncts to the standard manual medicine approach.

Corticosteroids (cortisone/steroids), typically used in combination with an anesthetic agent, may be injected into muscles, tendons, or ligaments *(trigger point injections)*, along nerves *(nerve blocks)*, or into joints *(joint injections)* when inflammation and swelling is suspected to be contributing to the cause of the pain. The type of injection utilized depends on the problem being treated.

Hypermobility or ligament incompetence can be treated with prolotherapy, also known as proliferative therapy, sclerotherapy, or regenerative injection therapy. Prolotherapy promotes healing of damaged tissues by initiating a controlled inflammatory response at the injection sites. Inflammation is necessary for healing to occur, and prolotherapy is an attempt to get the process started and stimulate proliferation of tissues necessary for repair. As the healing process continues ligaments and tendons increase in size and strength. These tissues gradually contract, eventually tightening the loose joints. The end result is better joint mechanics, less joint and muscle irritation, and ultimately less pain. Patients many times note a reduction of the "cracking" or "popping" that they started experiencing after their accident.

Typically, individuals experience significant improvement in their symptoms after three treatments. In some cases, because of nutritional, metabolic, or hormonal abnormalities, the body is not able to mount an adequate healing response. Under such circumstances, testing may be necessary to determine whether a correctable abnormality exists. Once the problem is addressed, prolotherapy may be resumed.

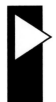

If You Want To Know More

1. Barnsley L, Lord SM, Bogduk N. *Whiplash injury.* Pain 1994; 58: 283–307.

2. Daum WJ. *The sacroiliac joint: an underappreciated pain generator.* Am J Orthop 1995; 6: 475–8.

3. Dreyfuss PH, Tibiletti C, Dreyer S. *Thoracic zygapophyseal joint pain patterns: a review and description of an intra-articular block technique.* Pain Digest 1994; 4: 46–54.

4. Koelbaek Johansen MK, Graven-Nielsen T, Schou Olesen AS, et al. *Generalised muscular hyperalgesia in chronic whiplash syndrome.* Pain 1999; 83: 229–34.

5. Maigne R. *Low back pain of thoracolumbar origin.* Arch Phys Med Rehabil 1980; 61: 389–95.

6. Pickin M. *A discussion of whiplash injury to the cervical spine.* J Ortho Med 1995; 17: 15–23.

7. Radanov BP, Sturzenegger M, Di Stefano G. *Long-term outcome after whiplash injury. A 2-year follow-up considering features of injury mechanism and somatic, radiologic, and psychosocial findings.* Medicine 1995; 74: 281-97.

8. Sehgal N, Fortin JD. *Internal disc disruption in low back pain.* Pain Phys 2000; 3: 143–57.

9. Schwarzer AC, Derby R, Aprill CN, et al. *The value of the provocation response in lumbar zygapophyseal joint injections.* Clin J Pain 1994; 10: 309–13.

10. Sterling M, Jull G, Vicenzino B, et al. *Sensory hypersensitivity occurs soon after whiplash injury and is associated with poor recovery.* Pain 2003; 104: 509–17.

Children & Men With Fibromyalgia

Women do not have a monopoly on fibromyalgia. I see many children and men with fibromyalgia in my practice. As a man with fibromyalgia (who has been told he frequently acts child-like!), I can appreciate that the "minority" hurts too and their lives are disrupted by fibromyalgia. As you've come to appreciate by now, not everyone with fibromyalgia is affected the same, and there are some unique differences among children and men that require some different strategies.

Children With Fibromyalgia

Top Ten Signs That Your Child May Have Fibromyalgia

1. Has growing pains without actual growth

2. Says your perfume makes him "puke his guts out"

3. Says when she grows up, will consider numerous jobs as long as they are classified as sedentary

4. Only kid in the school history to flunk gym

5. Volunteers in school to be in a sleep study

6. For Christmas, all he wants is a hot tub

7. Selective memory loss (can't remember homework assignment)

8. Complains of constant hairballs in her throat

9. Gets upset if you don't park exactly between the lines, gets completely embarrassed and refuses to get out of car if you straddle a line

10. Spends more time in the bathroom than the classroom

I see a number of children in my practice who have fibromyalgia. The youngest I have seen was a boy aged 3. I also see many teenagers, often children of a parent with fibromyalgia.

A child who has a parent or sibling with fibromyalgia or connective tissue disease is at risk. If this child at risk is involved in a competitive sport that stresses the muscles—tennis, dancing, gymnastics—risk is increased. Children can get post-traumatic fibromyalgia, especially those who have a hereditary vulnerability. A number of young female patients in my practice have been involved with dancing, gymnastics, or baton twirling for many years. Hours of practice and competition have been involved. Symptoms of pain appear and ultimately fibromyalgia develops.

Other risk factors I've identified in children include the presence of scoliosis (curvature of the spine) or forward posturing (rounded shoulders). Postural changes cause more strain on the back muscles which over time can lead to traumatic changes that trigger fibromyalgia. Girls are more likely to have scoliosis than boys (genetic risk). I see many youngsters who have intermittent back strains related to postural changes, and some have gone on to develop "full blown" fibromyalgia. There is no way to predict who will develop clinical fibromyalgia in those who are at risk, especially in those who are completely symptom-free.

In children, girls still outnumber boys, but the gap is smaller, about 60% girls and 40% boys in a survey of children with fibromyalgia in my practice. This is consistent with the research reported by Dr. Buskila. Causes of fibromyalgia in children are similar to the causes in adults: genetics, trauma (either a major trauma such as a fall or car accident or cumulative type trauma as with certain competitive sports), infections such as mononucleosis or other viral infections, or infections secondary to another condition. Primary fibromyalgia is more common.

In children there may be generalized widespread pain, but usually there are some common initial symptoms that may be part of the prodromal state that can ultimately turn into fibromyalgia. These symptoms include:

1. **Leg pains (may be called growing pains).** This appears to be a form of restless leg syndrome in children and is especially bothersome at night.

2. **Fatigue.** Episodic bouts with extreme fatigue may occur and the child will not want to do anything when this happens.

3. **Sleep problems.** Difficulty falling asleep and frequent awakening may occur.

4. **Headaches.** Frequent migraine headaches or tension headaches may occur with neck and shoulder pain or even in the absence of any other pain. Allergies and dry eyes may be present and contributing to the headaches.

5. **Abdominal pain.** Frequent stomach aches and stomach pain, possibly accompanied by nausea. This may be early irritable bowel syndrome.

6. **Cognitive difficulties.** This can include difficulty with concentration and attention in school, difficulty focusing on a topic, difficulty with reading and reading comprehension, and complaints about vision. School teachers will often notice these difficulties first and mention them to the parents.

Certain aggravating factors may cause fibromyalgia to flare-up in children. I find that many children will experience increased pain or more widespread pain during growth spurts. Perhaps fibromyalgia is thrown "out of balance," so to speak, as growth is occurring more rapidly than the fibromyalgia can adjust, hence the increased pain. The stress of growth may aggravate fibromyalgia symptoms, or perhaps the nerves grow at a slower pace than the rest of the body and they signal more nerve pain. Girls may notice increased pain when their menstrual cycles start, and they have exaggerated premenstrual symptoms from the very beginning. Children are not free from stresses, at school or home, particularly if there is marital discord between the parents. All of these factors can contribute to flare-ups of fibromyalgia in children.

Many times when I see these children with various symptoms or associated conditions, I find they have numerous painful tender points and ropey muscles with localized spasms. The diagnosis of fibromyalgia may be made if the criteria is met.

Minimal Invasiveness

I will approach children (say under 16 years of age) with fibromyalgia a little differently than adults. I want to make sure there is no underlying problem other than fibromyalgia that could be causing symptoms. Usually I will obtain some lab work including blood counts, sedimentation rate, and possibly thyroid studies. If cognitive difficulties are a problem, I will consider neuropsychological testing to specifically test memory, auditory comprehension, reading comprehension, and other integrative skills of the brain.

My treatment philosophy with children is mainly "let kids be kids." Children are active, they tend to sleep more, and they can be moody. Sometimes parents' concerns are based more on the parents' experience with fibromyalgia and fear that the child may be going through the same thing. I address these concerns and try to offer encouragement. I believe that minimal invasiveness is required. The main treatment may simply be a matter of reassuring the child and parent that there is no serious medical condition, but rather there is some evidence of fibromyalgia which can be handled with education, and tailoring an activity program to include stretches and specific exercises, nutritional approaches, and long-term monitoring.

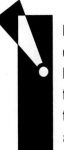

If gymnastics, tennis, or any other competitive sport activity appears to be a major factor in the cause of fibromyalgia and of flare-ups, I will tell the young athlete to think about a different competitive sport.

If there is a functional impairment as a result of fibromyalgia, such as the child is missing school or important school activities, or is unable to participate in sports because of pain and fatigue, I will treat more aggressively. Treatments could include specific, prescribed medicines such as Klonopin, Nortriptyline, or a mild pain medication. I may prescribe a therapy program to try to find out what works and to develop a successful home program. Nutritional strategies, education, manual therapy and stress management are other treatments to consider.

School modifications such as the following may be necessary on a temporary or ongoing basis.

1. Rescheduling student classes so the student may be able to arrive later and leave earlier and have a study hall/rest time in the middle of the day.

2. Physical adaptation, such as using a back pack or luggage cart, avoiding steps and using the elevator, and having another locker on another floor to decrease the need to carry a lot of books at any given time.

3. Excuse from school gym for the time being.

Sometimes it is necessary to temporarily remove the child from school and use a home tutor. If the process of getting to and from school is extremely difficult because of pain and fatigue, this may be a reluctant but necessary option.

I review the physical risks with each individual. If we determine that a certain athletic activity or a competition is the culprit in causing and aggravating fibromyalgia, I advise the child athlete on ways to modify or avoid the offending activity altogether. Several of my female patients were interested in a dancing major in college, but they developed fibromyalgia along the way that was made worse by repetitive dancing. I advised them about changing their major to one that was more realistic and did not involve activities that aggravate the fibromyalgia. Dancing could still be pursued as recreation, but fibromyalgia would probably not allow it as a career.

If gymnastics, tennis, or any other competitive sport activity appears to be a major factor in the cause of fibromyalgia and of flare-ups, I will tell the young athlete to think about a different competitive sport. First, they will back off from the activity, get the fibromyalgia under the best control possible, and then see what happens when the activity is resumed. If the fibromyalgia flares up quickly, it is a good indicator that the continued activity will not be tolerated well. We need to look at this honestly and realistically.

I find that kids are more resilient and adaptable to change than adults. Their youth gives them a better chance at controlling the fibromyalgia and maintaining a stable baseline or remission. I remind the parents not to project their fears onto their child, because each child is unique and the fibromyalgia has a unique identity as well. Even if the mother is having a difficult time with her fibromyalgia, the child can reach a stage where the fibromyalgia is hardly a bother. Most of the children I've seen have done better over time, and I am hopeful that they will continue to do well.

Men With Fibromyalgia

Men get fibromyalgia, too. In adults, women outnumber men by at least 6 to 1, but if 5% of the population has fibromyalgia, nearly 15% of those are men. Men seem to comprise a large number of the "undiagnosed fibromyalgia" category. If we go out and look for fibromyalgia, we will find it in men who have never gone to the doctor. In people younger than 18, the ratio of girls to boys is 3 to 2, so young men commonly get it too.

Differences Between Men & Women

Men with fibromyalgia react differently than women with fibromyalgia. The central nervous system responds differently to pain in each sex. Hormone differences, learned behaviors, and even gender stereotyping are all factors that make pain experiences different between men and women.

Men have lower concentrations of oxytocin (primary "bonding" chemical) and serotonin (calming, pain-regulating hormone) than women. This makes men less biochemically in tune with essential details and emotional components of pain. Plus, men have higher concentrations of testosterone and vasopressin than women; these male hormones contribute to the territorial, competitiveness, and group hierarchy instincts. In the real world, these instincts can be displayed as self-worth and identity being linked to job skills, being a workaholic, or being a yard "warrior."

Gender stereotyping and learned behaviors in our society further reinforce the biochemical signals. The male gender is not supposed to complain of pain so as not to be perceived as "feminine." Women are "allowed" to complain of pain and be feminine. Women learn how to read non-verbal cues and notice others' feelings. Women have deeper, more intense experiences and talk about them. Men talk about physical accomplishments or conquests and don't discuss emotional experiences or pain.

If you take this "male program" and have fibromyalgia, you will see a lot of frustration, anxiety and maladaptive behavior in affected men. The man with fibromyalgia is no longer able to say, "I don't hurt," because he does, but if he admits he hurts, he may be viewed as a "whiner," especially by other men. The pain causes more anxiety and fear, but the man has poor expression and articulation skills regarding painful emotions so the affected male may withdraw more and become more depressed.

Fibromyalgia attacks the very core of man: his prideful ability to be the breadwinner of the family. The pain may prevent him from working as his pillars of strength and stamina crumble. Men can try to hide their fibromyalgia problems and hold it together more than women, but they also can fall harder because of their fibromyalgia.

> ## FLAWS (Famous LAst WordS just before a flare-up)
>
> "Forty bucks to install! Forget it, I'll do it myself."
> "Game of one-on-one, old man?"

Men have some other "unique" characteristics with their fibromyalgia compared to women.

1. I have found that men are more likely than women to get fibromyalgia from trauma. When comparing the population of men and women with post-traumatic fibromyalgia, I found that men account for about 30% of this group, so the ratio of women to men is 7 to 3, compared to 6 to 1 in the overall fibromyalgia population.

2. Men are less likely to seek medical attention for pain problems. Men who finally present to the doctor and are diagnosed with fibromyalgia usually have a more severe form. Women are more likely to seek medical attention sooner, and thus are more likely to be diagnosed earlier with milder stages of fibromyalgia than men.

On exam, men, like women, have painful tender points, localized spasms and trigger points. Men seem to have fewer painful tender points overall than women, but they seem to have more overall impairment than women once they get to the doctor. Their tests give the same results (except their estrogen levels are much lower!). They can benefit from the available treatments; I don't find any unique medications or treatments that work better for men than women, although theoretically there could be differences in the responses to centrally acting medicines because of the differences in the central nervous system.

Men have specific issues and concerns regarding their fibromyalgia that may be different from those of women. Some of these issues include:

1. **Self-image**. Often it is difficult for a man to see a doctor to discuss chronic pain. As I mentioned, men have the stereotypical notion that they should be able to handle pain and should not complain. The mere fact that they have reached a point where they have to see a doctor can be perceived as both a failure on their part and an indication of just how severe the pain has become.

2. **Job and financial issues**. Men who have difficulty performing their jobs because of pain may experience a lot of fear and anxiety about whether they will be able to continue their livelihoods. Men take a lot of pride in their abilities to use their bodies to perform jobs in skillful manners, bring in income, and pay the bills. The thought of losing this, or the actual loss, can be very difficult for men.

3. **Disability**. Men may feel they have to pursue disability because their fibromyalgia prevents them from working. It is usually not possible or practical to simply find another job. Many job skills require physical abilities, and if fibromyalgia interferes, job skills cannot be performed. This creates a paradox where a man can no longer be proud of his abilities, but rather is forced to highlight his inabilities and failures.

4. **Interpersonal and intimacy problems**. Many men report erectile dysfunction or loss of libido because of pain and emotional issues that accompany a chronic pain disorder, or as a side

effect of medicines. Interpersonal relationships may be strained. Many men admit that pain causes a lot of frustrations that may be physically expressed—anger, yelling, irritability, throwing things, and feeling like they are ready to beat up someone at the slightest provocation.

These specific male issues need to be addressed as part of the overall fibromyalgia treatment. It can be challenging for men to get out of the disabled or victim mode once they have entered it. I try to use encouragement and to teach mental management strategies. Additional professional counseling may be needed. Education is crucial, and involving the spouse or significant other in a supportive role can help keep a man's goals and initiatives in focus. Life-style and vocational changes are part of coping with the fibromyalgia.

David Squires of *To Your Health* in Arizona is a great example of a man who has overcome severe fibromyalgia to reshape his life and accomplish a successful lifestyle change. Even with his condition, he has a positive approach to life and work. He runs his own business and devotes many hours to helping others with fibromyalgia. David has been active in support groups and is particularly interested in getting men with fibromyalgia to seek help and support.

I have the pleasure of knowing David and working with him at 2 support group workshops FOR MEN ONLY! It is apparent from these workshops that men have unique issues and concerns in dealing with fibromyalgia and that many have a difficult time. Since men are the minority, it is difficult for them to gather in numbers for a support group. Usually the men at fibromyalgia support groups are spouses of a woman with fibromyalgia. No one is present who can truly connect with the severe daily pain from a man's perspective. Also, support group facilitators are usually women, and men can feel uncomfortable being surrounded by women, although they certainly can benefit from support groups even if all the other members are female.

Men with fibromyalgia need to have supportive people around them to help them cope successfully with their condition. Gender support is even more important since there are fewer men with fibromyalgia than women. Many of my male patients have been able to find online support groups for men where they can discuss their unique problems and provide therapeutic support for one another.

Affected men represent the "silent minority" in fibromyalgia. As a male professional with fibromyalgia, I can relate to the men and appreciate that men hurt and have their lives disrupted. They often suffer silently, though. Our challenge is to reach out to this segment and help them connect. Men should feel comfortable expressing their pain and concerns and ultimately learn to cope better with fibromyalgia.

▶ If You Want To Know More

1. Buskila D, Press J, Gedalia A, et al. *Assessment of nonarticular tenderness and prevalence of fibromyalgia in children*. J Rheumatol 1993; 20: 368–70.

2. Pellegrino MJ. *Inside fibromyalgia*. Columbus OH: Anadem Publishing, 2001.

3. Pellegrino MJ, Waylonis GW, Sommer A. *Familial occurrence of primary fibromyalgia*. Arch Phys Med Rehabil 1989; 70: 61–3.

4. Romano TJ. *Fibrositis in men*. WV Med J 1988; 84: 235–7.

5. Yunus MB, Khan MA, Rawlings KK, et al. *Genetic linkage analysis of multicase families with fibromyalgia syndrome*. J Rheumatol 1998; 57 (suppl 2): 61–2.

When The Pain Worsens

All individuals with fibromyalgia will experience worsening of their pain from time to time; that is a fibro fact! Usually the worsening is temporary, perhaps a flare-up that settles down with treatment. Sometimes people do not respond as hoped to treatments directed at their fibromyalgia despite everyone's best efforts. They may have tried multiple treatments including medicines, therapies, supplements, but they continue to report a high level of pain interfering with function. What causes one's pain level to worsen or not get better? This chapter reviews those factors involved when the pain worsens or doesn't settle down.

Handling Flare-ups

We can't stop flare-ups from happening. We strive for a stable baseline as long as possible, but inevitably the ugly flare-up head will rear itself. Some have frequent flare-ups, others stay in remission practically all the time (and they'd better not brag about it if they want to stay in remission!). All flare-ups have a cause even if we don't know the cause for a particular one. Usually we can identify a specific cause of our increased pain, but if we can't find a specific reason, the flare-up may be called "spontaneous" or "idiopathic." One of the most frustrating complaints I hear is that flare-ups occur in spite of doing "everything" right. We must simply deal with them as they occur and try to accept these periodic, uncontrolled intrusions as part of this condition.

What exactly is a flare-up? How does one know if it is a flare-up due to fibromyalgia or if it is a new problem? What should we do during a flare-up; should we exercise, do our regular work duties, attend social events? These are frequent questions asked by individuals suffering from fibromyalgia.

My definition of a fibromyalgia flare-up is as follows: Increased regional or generalized pain or fatigue, when compared to a stable baseline level, that persists for at least three consecutive days and interferes with usual daily activities. General causes of flare-ups include:

1. Physical factors: physical activities, trauma, too little activity, severe fatigue
2. Infections: colds, flu syndromes, bladder infections, yeast infections
3. Hormonal factors: menstrual cycle, menopause, thyroid or growth hormone changes
4. Environmental factors: cold damp weather, hot humid weather, air conditioner drafts
5. Psychosocial stresses: job changes, marital stresses, depression, loss of loved one, moving

Flare-up causes can also be causes of the initial fibromyalgia. Many of my patients have the misfortune of having 2 injuries impacting their fibromyalgia. The first injury caused the fibromyalgia, then a later injury made it permanently worse.

A stable baseline is not a perfect state. We all experience increased pain on a daily basis. Fluctuations above and below our baseline state are typical—some days we feel better, other days we feel worse, and our pain moves around to different locations. Certain activities may cause a person to hurt more for a few days, but if the pain resolves or decreases to baseline, we would not consider this a flare-up. Each of us has a unique realistic baseline.

Our tender points always have some degree of spontaneous soreness responsible for that constant ache. Palpation of these tender points will cause increased pain, or certain activities will increase the pain, but the pain should quickly return to baseline. Flare-ups occur when the tender points become more persistently and painfully sore. We need to specifically address our flare-ups and ask various questions:

1. **Describe the pain**. Where is the pain? Is it localized to a region or is the whole body affected? When does it hurt? Is the pain constant or intermittent? If the pain is intermittent, does it occur regularly in the morning, during the day, after exercise or at night? Intermittent pain can still meet the definition of a flare-up if it is "persistently intermittent" and interferes with daily functions.

2. **What caused this increased pain?** Many factors can cause a flare-up, including physical, emotional, environmental and idiopathic reasons. Not all pain is related to fibromyalgia, since other unrelated conditions can be present. If the pain is mostly in the morning, the factors may be related to poor sleep or poor sleep positioning. Increased pain during the day may reflect work activities, household activities, or improper body mechanics. Pain after exercise may indicate that the person is overdoing activities or doing new and unusual activities, or not adequately stretching and warming up before the exercise. Increased pain at night might reflect accumulated strains during the day from job activity, or may reflect strenuous leisure activity. Increased fatigue at night often causes increased pain. A person in constant pain may have a combination of factors involved.

3. **What type of treatments can the individual do on his or her own?** If the cause or causes can be identified, they should be removed, altered or modified. Various stretches and exercises, resting certain body parts and restricting certain activities are all a part of the personal strategies in dealing with a flare-up. Increasing the use of home remedies or over-the-counter medications may help.

4. **When should your doctor be consulted**? The patient can consult with the doctor at any time he or she has increased pain. People who have had fibromyalgia for awhile may decide to try a home program first. However, even experienced fibromyalgia sufferers will get new pains or problems that require further medical evaluations, so one is never discouraged from consulting with a doctor. If you first try to manage the flare-up on your own and it does not improve, you will need to follow-up with your doctor.

When I evaluate increased symptoms in my patients, I always try to determine the answer to a basic question: Is this a fibromyalgia flare-up, or is a new condition involved? I perform a clinical evaluation and determine if any specific diagnostic tests are needed. My doctor-directed treatment might include prescription medicines, trigger point injections, therapy orders, manipulations,

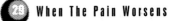

adjustments and specific instructions. Hopefully, the program instituted will resolve the flare-up, reestablish a stable baseline, and enable the home program to be resumed successfully.

Flare-ups are a part of fibromyalgia, probably the most aggravating part (no pun intended!). These flare-ups unpredictably (sometimes predictably) come to visit us from time to time. Our job is to make their visit as short as possible!

Resistant Fibromyalgia

This category represents those with fibromyalgia who do not respond to any treatment or get worse. They may have had brief responses to treatment, but nothing has made a long-term difference. The baseline pain remains very high and flares up frequently. There are various reasons why pain levels stay high and flare up easily.

Trauma. A new trauma may be superimposed on a previously stable fibromyalgia. This new trauma can cause permanent escalation of the baseline level of pain and involve new areas not previously painful. New traumas can occur with a single event such as a work injury or a car accident, or it may result from cumulative trauma such as repetitive activity from a job.

Worsening due to another condition. Worsening can also be related to another condition that is progressive, such as arthritis or neurologic diseases. Anyone who has fibromyalgia secondary to another condition (subset 8) or existing with another condition (subset 7) can be at the mercy of the other condition. If the other condition progresses over time, the fibromyalgia can worsen as well. Fibromyalgia is notorious for being easily aggravated with only mild increases of disease activity of another condition.

Like a virus, fibromyalgia can "mutate" to resist treatment, particularly in unstable fibromyalgia.

Fibromyalgia "mutates." Like a virus, fibromyalgia can "mutate" to resist treatment, particularly in unstable fibromyalgia. There may have been a window of improvement with a particular treatment, but the fibromyalgia always finds a way to break through and cause increased pain. Needless to say, this is very frustrating and people become discouraged. I have several patients who felt so great with a particular product that they began selling the product (nutritional supplements, magnets). But, the improvements did not last. Over time the fibromyalgia pain gradually took a renewed hold on them, and they had a hard time running their businesses, causing further pain.

As a physician it is difficult to address the issue of resistant fibromyalgia, and it needs to be handled with compassion and hope. I try to emphasize that their pain is not their fault or caused by something they are doing wrong.

It is hard enough for the patients to accept fibromyalgia, but they have to try to accept a persistently higher level of pain that is resistant to treatment. There are no easy answers. Sometimes I have to say, "I don't know" when asked what the future will hold. I emphasize the importance of continuing with a regular program in spite of pain. We try different things, and if new treatment strategies are reported or discovered, we are open-minded in trying these.

I rotate treatments. Sometimes an initial treatment works and then stops working. Then we will try another treatment that may work and rotate back to the first treatment at a later time. The more therapeutic options that are available, the more opportunities to find successful programs that can be rotated.

Individual job situations need to be addressed. Preserving the job or some modified version of it is a high priority, but at times the person with fibromyalgia is disabled. My goal is to keep the person active and gainfully employed for the longest time possible.

Patients Who Have Inappropriate Or Unrealistic Expectations

From time to time I see patients with chronic pain who come to my office for a specific reason other than treating fibromyalgia or trying to improve their quality of life. Examples of specific reasons include:

- Seeking narcotics or other drugs
- Want to be declared totally disabled
- Want me to state that a specific injury caused their problem

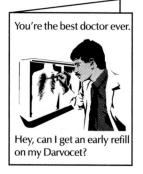

You're the best doctor ever.

Hey, can I get an early refill on my Darvocet?

These patients do not come right out and say "I need narcotics," or " I need you to write a good report so I can get disability." During the history taking, these patients will usually reveal clues as to the underlying motive or agenda for their visit with me. For example, patients who are seeking narcotics may say they have been to numerous doctors and no one could help them, and may be very vague about the details of who they saw, what medicine was prescribed and why they are no longer seeing these doctors. They report trying a number of medicines and may say they are allergic to all pain medicines except Percocet.

Patients who are seeking disability may say they have tried different jobs but can't stay at any job because of pain. Or they may say that someone else has suggested that disability should be looked into. They may say a primary care doctor steered them to me for disability or that disability was pursued and denied and they need a report from a specialist.

Patients who claim to have been injured may indicate repeatedly that the chronic pain was caused by an injury and that their attorney needs a doctor to make that association to help with the lawsuit. As an experienced physician, it is my job to spot these telltale clues and be able to factor in any hidden agenda (not so hidden!) and try to ascertain the true motive for seeing me.

I am not saying that these patients do not have pain or that they do not have fibromyalgia. In my experience, a true malingerer (someone who deliberately fakes an illness or injury for the purpose of a consciously desired end) is rare. I believe that patients are hurt but they have misguided or inappropriate expectations regarding their consult with me. My practice style is NOT to be the next doctor in line to prescribe heavy narcotics to a drug seeker. My style as a rehabilitation doctor is NOT to declare someone totally disabled on their first visit with me simply because the patient does not feel he or she is able to work. I focus on abilities despite a chronic illness.

I will NOT make a diagnosis because it will "help" a patient's case nor will I place restrictions on someone if I feel he or she is capable of doing a specific activity. I strive to be credible as a fibromyalgia specialist, and I am honest in my approach (I call it as I see it), even if the occasional patient is less than honest with me. As a consulting and treating physician, I need to make decisions and recommendations that I am comfortable with and that I feel will be beneficial to my patients.

I will always explain to the patient my treatment style and philosophy, and try to offer helpful strategies that I feel are realistic, even if they don't include narcotic medication. Most patients accept my recommendations and understand my philosophies and comfort levels. However, some are adamant about needing a specific narcotic in order to function, or have some other "need" and anything less than that would be unacceptable to these patients.

Sometimes this type of patient becomes very angry with me when they realize I'm not handing over a Oxycodone prescription. No matter what I say, they still equate my refusal to prescribe a narcotic or to declare them totally disabled as a sign that I don't care and that I won't help them. I may have offered much advice, recommendations and strategies to try, but all they heard was, "I'm not comfortable prescribing any narcotic medicine for you at this time."

I've gotten some detailed letters from some of these angry disappointed people. One lady told me that Satan was working through me! Does that make me a devil's advocate?

I always feel badly when this happens (when I disappoint these patients, not when Satan works through me!) because I was not able to help these patients. But the "help" they wanted was unrealistic. Patients need to be responsible and honest to hold up their end of the patient-doctor relationship and sometimes this doesn't happen and a therapeutic rapport cannot be established. When one deals with a chronic pain population, this situation 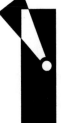 **I will always explain to the patient my treatment style and philosophy, and try to offer helpful strategies that I feel are realistic, even if they don't include narcotic medication.**
comes up from time to time, but fortunately they are vastly outnumbered by the "good" patient-doctor encounters. In my experience, most of the patients in this "unrealistic" category will continue to report persistent pain that never settles down regardless of the treatment.

Chronic Pain Syndrome Associated With Fibromyalgia

Some individuals develop a condition known as chronic pain syndrome. This is defined as a state of overwhelming chronic pain that interferes with the person's physical, emotional, and psychological functional abilities and causes depression in everyday life's activity. This condition is more overwhelming than fibromyalgia alone. Dr. Keefe (1982) described characteristics of a person with chronic pain syndrome. They include:

Significant subjective and functional limitations out of proportion to the objective physical exam findings. TRANSLATION: Patients will report they are unable to do certain activities, but the doctor would expect they could do these activities based on the physical exam. For example, patients may say they cannot put on shoes even though they demonstrate the abilities to bend their back and move their arms in a manner required for that activity.

Dependency and addictive behaviors. This includes the use of excessive narcotic or opioid medications, increased alcohol or nicotine consumption, and an increased dependency on others to assist them in everyday activities.

Well-defined pain behaviors. Examples of pain behaviors include slow, deliberate movements, walking with an inconsistent limp, exaggerated flinching upon palpation, frequent facial grimacing and sighing, and frequent indications of "I can't" when asked to perform a certain movement or physical task.

Most people who have severe pain from fibromyalgia do not develop chronic pain syndrome. However, it does commonly develop from fibromyalgia. In my experience, about 2% of people with fibromyalgia develop chronic pain syndrome. These patients will give a history of terrible pain which continues to get worse, although everything has been tried. The patient may report that he or she spends most of the day in bed, and often complains of feeling depressed, frustrated, and anxious, and describes himself or herself as disabled. Typically, the physical examination is difficult because of pain behaviors. There is difficulty examining the muscles, because light palpation results in significant pain responses. Neurologic testing, particularly muscle strength testing and muscle sensory testing, may be impossible because the patient is not able to cooperate reliably.

The person has true pain. The person with chronic pain syndrome has true pain. A psychological reaction to the pain has occurred, however, resulting in the syndrome described above. In this situation both fibromyalgia and chronic pain syndrome are present, even though it is usually difficult to isolate specific painful tender points because the patient complains of diffuse pain wherever touched.

Treatment of chronic pain syndrome, in my experience, is very difficult. It's hard to achieve consistent high success rates with treatments. This difficulty stems from the fact that in chronic pain syndrome, fibromyalgia is no longer the main condition causing symptoms. Rather, the chronic pain and pain behaviors become the primary conditions. Chronic pain syndrome is a separate disease entity that requires its own separate treatment. It is a very complex condition and the patient is actually more resistant to treatment.

A comprehensive multidisciplinary approach with knowledge-able personnel is once again necessary. The evaluation process includes core personnel of the chronic pain management team, *i.e.*,

Chronic pain syndrome is a separate disease entity that requires its own separate treatment. It is a very complex condition and the patient is actually more resistant to treatment.

physician, psychologist, physical therapist, occupational therapist, social service counselor, rehabilitation nurse, vocational counselor, pharmacist, and dietician. The treatment emphasizes modifying and reducing medications, behavior management of pain by modifying pain behaviors and how pain interferes with one's life, addressing psychosocial and vocational issues, and increasing physical activity and vocational abilities. This type of intensive multidisciplinary evaluation and treatment with emphasis on behavior modification is probably the best.

Top Ten Pain Behaviors To Let The Doctor Know You Hurt

1. Keep saying, "this pain is killing me."
2. Limp out of the office
3. Slouch and walk slowly into the exam room
4. Cry out loudly as soon as the doctor touches your skin
5. Sigh frequently during the interview
6. Squirm and fidget in the chair
7. Begin hyperventilating halfway through the physical exam
8. Grab the doctor's hand when ever he tries to press on your muscles
9. Grimace whenever touched (watch so you don't strain your face muscles)
10. When asked to bend forward, move a few inches and say "that's it."

The Patient Who Lacks Resources

Unfortunately, patients with fibromyalgia sometimes find themselves without insurance or funds, which results in very limited abilities to get medically necessary treatments for their painful condition. This is another reason why patients may not improve.

The reality with fibromyalgia is this condition has a better chance of improving or stabilizing with appropriately prescribed treatments. Not everyone needs prescribed medicines or therapy, but most people, in my experience, need some type of prescribed medical intervention during their course of fibromyalgia.

The goal is to minimize any need for prescribed treatments, but the fibromyalgia has to be addressed, and the more treatment options available, the better the chance of successful treatments, successful home programs, and minimal use of insurance for treatments. Those who have no insurance coverage, no treatment benefits with their plan, or poor financial situations will have more limited treatment options available. These patients will not be able to afford medicines, massages, chiropractic treatments, supplements, etc. and their fibromyalgia will not have the "opportunity" to respond to these treatment options.

> Not everyone needs prescribed medicines or therapy, but most people, in my experience, need some type of prescribed medical intervention during their course of fibromyalgia.

For these patients, I try to provide as much as information to them as possible and guide them to free resources at the library or online to enhance their fibromyalgia knowledge. We discuss home strategies, *e.g.*, heat, cold, stretches and exercises, and I give them handouts. We offer a 6 week fibromyalgia course and I will provide "scholarships" to financially challenged patients so they can benefit from education and support. Patients are encouraged to reach out and connect with other fibromyalgia peers via support groups or other means.

Community and hospital clinics may offer physical therapy programs for qualified patients. Drug companies may offer coupons, vouchers or other programs for financially distressed patients. In our practice, we try to be generous with our time and services for individual patients who may benefit from them. Hopefully patients can improve from available resources to better control their fibromyalgia and help the pain settle down.

Summary

Unfortunately there are a number of patients who have had multiple treatments but continue to be bothered by significant pain. The pain is disabling for them, and they are not able to carry out their daily activities or job functions. They have fluctuations of pain above and below their baseline, or have frequent flare-ups, but at their baseline level they continue to have severe disabling pain.

What causes one's pain level to worsen or not improve? There may be ongoing trauma or stresses that worsen the fibromyalgia or another condition such as a progressive arthritis. The individual may be resistant to treatment because of well-ingrained disability and pain behaviors. The person expects to hurt and not get better. The patient may remember what it was like to have less pain, and this "remembered standard" is what is expected of successful treatment. If this standard is not reached, the perception is that the treatment is failing. There may be increased anger, frustration, anxiety, and depression contributing to the increased pain. Sometimes the person is just unlucky and has a more severe, resistant form of fibromyalgia. Even with patients who have not been compliant with the recommended treatment program, I do not confront them, but give them their options and respect the choices and decisions they wish to make regarding their fibromyalgia.

I'll also review any additional treatment considerations for the patient whose severe pain has not settled down. New medicines or medicine combinations, chronic pain and stress management programs, other medical professionals, supportive counseling, reassurance, or addressing work or disability issues are various treatment considerations. Hopefully different approaches can help overcome the persistently painful situation and enable patients to get to a more stable baseline level of pain.

If You Want To Know More

1. Keefe FJ, Block AR, Williams RB, et al. *Behavioral treatment of chronic low back pain: clinical outcome and individual differences in pain relief.* Pain 1981; 11: 221–31.

2. Pellegrino MJ. *Inside fibromyalgia.* Columbus OH: Anadem Publishing, 2001.

3. Weitz SE, Witt PH, Greenfield DP. *Treatment of chronic pain syndrome.* N J Med 2000; 97: 63–7.

SECTION V—UNDERSTANDING POST-TRAUMATIC FIBROMYALGIA

Post-traumatic fibromyalgia, or fibromyalgia caused by trauma, is a special interest of mine. I feel it is important enough to warrant its own Section and Chapters. I think it fits right here between specific fibromyalgia-related problems and unique situations, and I've designed this section to be a mini-book within the book.

What Is Trauma?

Post-traumatic fibromyalgia (PTF) is a common type of fibromyalgia, in my experience. Simply defined, PTF is fibromyalgia caused by trauma. Some type of trauma started a chain reaction that ultimately led to fibromyalgia in each patient with PTF.

We all have multiple experiences with trauma throughout our lives. They may be sudden forceful injuries or may be subtle everyday wear and tear changes. Most traumas are minor, but some do major damage to the body. The human body is composed of delicate biological tissues, and when these tissues encounter concrete, wood, metal, and various physical forces, the tissues lose!

Traumas can be defined into two categories: acute and chronic.

Acute Trauma

Acute trauma is when a sudden forceful injury causes pathological changes to body tissues. An acute injury can occur with a direct blow, a penetrating object, a fall, an abnormal twist, jerk or bend, or a jam. Categories of acute injuries include:

- Bruises or contusions
- Sprains
- Strains
- Dislocations
- Fractures

Bruises occur when small blood vessels under the skin tear or rupture. Blood leaks into the tissues under the skin and causes the classic black and blue color. Gravity can pull blood downward so leg bruises can end up discoloring the foot.

Severe bruising can cause immediate pain and swelling within 30 minutes of the injury and this often indicates a more serious injury such as a sprain, strain or fracture. Bruises heal faster on the face than on the arm and heal slower in the legs. Bruises should heal within a few weeks.

Some people bruise more easily than others. Older adults and women tend to be more prone to minor bruises. Many of my patients with fibromyalgia complain of easy bruising as well.

A sprain is an injury to a ligament, either by stretching or tearing. The severity of the injury will depend on how many ligaments are involved and whether the tear is complete or partial. A fall or sudden twist can cause an over-stretching of the ligament supporting a particular joint and tearing or sprains can result.

If one twists a knee, turns an ankle, falls and lands on an outstretched arm, a sprain can occur. The most common site of sprains is the ankle. Wrist and shoulder sprains are common when people fall and land on an outstretched arm. The usual symptoms of sprains include pain, swelling, bruising and loss of mobility in that joint. Sprains usually heal within two–six weeks.

A strain is similar to a sprain but it affects the muscle or tendon. Strains can be acute or chronic. An acute strain is caused by lifting heavy objects or performing unusual activities, or in an athlete who runs without proper warm-up. Chronic strains are usually the result of overuse of the muscles and tendons.

Two common sites for a strain are the back and the hamstring muscles. Symptoms of a strain include pain, muscle spasm, some swelling, and loss of muscle function. More severe strains can result in complete tearing of the muscle or tendon and are often very painful. Strains can heal within a week to a few months depending on the severity.

The treatment of sprains and strains includes reducing swelling and pain. RICE therapy may be advised by a treating doctor.

RICE therapy includes:

Rest: Reduce regular exercise or activities of daily living as needed. Depending on the area injured, you may be advised to not put any weight on the area or use crutches or a cane.

Ice: Apply an ice pack to the injured area for 20 minutes at a time, 4–8 times a day. A cold pack, ice bag, or plastic bag filled with crushed ice and wrapped in a towel can be used. To avoid cold injury and frostbite, do not apply the ice for more than 20 minutes.

Compression: Compression bandages such as elastic wraps, special boots, air casts, and splints may be recommended to help reduce swelling.

Elevation: If possible, keep the injured ankle, knee, elbow, or wrist elevated on a pillow, above the level of the heart, to help decrease swelling.

The next stage of treating a sprain or strain is rehabilitation where the goal is to restore function. An exercise program might be prescribed to improve flexibility, increase range of motion, and restore strength. Some people may require a physical therapy program. Despite best treatment efforts, some people may go on to develop PTF following sprains or strains.

Dislocations and fractures are more serious joint and bone injuries that usually require an orthopedic specialist to evaluate and treat. Orthopedic manipulation to reduce or fix a dislocation, casting, or even surgery may be required to treat these types of orthopedic injuries. The treatment goals are to restore the joint or bone to normal strength, normal mobility, and prevent any complications. Some people, however, do develop PTF following these orthopedic injuries.

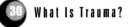
Acute injuries are waiting to happen everywhere. They wait at sporting events (especially contact sports), in work places (especially where a lot of bending and lifting is required), at home, in recreational facilities, on icy sidewalks, inside cars, and elsewhere. Many times a combination of different types of injuries all occur with one single acute trauma.

Chronic Trauma

The mechanism of chronic trauma is different from acute trauma. Chronic trauma is a more subtle, low-grade type that occurs over time from cumulative and repetitive actions of soft tissues such as tendons, ligaments, muscles and joints. Other names for chronic trauma include repetitive injury, overuse injury or overuse syndrome. In this injury, too much stress is placed on the soft tissues over and over again over time.

Categories of chronic injuries include:

- Tendinitis
- Bursitis
- Epicondylitis
- Carpal tunnel syndrome
- Stress fractures
- Degenerative arthritis

Tendons are the tough rope-like fibers that connect muscles to bones. They can be acutely sprained, and they are commonly injured through overuse. An inflammation of the tendon through overuse is called tendinitis and common areas of tendinitis include the shoulder, wrist, and knee. Those with wrist tendinitis are more prone to develop carpal tunnel syndrome where the carpal tunnel nerve (median nerve) gets squished by the swollen tendons around it.

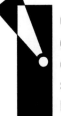

Chronic trauma is a more subtle, low-grade type that occurs over time from cumulative and repetitive actions of soft tissues such as tendons, ligaments, muscles and joints.

Bursitis is an inflammation of the bursa. A bursa is a fluid-filled sac that cushions and lubricates the area between one bone and another bone, a tendon, or the skin. Repetitive injury or continuous pressure over a bursa can cause bursitis. Common symptoms of bursitis and tendinitis include pain, swelling, redness, warmth and limitation of mobility. Bursitis is common in the shoulders, hips and knees, and often co-exists with tendinitis.

Epicondylitis is another type of inflammation affecting the tendons and ligaments adjoining the epicondyle of the elbow. There are two epicondyles at the elbow, the lateral epicondyle (outside elbow) and the medial epicondyle (inside elbow), where the muscles of the forearm attach to the elbow via a thick tendinous-type ligament. Inflammations of these areas are called a lateral epicondylitis or tennis elbow, and medial epicondylitis or golfer's elbow. Most people with epicondylitis are not tennis players or golfers however.

Treatment of tendon, bursa and epicondyle inflammation includes antiinflammatory medications, injections, splints, physical medicine and rehabilitation treatments. If bony involvement is occurring as part of the cumulative trauma (*e.g.*, stress fractures or degenerative arthritis), additional treatment considerations may include joint injections, or casting (for a stress fracture in the foot for example). The treatment goals are always to reduce pain, improve function, and to prevent further chronic trauma.

The number of cumulative trauma cases has increased, especially in the workplace. Improved technology has caused jobs to be more repetitive while work speed has increased. Work places have become more specialized, plus workers and physicians are more aware of symptoms of cumulative trauma.

Risk Factors For Work-Related Cumulative Trauma

Various risk factors are involved in developing cumulative trauma and PTF or aggravating pre-existing fibromyalgia. These risk factors include:

1. **Repetitions.** Jobs that require a lot of repetitive put continuous strain on soft tissues. Many manufacturing, assembly line, and secretarial jobs involve frequent use of the hands and arms and are examples of jobs that are risky.

2. **Excessive force.** Jobs that require excessive force also increase the risk. Activities such as power-gripping or movements against gravity (lifting objects off the ground or pushing up on tools) are examples of activities requiring excessive force on soft tissues.

3. **Unnatural positions.** If joints are not in the neutral or natural position, more strain is exerted on them and on soft tissues. The arms outstretched or overhead, elbows away from the body, wrists bent up or down, palms facing up, or leaning forward and bending are various unnatural positions that increase the risk of injury and subsequent post PTF.

4. **Cold, damp environments.** Jobs that require a lot of outdoor exposure, particularly in the wintertime, or frequent changes in temperature within the workplace itself (going from a freezer to a refrigerator to a heated area at various times during the course of the day) will increase risk for cumulative stress and trauma and ultimately fibromyalgia.

5. **Stress.** Increased stress on the job can occur for a variety of reasons. Working long hours of overtime, working strictly night shifts, worries about job security or financial issues, and extra responsibilities or management positions are a few examples of stresses on the job that can increase the risk for injury or fibromyalgia.

No matter what type of injury or combinations of injuries, the body tries to completely heal all injuries. Sometimes complete healing does not happen and complications occur including PTF. Not everyone with an injury heals completely, and not everyone who heals incompletely develops fibromyalgia, but some do.

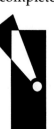

I have seen over 15,000 people with fibromyalgia, most of whom report a trauma of some sort that caused their condition.

When I first began private practice in my specialty of Physical Medicine and Rehabilitation in 1988, I saw many people who reported pain all over their bodies, pains that were chronic and often debilitating—fibromyalgia.

When I asked these people with fibromyalgia about their pains, I was surprised that a number of them were able to emphatically state the exact instant when their pains began: after they had an injury. The stories from this diverse group of patients of different backgrounds, ages, nationalities, and occupations began to weave a recurrent theme that I couldn't ignore: The person was pain-free until he or she sustained a trauma, and then developed pain that never went away. The pain often got worse over time, and eventually the person was diagnosed with fibromyalgia.

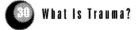

This association between trauma and fibromyalgia was further supported by my firsthand observations. Some patients I treated for acute injuries never got better, despite aggressive therapies. Right before my eyes, no matter what was tried, these people developed fibromyalgia. They never had any significant pain to speak of before the injury, and now they have a chronically painful condition for which there currently is no known cure.

Over the years I have seen over 15,000 people with fibromyalgia, most of whom report a trauma of some sort that caused their condition. In 1996, I published a book, *Post-Traumatic Fibromyalgia, A Medical Perspective* (Anadem Publishing) which included a review of 2000 records of fibromyalgia patients I saw between 1990 and 1995. Of those, 65% reported the onset of their symptoms of fibromyalgia after a traumatic event (PTF). Of this group, 52% (1,040 people), were involved in a motor vehicle accident and had a whiplash injury, 31% had work injuries that led to the fibromyalgia (both acute and chronic), and 17% had another type of trauma such as a sports injury, home injury or surgical procedure. Thus, the whiplash injury is the most common trauma I see that leads to PTF.

Personal Profile

by Mark J. Pellegrino, M.D.

I enjoy writing, and I like to write letters. Sometimes a situation involving fibromyalgia just screams for a "good" letter. This letter was originally published in *The Fibromyalgia Network* newsletter.

An Invitation to Those Who Don't Believe Trauma Causes Fibromyalgia

Dear Non-Believing Medical Colleagues:

I need your help. I am a Board-Certified Physiatrist who has seen over 15,000 patients with fibromyalgia. Over half the people I have diagnosed with fibromyalgia report that trauma caused their symptoms. This is consistent with what other doctors who see fibromyalgia tell me.

I know you don't believe in post-traumatic fibromyalgia, or fibromyalgia caused by trauma. You are always quick to deny any relationship between trauma and fibromyalgia, and repeatedly play your same trump card to defend your statements, the one that says "There is no scientific proof that trauma causes fibromyalgia." Is there any truth to the rumor that your are seeking to license a new motto "In Absolute Proof We Trust?"

Some of you are getting a little bolder and saying trauma cannot cause fibromyalgia rather than just saying there is not proof that it does. Just last week I got a report from one of you (I'll call him Dr. X) who did an independent medical exam on one of my patients with post-traumatic fibromyalgia. Dr. X wrote that my patient has fibromyalgia. He said he did not know what caused her fibromyalgia, but he is certain that it was not caused by trauma. I was amused by Dr. X's paradoxical position; he doesn't know but he does know. I think a more appropriate (and truthful) statement from Dr. X would have been something like this: "I don't believe in post-traumatic fibromyalgia, so I never make this diagnosis, and thus, have never seen it. I am the last person who should be asked to provide a knowledgeable opinion of whether trauma causes fibromyalgia, because I haven't a clue."

continued on next page...

Personal Profile

continued from previous page...

My amusement was short-lived however, because Dr. X's report hurt my patient by preventing necessary medical treatment. It seems the insurance company that requested the exam was so impressed by Dr. X's certainty that it halted all coverage of her fibromyalgia, for now. By the way, the insurance company paid Dr. X $450.00 for his exam and report. My patient's necessary treatments would have cost more than that, so I bet the insurance companies are glad they have people like you and Dr. X to send their patients to for these exams.

Not that you shouldn't get paid for your work. I am not trying to anger you, I really need your help. Here's my request I would like you to consider:

I would like you to design, carry out and publish a research project that proves trauma does not lead to fibromyalgia, as you always talk about. Since you are such fans of the absolute certainty/100% proof research criteria, I think this project would be perfect for you.

Imagine, a chance to actually back up what you say! You could finally shout to the medical world that your own research proves trauma does not cause fibromyalgia, rather than hiding behind the shield of scientific "uncertainty" and collectively whispering "there's no proof yet."

I hope you will consider my request. I am unable to perform this project because I am busy in my clinical practice. I'm one of these old fashioned doctors who listens to patients and tries to determine the cause of pain so I can help them as best as possible. I can offer you some guidelines and suggestions should you choose to embark upon this exciting research project.

1. Study design. You need to use the highest level of scientific evidence, the age-matched, double-blinded, placebo-controlled study. Double-blinded does not mean twice ignoring the excellent scientific research already published that establishes **probability** that trauma causes fibromyalgia within a reasonable degree of medical certainty. Double-blinded means you don't know who has been injured or not when you evaluate them for fibromyalgia over time. Since probability (greater than 51%) is not good enough for you, you need to be 100% sure, so set up the project right.

2. Subjects. You need two subject populations, a trauma group and a placebo-control group that are age matched and in large numbers, preferably over 200 people in each group. Avoid small samples because that's always easy to criticize, you know, the results may have been different if the sample were larger. . . .

    It is very important not to pay the subjects. You tell me all the time how you believe so strongly that people with pain after an injury only have pain because they may be compensated (insurance, disability, lawsuit). I suggest you avoid any payment whatsoever so no one will say the subject was seeking a financial "reward." I never understood how you put "reward" and "fibromyalgia" together in the same sentence anyway. So just avoid any confusion by making this project one of volunteer subjects only.

    The trauma group should have experienced documented physical injury. Different parts of the body may be more susceptible to injury so include injuries to all parts of the body including the neck. Since you are a particularly skeptical group at times, I suggest that you don't assume a person was injured just because he or she says so. You don't want anyone criticizing how some patients could have been faking an injury since they weren't documented and thus your whole study should be disregarded. Accept patients only if they can produce verifiable proof of injury,

continued on next page...

Personal Profile

continued from previous page...

i.e., unaltered videotape and photographic evidence, or eyewitness testimony. You should discuss among yourselves whether subjects should be required to pass a lie detector test first. Remember, common sense has no role in this research project so don't let it confuse you. Verify everything!

Controlling for placebo effect is a challenge here, but you have to do it right. It is possible that some patients who develop fibromyalgia after a trauma are only imagining that they do, and this could lead to fibromyalgia findings not due to actual body tissue injury. Your placebo group should believe they actually experienced a trauma even though they didn't. Maybe you can get cooperation from amusement parks, movie theaters or computer software companies with "virtual reality" technology. This technology could create "virtual trauma" on a group of people who could form the placebo group.

3. Gathering data. This should be easy. All you have to do is repeatedly examine these hundreds of subjects in both groups over time. Immediately after the trauma, real or virtual, each subject should be assessed for symptoms and tenderness. Frequent repeated exams are necessary over time because localizing generalized fibromyalgia can take many months to fully develop. You need to be available 24 hours a day as the subjects become available, so hold off on any vacation. Use both subjective tools (*i.e.*, Visual Analog Pain Scale) and objective evidence (Tender point score).

4. Interpreting data. When analyzing data, use accepted statistical calculation methods. Don't use consensus where you combine all of your individual opinions and pretend it's "research." Remember, the data is independent of any expectations of the insurance, legal or medical profession. If the data doesn't support what you expect and shows that trauma **does** cause fibromyalgia, don't be too disappointed. I am sure you will be able to find some way to criticize your own research and try to cast doubts!

I hope these suggestions are helpful. I would appreciate if you could hurry with this study. This absolute proof standard you require is scaring me. Suppose we have to approach everything we diagnose and treat in medicine using this standard. Since very little of what we do in medicine currently meets this strict evidence standard, I am afraid I won't be able to treat anything at all without the "proof." Thank you for your urgent attention to my request.

Sincerely (I think I'm sincere, but I've never seen any studies that "proves" sincerity exists.)

Mark J. Pellegrino, M.D.

PS—Until you've completed your project, I am going to continue taking care of patients with post-traumatic fibromyalgia because, well, no study yet has proven trauma does **not** cause fibromyalgia!

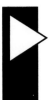

If You Want To Know More

1. Pellegrino MJ. *From whiplash to fibromyalgia*. N. Canton OH: ORC Publishing, 2002.

2. Pellegrino MJ. *Inside fibromyalgia*. Columbus OH: Anadem Publishing, 2001.

3. Pellegrino MJ. *Understanding post-traumatic fibromyalgia*. Columbus OH: Anadem Publishing, 1996.

The Whiplash Injury

Whiplash injury is the most common type of trauma that leads to fibromyalgia in my patients. Patients' symptoms, physicians' experiences, scientific publications and ongoing medical research allow us to conclude that whiplash trauma probably leads to fibromyalgia.

Not that there isn't any controversy regarding whiplash and fibromyalgia. If I could pick two of the most "controversial" medical topics in my specialty today, they would be whiplash and PTF. Each one in itself is an explosive topic among physicians and attorneys. Put the two conditions together and you create spontaneous combustion within the dynamite.

Ever since humans have been stopped suddenly while traveling inside or on moving objects, there have been whiplash injuries. Whiplash has become a "street term" for a serious neck injury. As a physician specializing in pain problems, I have seen thousands of patients over the years who have hurt their necks after collisions involving cars, buses, taxis, motorcycles, mopeds, or bicycles, and one person who hit a tree while cruising down a hill in his homemade racer. Whiplash injuries frequently lead to chronic medical problems and disability.

The term "whiplash" was first used by Dr. Crowe in 1928 to describe the forced hyperextension and hyperflexion pattern of neck injury in a rear-end collision, the so called "whipping" motion that occurs to the cervical spine. "Whiplash" is often perceived to be synonymous with any neck injury occurring after a motor vehicle accident. Yet the term "whiplash" is actually a description of an injury mechanism where the head and neck undergo complex motions (NOT like a whip) in response to collision forces. Injuries can occur to many different parts of the body, not just the neck, and a person can suffer from "whiplash" injuries without being involved in a rear-end collision. Despite any confusion regarding injury mechanisms versus injury symptoms, one thing is clear: "whiplash" is a common problem in the world, and many who have a "whiplash" are left with chronic and debilitating pain.

The Western world has seen an epidemic increase in the number of whiplash injuries in the past century. Dr. Erichson wrote in 1882 of train passengers who suffered from "concussion of the nervous system" when the train was struck from behind. As we've hurtled through time in trains, cars, and other moving objects, we've also been hurtled forwards and backwards suddenly, unexpectedly, and often painfully. The National Safety Council estimated there were nearly 12.7 million motor vehicle accidents in the United States in 1998 involving about 21.3 million drivers (about 1 in 9 licensed drivers). How many of these accidents (whiplash "opportunities") led to actual whiplash injuries are not able to be determined exactly.

Since whiplash injuries are not fatal, rarely require hospital admissions, and oftentimes do not result in an immediate visit to a hospital emergency department, reliable medical records on who sustained whiplash injuries are not readily available. People with pain following a collision usually seek medical care, as I have seen firsthand thousands of times. The injured person may see a private physician instead of going to the hospital emergency department, or may wait a few days then go to a hospital emergency department. In these instances, the medical records may not contain the specific information about the accident needed to study the relationship of the trauma to the symptoms.

In 1992, Dr. Evans estimated the annual incidence of new whiplash injuries in the United States to be 391 per 100,000 population. In the United Kingdom, Dr. Galasko, *et al.,* calculated the annual incidence of new whiplash injuries in the United Kingdom to be 417 per 100,000 population. Other studies of the Western world's rate of whiplash injuries per population concludes the same ballpark figure, about 400 injuries per every 100,000 people.

If we combine the number of accidents per USA population (12.7 million per 273 million population) with the incidence of new whiplash injuries (400 per 100,000 population), the number of whiplash injuries per motor vehicle accidents can be estimated. The number turns out to be about 1 whiplash injury per every 12 accidents (8.3% of the time). This figure is an estimate because some accidents may cause more than 1 whiplash injury. Over a million whiplash injuries a year occur in the United States, roughly 1 every 30 seconds. The costs are staggering, estimated in the billions of dollars.

Laws Of Physics

The most important factor regarding motor vehicle collisions and injuries is how much (or how little) of the collision force is absorbed by the occupants. Regardless of the number of variables involved, the key question is always: what happens to the forces generated by the collision?

Laws of physics allow us to determine what happens to the collision forces. Momentum (M) is the term for "motion energy" and equals the mass of an object (m) times its velocity (v), or $M = mv$. Any object that is not moving has no momentum, no matter how heavy it is (if $v = 0, M = 0$). Momentum is proportional to force; the more the momentum, the more the force (or energy). If a car weighing 1 ton accelerates from 10 mph to 20 mph, the car's momentum has doubled. (twice as much motion energy going 20 mph compared to 10 mph). A 3 ton bus going 10 mph, a 2-ton truck going 15 mph, and a 1-ton car going 30 mph all have the same momentum, or the same amount of motion energy.

If any of these moving vehicles collide with an object, Newton's Third Law of Motion states that the momentum must be conserved. Any energy that exists before the collision must exist after the collision. Energy (force) can be transferred from one object to another, or be converted to a different form (*e.g.,* heat, sound), but it must be conserved.

Let's review two examples of Newton's Third Law of Motion. Say an empty car accidentally left in neutral rolls down a hill and collides with a telephone pole. The car has momentum, or motion energy, when it hits the pole. Just before the impact, the inert pole had no momentum, and it would not have moved on its own unless something moved it. The car's total motion energy (determined by its weight and traveling speed) must be conserved after the collision. The collision causes energy to be transferred to the telephone pole. The pole is actually moved from the car's momentum, accelerating quickly from rest and ending up at rest again in a different position.

Some of the energy is absorbed by the front of the car when it crumples, and other energy is transferred to heat (friction) and sound (noise) from the crash. Some energy may be absorbed by the pole, causing the pole to break. When the crash sequence has ended, and both the car and pole are at rest again, we would be able to determine that all the energy present before the collision equaled the energy present after the collision; thus the momentum was conserved.

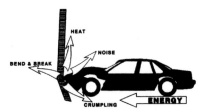

Energy before collision = Energy after collision

Let's review a second example, a rear end collision. Car A, stopped at a red light, is suddenly rear ended by Car B. As in the first example, the total energy must be conserved before and after the collision. The difference in this example is that a driver is present in each car. Thus, human biologic tissue is in the pathway of the energy transfers.

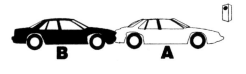

When Car B hits the rear of Car A, momentum is transferred from B to A. The energy from the rapidly decelerating Car B is transferred to Car A, which rapidly accelerated from rest to move a short distance, then both cars come to a complete stop. The drivers each undergo rapid violent movements in response to the collision. Some of the energy is absorbed by crumpling metal, and some is transferred to friction and noise. Some energy, however, is absorbed by each driver. The total energy before and after are equal, but the small portions of energy that were diverted into the human bodies could have wreaked havoc on the sensitive biologic tissues.

Whiplash injuries are the result of rapid and violent acceleration and deceleration movements of the human bodies, especially the head and neck, from a stationary position to a new position. The human body is simply participating in the laws of physics, yet it can pay a heavy price for its role in absorbing some of the collision forces.

FLAWS (Famous **LA**st **W**ord**S** just before a flare-up)
"That car is coming awfully fast, I don't think it is going to stop in time."

Organic Vs. Inorganic

Organic living tissue is much more vulnerable to injury when exposed to collision energy than inorganic non-living objects. This may seem like an obvious statement, but I frequently hear patients, doctors and attorneys discuss the potential for bodily injuries to be directly related to the amount of visible damage done to the car. I have witnessed attorneys show jurors pictures of cars with no visible damage and proclaim that no injury was possible based on the photo "evidence." The erroneous perception is often: minimal damage to vehicle = minimal risk of injury. Yet large amounts of energy can be transferred at very low speed collisions, leading to tissue injury.

Consider the example of unbroken eggs in an egg carton. The eggs represent the biologic tissue, and the carton the inorganic tissue. If I were to drop this carton of eggs to the floor from waist height (which I have done, both purposefully in the name of scientific observation, and accidentally in the name of clumsiness), I could look at the egg carton and notice minimal damage on the outside. There may be some indentation where the carton hit the floor, but the carton is functional and reusable. Yet when I open the carton, I find some broken eggs.

I could use the energy calculations and determine the momentum of the egg carton and eggs was conserved. Most of it went to moving a small part of the impacted floor a small distance, and the rest was absorbed by the carton and eggs, or turned into heat and noise. The part absorbed by the eggs was enough to seriously damage some of them, yet the carton was hardly scathed.

If I dropped the carton from above my head, more damage would occur, both to the carton and to the number of eggs broken since more momentum was achieved by the faster moving egg carton before it hit the floor. If I reinforced the egg carton with tape and a steel wire mesh, and dropped it to the floor from either waist or shoulder height, I probably wouldn't see ANY damage to the carton. Upon opening the carton however, there will be at least 1 egg broken virtually 100% of the time.

The reason the egg can sustain severe damage without damage to the carton is due to the different properties of the two objects. Organic objects, including living tissue, have different molecular properties that render them fragile, delicate and vulnerable to injury. They have less tensile strength (greatest stress a substance can bear without tearing apart) and less density (mass packed per volume) than their inorganic counterparts, like metal. Thus, organic tissue is weaker. Ligaments and muscles can be stretched to some extent, but they will tear if too much force is exerted on them.

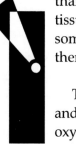

The erroneous perception is often: minimal damage to vehicle = minimal risk of injury. Yet large amounts of energy can be transferred at very low speed collisions, leading to tissue injury.

The human body is a potpourri of different organs, tissues and cells intimately interconnected to allow bioelectrical signals, oxygen and nutrients to sustain life. Molecular uniformity and tight cohesive molecular bonds are not part of living tissue as they are in steel, aluminum, fiberglass, and glass. An accident that dents a fender, shatters a headlight, and rips off a piece of bumper is not likely to prevent the car from being driven. These same collision forces absorbed entirely by a human being would probably be fatal. A small amount of that force transmitted to the human body could be life threatening, or tissue damaging.

Energy (momentum) forces transmitted to the occupants of colliding vehicles can cause severe tissue damage independent of the vehicle damage. Cars are designed to withstand impacts better, with stronger bumpers and sturdier frames. Crumpling does not occur much when modern cars collide. Whereas this may be good for the cars, it means less momentum is "dissipated" through the crumpling metal, and more momentum is still available to be transmitted to the vehicle occupants during a collision.

It appears that the less a struck car is damaged in a collision, the more it was caused to accelerate, and the greater the risk of injury. In 1968, Dr. Schutt reported in *JAMA* that severe tissue damage to the neck can occur when the offending car is traveling 7 mph. Dr. Brault's research in 1998 showed even slower speeds could cause damage, because nearly a third of healthy subjects reported injuries from collisions of just 2.5 mph. Theoretically, a vehicle moving only 1 mph could cause a whiplash injury, especially if that vehicle were a semi-truck loaded with steel beams.

This research supports the lack of a relationship between vehicle damage and tissue injury. Tissue injury is related to momentum. In order to reduce the risk of injury, the momentum must be reduced or redirected away from the occupants. What would hurt the most, falling and landing on, a: a wrestling mat, b: a carpeted floor, or c: a hardwood floor?

To understand the importance of "crumpling" or other means of absorbing momentum and reducing the risk of injury, think of the sand bags or sand "barrels" strategically placed in front of concrete dividers, or "breakaway" aluminum lamp poles, or airbags. It is not technically feasible or safer to design cars that crumple like an accordion upon impact. Many laws have been passed to regulate safety requirements for vehicles. No matter how safe a vehicle is designed, there will still be fatalities and injuries because of the omnipresent momentum and the natural laws that govern it.

Variables

Despite our knowledge of whiplash mechanics and laws of physics, it is impossible to determine exact forces present in a specific motor vehicle accident because so many different variables are present, and they are all different for each collision. Certainly size and speed of the involved vehicles are major factors that can be measured, but ultimately, multiple other variables are the difference between a high speed collision that results in no injuries, or a low speed collision that results in a serious whiplash injury. Although we can't determine "exact" forces, we are able to analyze actual variables present for a given collision and determine accurate estimates of forces and risks.

Numerous variables include:

1. **Type of collision.** Was it head-on, rear-end, sideswipe, or T-bone? A study of over 1000 cases of whiplash injuries in Munich (Dr. Schuller, *et al.* 1999) found the following distribution of accident types:

   Rear-end collision 59%

   Head-on collision 16%

   Side glance collision 11%

   No collision (braking, swerving, bump) 9%

   Side collision (T-bone) 5%

   The rear-end collision is the most common type causing whiplash injuries. Whiplash injuries can occur with no collision. Collisions from an angle can be risky because more spine twisting and rotation can occur.

2. **Occupant morphology.** The weight, height and build of the vehicle's occupant(s) are important variables. Taller people whose head and shoulders extend beyond the top of the seat are more at risk because of increased "free space" for the head and neck to "whip" into. Shorter heavier people may have poorly "fitted" seat belts that increase the risk for seat belt-type injuries. Those with shorter thicker necks are less vulnerable to whiplash trauma than those with longer thinner necks.

3. **Occupant gender and age.** Females have a greater risk of injury than males, presumably because of less muscle mass in the female neck. Older drivers have a greater risk of injury than younger drivers, probably because of stiffer, older neck soft tissues and bones which render them more vulnerable to whiplash-type injuries.

4. **Occupant head position.** Whether the person was looking in the rear view mirror, looking down, or turned to the side makes a difference in whether whiplash injuries occur. The neutral position (looking straight-ahead, neck slightly bent forward) is the most natural protective position of the head and neck in case of a collision. The more the head is out of

this position at the time of impact, the greater the risk of injury, especially when the head is turned to the side.

5. **Occupant awareness.** Awareness of the impending impact has a protective effect on the severity of the initial injury. This allows the person time to "brace" the neck muscles, a protective measure, prior to the impact. The occupant who is surprised by the impact does not have time to voluntarily brace the muscles before the collision forces have already done their damage. Since the cervical muscles take 150–200 ms (.150–.200 seconds) to contract, and the damage is probably done within the first 75 milliseconds (.075 seconds) (Dr. Ryan, 2000), it is not likely that the muscles can provide any protective effect during an unexpected rear-end collision.

6. **Headrests.** Headrests are actually restraints designed to decrease the hyperextension of the head in case of a rear-end collision. If the headrest is not positioned so the back of the head touches it (*i.e.,* it's too low, or angled too far back), it will not help decrease injury from hyperextension. A headrest that is too low can act as a pivot on the backwards moving head during a whiplash event, increasing the risk or severity of an injury.

7. **Seats.** Seats angled too far forward may position the head too far from the headrests. Seats angled too far back may "slide" down the torso during a rear-end collision and focus more force on the neck. Stiffer seats transmit more force to the occupant.

8. **Seat belts.** Seat belts cause soft tissue damage to the chest, ribs and shoulders and transmit force to the body when they restrain and lock-up during a collision. However, seat belts definitely save lives. Some people don't wear the shoulder strap, or wear the belts too loosely, or simply don't "fit" them well, and are at more risk for injury.

9. **Secondary impacts.** If the vehicle struck from behind gets pushed into a car in front, a second collision occurs and contributes to the crash dynamics. Likewise, secondary impacts with other objects such as trees, poles, curbs, or barriers will increase the risk of injuries. Direct occupant impacts (*i.e.,* hitting the windshield, steering wheel, or dashboard) can cause additional serious injuries.

10. **Road dynamics.** If the drivers were braking at the time of impact, the injury risk decreases (less velocity = less momentum). Icy or wet road surfaces can increase the amount of car motion after an impact, causing more severe injuries.

11. **Pre-existing medical conditions in the occupants.** Certain disorders of the cervical spine, such as degenerative disc disease, arthritis, or stenosis can predispose a person to whiplash injuries, or more severe injuries.

Other Whiplash-type Injuries

Different types of whiplash injuries, like different variables, are possible. Although the "whiplash" was described for rear-end collision consequences of the neck, one can suffer from a whiplash injury without being involved in a collision. I mentioned above how whiplash injuries occur 9% of the time with no collision involved, after a sudden "avoidance" swerve or sudden braking while driving. I've had patients develop whiplash trauma after going off the road and up an embankment, or riding over a big bump and bouncing unexpectedly, hitting the top of their heads on the inside car roof. Motion energy is present in any moving vehicle, and the potential is always there for this energy to be suddenly transmitted to the occupant.

Other kinds of whiplash "opportunities" occur without the need for a moving vehicle. A common one is a fall to the ground unexpectedly. If your feet suddenly go out from under you while walking on ice, you could fall on your back and end up with a whiplash injury. Your falling body gains momentum, and depending on the sequence of impacts, much of this energy can be transferred to the neck structures and injure them, as in a rear-end collision.

A backward fall is riskier, especially if the head accelerates down and ricochets off the ground. Forward falls, twisting sideways falls, fainting falls and falling down the stairs can all lead to whiplash-type injuries.

I once saw a woman who sustained a whiplash injury after a mail cart was accidentally pushed into the back of the office chair she was sitting in. A male construction worker hurt his neck after he slipped off the scaffold and grabbed a metal rod to arrest his descent to the ground. I've seen patients who suffered whiplash-type injuries from altercations or physical abuse.

Specific Whiplash Injuries

Wherever there is momentum, there is a potential for tissue injury. Injuries are the result of actual tissue damage. Collision forces disrupt cell integrity and function, and multiple areas of damage occur with a single accident. The study of abnormal physiologic processes occurring after exposure to whiplash forces allows us to determine the pathophysiology (distinct abnormalities) of whiplash injuries.

Researchers have done autopsies on victims of fatal accidents to examine injured tissues and help us extrapolate from these findings the sort of damage a non-fatal whiplash injury may cause. Experimental animals have also shed light on specific injuries and tissue damage. Medical imaging technology (CAT scan, MRI, PET scan, SPECT scan) allows us to examine the actual anatomy and function of injured tissues in a whiplash sufferer and gather clues to the pathophysiology.

Tissues frequently injured in a whiplash include:

- Muscles
- Ligaments
- Intervertebral discs
- Vertebrae
- Facet joints
- Nerves
- Spinal cord
- Brain

Muscle Injuries

Whiplash can cause injuries to muscles ranging from micro-hemorrhages (when viewed under a microscope) and minor tears or strains, to severe tears and disruption of function. Commonly injured muscles include the front neck muscles (sternocleidomastoid) and the muscles in the back of the neck (scalene, splenius capitis, longus collis, cervical paraspinals, and trapezius).

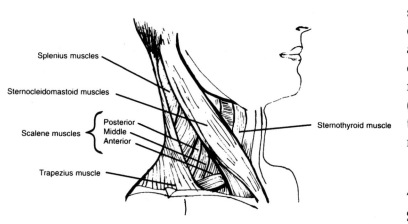

Splenius muscles
Sternocleidomastoid muscles
Scalene muscles { Posterior Middle Anterior
Trapezius muscle
Sternothyroid muscle

The sudden stretch of normal relaxed skeletal muscles by the collision forces overwhelms the muscles' abilities to expand and absorb the force. Internal muscle cell damage and tissue disruption occurs, with resultant hemorrhage (bleeding) and edema (swelling). There may be no visible bruises on the outside, but painful symptoms are usually noticed immediately.

Neck muscles aren't the only ones that "feel" the collision forces and become injured. Shoulder muscles (including the trapezius which is both a neck and shoulder muscle), mid and low back paraspinals, and jaw (TMJ) muscles can also be injured during a whiplash. The neck muscles, recipients of the most force, usually suffer the most trauma. Hence the neck pain may be noticed the most initially, but patients often complain of muscle pains in multiple locations.

Ligament Injuries

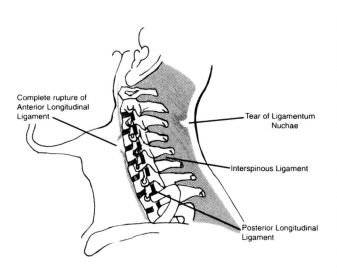

Complete rupture of Anterior Longitudinal Ligament
Tear of Ligamentum Nuchae
Interspinous Ligament
Posterior Longitudinal Ligament

Spinal ligaments hold the vertebrae in place. In whiplash injuries ligaments may be stretched, partly torn, or completely ruptured. Key ligaments include the anterior longitudinal ligament, posterior longitudinal ligament, ligamentum nuchae, and interspinous ligaments.

The anterior longitudinal ligament runs vertically along the front of the vertebrae. It is a paper thin ligament that is vulnerable to injury with sudden backward movements of the head (hyperextension). Indeed this hyperextension action is one of the most forceful movements caused by the whiplash. Without much help from the sparse front neck muscles (sternocleidomastoids), this ligament is limited in its defense from the collision forces, and frequently stretches, tears or ruptures.

The posterior longitudinal ligament and the ligamentum nuchae are in the back of the neck vertebrae and are at risk for injury during the rapid forward movement of the head (hyperflexion phase). These ligaments are thicker and guarded by more muscles than the anterior ligament counterpart. Plus, excessive flexion is limited by chin contact to the chest, a built-in safety measure for the posterior ligaments. Stretches, tears and ruptures of these ligaments are not likely to be as severe as the anterior ligaments.

The interspinous ligaments, like their name implies, interweave the vertebrae and hold them together. They are subjected to crushing, twisting, and stretching forces during the whiplash. Any injury to these ligaments can destabilize the spinal integrity.

Ligaments in the cervical (neck) and thoracic (mid back) areas are most likely to be injured during a whiplash. If ligaments sustain an overstretch injury, like a rubber band being overstretched, they become too loose and are not able to spring back to their original shorter size. The damaged ligaments are not able to hold the bones or joints tightly anymore, and these lax, wobbly areas can become sources of chronic pain. Part of fibromyalgia's genesis is unstable loose areas causing persistent pain generators.

Intervertebral Disc Injuries

The discs lie between two vertebrae and cushion them. The discs consist of two parts, the inner gel portion called the nucleus, and the outer ligament layered shell called the annulus. Think of the popular gel-filled soft licorice balls as an example of the discs' structure.

Post-mortem and MRI studies of the discs reveal frequent injuries to them. Several types of disc injuries can occur when the momentum reaches these gelatinous-filled ligaments. During the extension phase of the whiplash, the anterior longitudinal ligament can rupture and the front part of the disc can be torn from the rim of the vertebra (see FIGURE A).

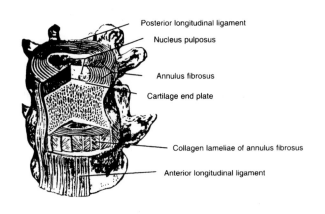

FIGURE A and B detail diagrams with labels:
Posterior longitudinal ligament
Nucleus pulposus
Annulus fibrosus
Cartilage end plate
Collagen lameliae of annulus fibrosus
Anterior longitudinal ligament

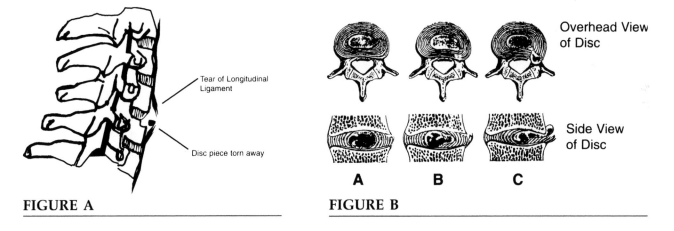

Tear of Longitudinal Ligament

Disc piece torn away

FIGURE A

Overhead View of Disc

Side View of Disc

A   B   C

FIGURE B

Once the flexion phase occurs, downward compressive forces are placed on the discs throughout the spine, especially in the neck, and may be sufficient enough to cause rupture of the discs. The discs may rupture backwards and to the side (into the spinal canal), or straight back through the vertebral end plate, depending on which part of the disc's outer ligament rim (the annulus) tears first. A rupture of the disc is called a disc herniation. This is the equivalent of a hole in the soft licorice candy from which the inner fruity gel oozes out (see FIGURE B).

If the disc rim does not tear completely, the internal gel portion of the disc (the nucleus) may still be abnormally shifted to different positions and put pressure on the annulus and cause disc pain (see FIGURES A & B). Imagine the soft licorice candy has been smashed on one side and the fruity gel shifts to the other side, but not breaking through. An MRI can show this nucleus shift and may also show disc bulging (instead of a herniation). This condition is known as intervertebral disc dysfunction.

The outer part of the annulus is richly supplied by pain nerves, so any tears, ruptures, bulges or pressure will usually hurt.

Vertebral Injuries

The spine is comprised of individual bones known as vertebrae. When the anterior longitudinal ligament tears during hyperextension, pieces of bone may be ripped from the cervical vertebrae where the ligament connected into the bone. Fractures can occur in the spinous processes (see FIGURE C). Wedge-shaped crush fractures, known as compression fractures, can result from the crunching compressive forces created when the head is propelled forward and downward (hyperflexion phase). Older women with bone thinning (osteopenia or osteoporosis) are more vulnerable to compression fractures.

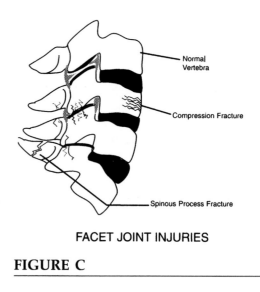

FACET JOINT INJURIES

FIGURE C

Facet Joint Injuries

The zygapophyseal facet joints, known more simply as "facet joints" are believed to play a major role in causing whiplash pain (Dr. Bogduk, *et al.*). These oval-shaped structures in the back of the vertebrae are true joints, comprised of a joint capsule, synovial membrane and fluid, and covered by joint cartilage. Each facet joint combines the inferior (or lower) part of one vertebra's facet surface with the superior (or top) of the next vertebra's facet surface (see FIGURE D).

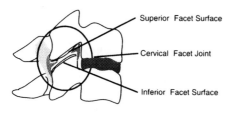

CERVICAL FACET JOINT

FIGURE D

The cervical facet joints have a complicated role in protecting the cervical spine and allowing it to have mobility. They stabilize the neck from moving too far forward, and they resist weight bearing or compressive forces that push down and back on the head. The facets glide across each other in unison and permit the neck to bend forward, backward, sideways, and to rotate around. This delicate balancing act of protecting-permitting works beautifully nearly all the time, except when whiplash forces rush through.

The forced straightening of the cervical spine at the time of impact (within the first 75 ms (.075 seconds)) just before the actual cervical extension occurs (head moves backward) results in significant downward compressive forces on the cervical spine and facet joints (Dr. Ono, *et al.*, 1997). Injuries to the facet joints include capsular ligament tears, small impaction fractures, rupture of the joint surface, and joint hemorrhages. Since facet joints are abundantly represented by pain nerves, injuries to these joints will result in neck pain and referred pain to the shoulders.

Because of the downward propagation of the whiplash forces, the rest of the spine can sustain damage, including thoracic and lumbar facet, ligament and disc tissues. Cervical injuries predominate, but the whole spine is vulnerable to injury and potential chronic pain generation.

Nerve Injuries

Nerve tissue can experience injuries as the result of blunt trauma, stretch injuries, disruption of blood supply, or pressure from hemorrhage, swelling or damaged tissues. All pain is conveyed through nerves, whether it arises from injured nerves or from injured tissues sending pain signals through "normal" nerves.

Nerve roots arise from the spinal cord and pass through small bony openings in the vertebrae. These roots can bang up against the bone during a whiplash. Any pre-existing arthritis that narrows the bony passages will increase the risk of nerve root injury during a collision. Intervertebral disc ruptures can pinch the nerve roots, causing swelling and pain.

Peripheral nerves supply sensory and motor signals to various organs including muscles. Bundles of nerves or individual nerves can be damaged during a whiplash, and more vulnerable ones include the brachial plexus (bundle of shoulder nerves) and the spinal accessory nerve (nerve to the sternocleidomastoid and trapezius muscles).

The cervical sympathetic nerves are located deep in the neck along the carotid artery and jugular vein. These nerves are important relay centers for monitoring and controlling pain signals, blood flow, heart rate, blood pressure, and much more. They can be stretched and damaged during a whiplash, leading to considerable pain and altered nerve signals. As we'll review in more detail later, the sympathetic nerves probably play the greatest role in causing chronic pain to develop in fibromyalgia.

A specific condition known as reflex sympathetic dystrophy sometimes develops as a complication of nerve injuries or soft tissue trauma. This condition is characterized by overactive small sensory and autonomic nerves which causes extreme pain, burning, and swelling in the affected limb (*e.g.*, arm). Causalgia is another term used to describe persistent painful burning and tingling after a nerve trauma.

Spinal Cord Injuries

The spinal cord is housed in the protective bony canal of the vertebrae. It is subjected to momentum forces during the whiplash, but the protective structures (muscles, ligaments, discs) do everything they can to absorb or redirect the forces to guard against spinal cord trauma. Despite these guardians' valiant efforts, the spinal cord can be subjected to stretching, bruising, shock waves, or impactions during a whiplash.

Any damage to the sensitive spinal cord tissue can cause various symptoms of pain, numbness, weakness, or bowel and bladder disturbances. Different syndromes of spinal cord injury are listed in the chart below. Severe spinal cord injuries are uncommon following a whiplash event. Elderly people with cervical spine arthritis are more prone to severe spinal cord damage. Symptoms may be temporary or permanent, depending on whether the neural tissue undergoes irreparable damage.

SYNDROMES OF SPINAL CORD INJURY

Central Cord Syndrome: Affect pain, temperature and motor functions of the arms more than the legs.

Anterior Cord Syndrome: Immediate and complete motor paralysis with preservation of some light touch sensation below injury level.

Brown-Sequard Syndrome: Immediate motor paralysis of one side of body, loss of sensation on other side of body at level of cord injury.

Cauda Equina Syndrome: Weakness in legs, arms not affected.

Brain Injuries

Brain injuries can occur during the whiplash. Loss of consciousness may result if the head hits the windshield, steering wheel, dashboard, or another object inside the car. Brain injuries can occur without blunt trauma to the head, and concussions can happen without loss of consciousness.

The brain is suspended in a fluid medium within the rigid skull. To appreciate what can happen to the brain during a whiplash, imagine a common activity we've all done: shaking a rattle. When we rapidly move the rattle down, the small ball inside the rattle stays in place at first, being impacted by the top half of the rattle. Then the ball overcomes inertia and moves down, but this time the rattle is on the upswing of the shake cycle, and the downward moving ball meets the upward moving lower rattle half.

The brain, acting as the ball, gets banged from the front part of the skull during the hyperextension phase of the whiplash. The brain is also overcoming inertia and accelerating back to catch up with the already backwards moving skull.

But the brain is in for a surprise. After moving full speed to catch up with the skull, it encounters the back of the skull heading in the opposite direction. The skull is now in its hyperflexion phase of the whiplash, unbeknownst to the brain. The brain takes its obligatory bash, and reverses its momentum to speed toward the front of the head.

Meanwhile the head is moving forward until its progress is abruptly halted when the chin wedges into the chest. The brain is following momentum orders and racing full speed to the front of the head, only to be suddenly stopped (and smashed) once again.

The brain is bonked three times by the skull, but it abruptly changes directions four times. The sudden slowdown, stop, and re-acceleration when the brain hits the back of the skull (at the end of the head hyperextension phase) counts as two direction changes. No direct blow to the head occurred, yet the brain was traumatized. Concussions and loss of consciousness can result.

Contrary to what one might expect, the brain does not act like a soft rubber ball inside the skull when exposed to whiplash forces. Rather, it acts more like a deck of cards. Different parts of the brain can shift more than others, causing irregularities, like cards that have been unevenly stacked. These irregularities can cause microscopic disconnections of cellular-nerve bonds in the brain, a damaging process known as diffuse axonal injury.

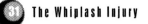

Dr. Radanov of Switzerland recently reported that any whiplash trauma which leads to an unconscious period of less than ten minutes, or an amnesia period that spans less than four hours (minor concussion) is not likely to cause any lasting brain damage or dysfunction. In these situations, the brain injury was reversible and not permanent. If more severe damage occurred, or a coexisting loss of blood supply (stroke) or bleeding (hemorrhage) was present, the brain damage will likely be permanent.

A condition known as post-concussive syndrome is common after whiplash-type injuries where a concussion occurred. Symptoms of post-concussive syndrome include headaches, difficulty with memory, poor concentration, dizziness, fatigue and irritability.

Statistics

Dr. McLean, in a 1995 published study, found a strong association between increased neck injuries and increased speed of impact and damage to the vehicle. That is not to say that all people involved in high speed crashes will become injured, nor will no injuries occur in low speed impacts. His study and others simply reflect the obvious: in high speed impacts, more injuries will occur compared to low speed impacts.

As I've previously mentioned, low speed impacts can cause severe injuries, even though fewer people are less likely to be injured. More people involved in high speed collisions are injured, but more total low speed collisions occur than high speed ones. In the German study (Dr. Schuller, *et al.*, 1999), 92% of the collisions causing whiplash were at speeds less than 10 mph, and only 8% were 10 mph or greater speeds. So the total number of people injured is far greater from low speed impacts (less than 10 mph), even though a much smaller percentage of people involved in low speed impacts are injured.

The Quebec Task Force report on Whiplash Associated Disorders (1995) reviewed 294 papers and summarized overall risk factors. About 35–40% of drivers in all rear-end impacts (the majority are less than 10 mph) suffer some form of neck symptoms and pain. The risk for females is 1.5 to 2 times that of males, and older drivers (over 25 years-old) have a risk 1.5 times that of younger drivers. Increased severity of impact is associated with increased symptom severity. If the driver is aware of the impending crash, the initial symptoms are usually less than those of a surprised driver.

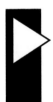 # If You Want To Know More

1. Barnsley L, Lord SM, Bogduk N. *Whiplash injury.* Pain 1994; 58: 283–307.

2. Brault JR, Wheeler JB, Siegmund GP, et al. *Clinical response of human subjects to rear-end automobile collisions.* Arch Phys Med Rehabil 1998; 79: 72–80.

3. Dwyer A, Aprill C, Bogduk N. *Cervical zygapophyseal joint pain patterns. A study in normal volunteers.* Spine 1990; 15: 453–7.

4. Evans RW. *Some observations on whiplash injuries.* Neurologic Clinics 1992; 10: 975–97.

5. Gurumoorthy D, Twomey L. *The Quebec Task Force on whiplash-associated disorders.* Spine. 1996; 21: 897–8.

6. Harder S, Veilleux M, Suissa S. *The effect of socio-demographic and crash-related factors on the prognosis of whiplash.* J Clin Epidemiol 1998; 51: 377–84.

7. Kaneoka K, Ono K, Inami S, et al. *Motion analysis of cervical vertebrae during whiplash loading.* Spine 1999; 24: 763–9.

8. McLean AJ. *Neck injuries severity and vehicle design.* In: Griffiths M, Brown J, eds. The biomechanics of neck injury-proceedings. Seminar, 1995; 47–50.

9. Melton MR. *The complete guide to whiplash.* Body Mind Publications, 1998.

10. National Safety Council 1992. www.nsc.org

11. Pellegrino MJ. *From whiplash to fibromyalgia.* N. Canton OH: ORC Publishing, 2002.

12. Pellegrino MJ. *Understanding post-traumatic fibromyalgia: a medical perspective.* Columbus OH: Anadem Publishing, 1996.

13. Radanov BP. *Controversy about brain damage following cranio-cervical acceleration-deceleration trauma.* J Musculoskel Pain 2000; 8: 179–92.

14. Ryan GA. *Etiology and outcomes of whiplash: review and update.* J Musculoskel Pain 2000; 8: 3–14.

15. Schuller E, Eisenmenger W, Beier G. *Whiplash injury in low speed car accidents: assessment of biomechanical cervical spine loading and injury prevention in a forensic sample.* J Musculoskel Pain 2000; 8: 55–67.

16. Schutt CH, Dohan FC. *Neck injury to women in auto accidents.* JAMA 1968; 206: 2689–92.

17. Severy DM, Mathewson JH, Bechtol CO. *Controlled automobile rear-end collisions, an investigation of related engineering and medical phenomena.* Can Serv Med J VII; 1955: 727–59.

18. Sturzenegger M, Radanov BP, DiStefano G. *The effect of accident mechanisms and initial findings on the long-term course of whiplash injury.* J Neurol 1995; 242: 443–9.

19. Tencer AF, Mirza S. *Whiplash mechanics in low speed rear-end automobile collision.* J Musculoskel Pain 2000; 8: 69–86.

Evaluation & Treatment Of Injuries

Following a whiplash injury, the person can complain of a number of symptoms. A typical story I hear from patients goes as follows:

"I was sitting at a red light when suddenly my car was rear-ended by another car. My neck jerked back and forth, but I don't think my head hit anything. I didn't black out, but I was stunned, almost like I was in shock. At first, I noticed pain in my right knee where it hit the dashboard, and my chest was sore from the seat belt."

Unexpected collisions are the usual for rear-end events. In the immediate aftermath, people feel confusion, shock, or disbelief. Initially, pain may not be noticed anywhere, leading one to believe he or she has escaped injury. If pain is noticed immediately, it may be limited to areas banged up against something (*e.g.,* knees, ribs). Immediate neck, shoulder and back pain can occur.

"When I got out of the car, I felt shaky and noticed burning in the back of my neck. My head felt funny. By the time the police got there, my neck and head were hurting. My back felt stiff. The paramedics were called and I was put in a neck brace and taken to the hospital emergency room."

Pain in the neck is a hallmark of whiplash injuries. Its onset can be immediate, but more often is delayed for a few minutes, hours, or even days. Neck stiffness or spasms can occur.

Headaches can be seen in up to 80% of patients, depending on the severity of the injuries sustained (Dr. Norris, 1983). They can be one-sided, or affect both sides of the head equally. Jaw pain or temporomandibular joint (TMJ) damage resulting from whiplash forces through the jaw hinged-joints can cause pain in the face and head areas. Blurred vision, ringing in the ears, memory loss, and dizziness can accompany the headache and TMJ problems, or develop later on.

Pains are frequently reported in the shoulders, jaws, arms, chest, ribs, and low back. Low back pain occurs in the majority of rear-end collisions (Dr. Norris). Pains can radiate down the arms or legs from the spine, especially if nerves are injured.

Because neck or spine pain after any accident could indicate a spine fracture or potential for spinal cord injury, spine stabilization precautions are followed by the paramedics. Bracing the neck or back and transporting the patient on a backboard are standard procedures when bringing a patient with spine pain from the accident scene to the hospital emergency room. The hospital physician decides when the brace can be removed after an assessment is performed.

The Emergency Room Evaluation

The ER physician will take a brief history and perform a clinical examination. The main goal of the first medical evaluation of anyone who has been injured is to determine if any life threatening organ or structure damage is present. Brain hemorrhage, spinal cord injuries, fractures, spleen rupture, and lung collapse (pneumothorax) are examples of serious conditions that could threaten life. These complications from whiplash accidents are less common.

The majority of the time the ER physician encounters a frightened patient with non-life threatening whiplash injuries who is complaining of pain and stiffness. The clinical examination of such a patient usually reveals pain of the soft tissues in the neck, shoulders, back and other areas reportedly painful. Restriction of joint and spine mobility is often present. Swelling without visible bruising may be detected in painful soft tissues, especially in the neck and shoulder areas.

Any painful pre-existing condition, including pre-existing fibromyalgia, is at risk for becoming aggravated or severely worsened following any trauma.

Typical whiplash-injured patients do not have evidence of nerve damage in the ER. The reflexes react normally, the strength, sensation and coordination are normal. There may be complaints of tingling or numbness, or feeling of weakness because of referred pain that interferes with one's ability to contract muscles; but true neurological damage is usually absent.

X-rays are usually obtained if there is persistent pain to rule out any fracture or bony abnormalities. Plain X-rays of the painful areas such as the cervical spine or the lumbosacral spine serve 2 important purposes. They allow the physician to detect any traumatic changes such as fractures or abnormal straightening of the spine. Loss of the normal cervical curvature or lordosis is common in neck injuries where neck muscle spasms cause the spine to straighten, or lose its normal lordosis. A straight alignment of the vertebrae, instead of a normal lordosis, is an abnormal X-ray finding.

Rarely are fractures found, or at least ones visible on the X-rays. As mentioned in the previous chapter, small impaction or avulsion fractures can occur at the facet joints or vertebral edges that may be too small for X-rays to detect.

The second reason X-rays are helpful is to view the person's pre-existing spine status, or "baseline." Any evidence of arthritis (spurs, narrowing) or disc degeneration (disc space narrowing, calcifications) seen on the ER X-rays indicate changes that were present BEFORE the accident. These changes are not acute changes caused by acute trauma, but rather ongoing chronic changes that had to be there before the accident.

The presence of these pre-existing X-rays changes does not mean the person had pre-existing symptoms of arthritis or disc disease. A number of studies have shown the majority of people with evidence of radiographic degenerative changes are completely asymptomatic. In 1999, Swedish investigators discovered that asymptomatic aircraft pilots had a lot of degenerative changes on their cervical spine X-rays.

In those people who had neck pain from symptomatic cervical arthritis or disc disease before the accident, the whiplash trauma is more likely to cause more severe neck injury (Dr. Maimaris, 1988). Any painful pre-existing condition, including pre-existing fibromyalgia, is at risk for becoming aggravated or severely worsened following any trauma. Also, any pre-existing arthritis, whether or not it is causing symptoms, is at risk for worsening over time after a trauma to the spine.

Additional X-rays can be done, such as flexion/extension views to evaluate for cervical spinal ligament tears. If a disc rupture or hemorrhage is suspected, specialized radiographic studies such as a CAT scan or MRI might be obtained to clarify the extent of the injuries. Testing may be negative for fractures, disc herniations, bleeding, etc., but that doesn't mean the person has nothing wrong. On the contrary, the person typically has painful soft tissue injuries that are not detectable by X-rays.

If the ER physician is satisfied the patient does not have a serious medical condition requiring surgery or hospitalization, the patient is given a diagnosis, treatments and recommendations and discharged to home. I've reviewed perhaps hundreds of ER diagnoses over the years, and they vary from "whiplash" to "acute cervical sprains" to "spine sprains/strains" to "pain from MVA" or simply "neck pain."

Standard treatments initiated in the ER include medicines to reduce pain, (antiinflammatory medicines, muscle relaxants), a cervical collar, instructions to rest and apply ice and heat, and a recommendation to follow-up with the primary doctor or a specialist. The emergency room mission is completed, and the patient is hopeful that he or she will be feeling much better in the morning after a good night's sleep.

The Next Day

Typically, the patient's hopes and the body's realities are two completely different things. Instead of waking up the next morning feeling much better, the patient often wakes up feeling like he or she were run over by a truck during the night. Patients tell me they hurt all over and can hardly get out of bed. They are stiff and have difficulty moving. Their arms and legs may feel numb. The head and neck may still hurt the most, but the rest of the body is also painful.

Why does the person usually feel worse the next day? Several factors are probably involved:

1. **The adrenaline effect wears off.** After acute injuries, the body releases hormones (especially adrenaline) which blunt pain and put the body in a "fight or flight" state for several hours or more. The athlete who continues to play despite an injury demonstrates the effectiveness of adrenaline in masking initial pain. Once the initial "shock" subsides, the adrenaline returns to baseline, and pain is perceived more.

2. **Delayed reaction to injury.** Sometimes the body needs time to realize how severely it has been injured. Acute damage to tissues causes an acute inflammatory-injury reaction. Different inflammatory cells residing in the bloodstream and tissues respond in an orderly fashion to recognize, react to and begin repairing the damage. The reaction is a slowly progressing one that can become incrementally painful over hours and days. Hence, overnight the person becomes worse, but doesn't fully appreciate the increased pain until morning awakening, and awareness.

3. **Delayed additional tissue injury.** Sometimes the full injury evolves over time. Swelling occurs and can cause pressure or block blood flow. Tissues that were not damaged initially, or "borderline" injured can become damaged after a few hours or longer. The inflammatory-injury reaction can "sacrifice" some normal or undamaged tissue as part of the clean-up process.

The patient with persistent severe pain the next day will usually seek medical treatment. Some people will try self-treatments for the pain. Electric heating pads, microwave moist heating packs, ice packs, muscle creams, hot showers or baths, and over the counter pain medicines are examples of "home" treatments that are often tried. Bed rest, restricting activity level, seeing a massage therapist and other strategies may be tried. If these fail to relieve symptoms over time, a doctor visit is scheduled.

Doctor Evaluation

Patients will usually see their primary care doctor (internist, family doctor), a chiropractor, or a specialist (*e.g.,* physiatrist, orthopedist). As a specialist in physical medicine and rehabilitation (physiatrist), I see patients with whiplash injuries either early on for management of their acute injuries, or later on for evaluation and treatment of persistent and chronic symptoms.

Doctors who see these patients will perform a clinical evaluation that includes asking questions about current symptoms and how they occurred. The patient's medical history is a description of current symptoms (especially PAIN), when they occurred (from the whiplash?), what affects them, are they getting better or worse, what has been done so far, and are there any other related problems?

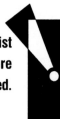

The longer the symptoms persist after a whiplash injury, the more likely specific tests will be ordered.

When I see patients with acute injuries from whiplash trauma, I inquire about different factors. I ask about vehicle type, vehicle speed at time of collision, seat belt, headrest, airbag deployment, awareness of impending crash, location of collision, position of head at time of collision, any secondary collisions, any objects struck in car, or any loss of consciousness. This information is recorded.

The medical history is not an informal narrative by the patient, but rather a specialized form of information gathering prompted by the physician. All symptoms are "subjective" or abnormal sensations perceived by the patient. Any physical sign or abnormality that can be seen, felt or heard by the physician is an "objective" finding.

The physical examination will try to detect any objective findings or abnormal signs. The physician inspects the patient for any abnormalities (bruises, swelling, redness, atrophy, etc.), palpates for any changes (spasms, nodules, stiffness, etc.) and determines if any neurological or joint problems, or any other problems are present. The physician uses his or her knowledge and skills to recognize various abnormal findings on the physical examination, and attach clinical meaning to them.

After the history and physical examination of the whiplash-injured patient, the physician will make a diagnosis. A whiplash-related problem certainly may be suspected based on the history alone, but the diagnosis must include the physician's interpretation of BOTH the history and exam. There may be more than one diagnosis made, and they may differ from the ones made by the ER physician. The patient's overall medical condition a day later, or a month later is often completely different from when first seen in the ER.

Additional tests may be ordered to help clarify the diagnosis. The physician will form his or her initial impression or diagnosis before the tests and clarify or "fine-tune" the diagnosis after the test results. For example, a patient with neck and arm pain may be suspected of having a herniated disc in the neck along with neck muscle and ligament injuries (cervical strains and sprains) from the whiplash injury. A cervical MRI is obtained and if it shows a herniated disc, the suspected diagnosis is confirmed by the physician; a negative MRI may allow the physician to discard the suspected diagnosis or "rule-out" the disc herniation.

The longer the symptoms persist after a whiplash injury, the more likely specific tests will be ordered. The reasoning is simple: if complete healing of uncomplicated injuries is going to happen, it does so predictably within several weeks. Additional tests are not necessary if the pain is disappearing. If pain is not disappearing within weeks, a more complicated injury may be present.

Specific Diagnoses

A medical diagnosis of "whiplash" is technically an incorrect one. "Whiplash" refers to an injury mechanism that, over time, has become associated with a medical diagnosis.

The soft tissue and bony injuries have very specific names, and each condition needs to be medically named or diagnosed. Just as we wouldn't call every family member by a single first name, we shouldn't do that with the various medical conditions that are part of the whiplash family. "Whiplash" may be the common cause (the same last name), but each condition has its own first name.

Depending on the clinical findings, specific whiplash-associated diagnoses typically include:

- Cervical strain (muscle injury) and sprain (ligament injury)
- Thoracic sprain/strain
- Shoulder sprain/strain
- Lumbosacral sprain/strain
- Spinal segmental dysfunction (cervical, thoracic, and/or lumbar spasm and restriction of mobility)
- Facet dysfunction (injury to the stabilizing joints between the vertebrae)
- Intervertebral disc dysfunction (painful tear of the inner disc)
- Tension and/or migraine headaches
- Post-concussive syndrome

Other diagnoses can be made if the clinical manifestations and testing support them, including herniated disc, radiculopathy, spinal cord syndromes, reflex sympathetic dystrophy, causalgia, PTF, and more. These diagnoses usually indicate a more complicated injury.

PTF, as you will see, is an example of a chronic painful complication of a whiplash injury that may be diagnosed months or even years after the original injury.

Doctor-directed Treatments

A variety of treatments may be prescribed for the patient with a whiplash injury or other acute injury. There is no one single treatment that eliminates all symptoms, but various treatments can help, often when combined. Each person's treatment program is individualized; what works for some may not work for others.

The goals of treating acute problems from a whiplash injury are to reduce pain, speed up healing, improve function, and minimize the chance of complications or persistent symptoms. Dr. Bogduk, in a recent review (*Journal of Musculoskeletal Pain*, 2000), concluded that the combined data showed active intervention such as physical and manual therapy was superior to just resting and taking pain pills in decreasing symptoms of acute whiplash injuries.

The goals of treating acute problems from a whiplash injury are to reduce pain, speed up healing, improve function, and minimize the chance of complications or persistent symptoms.

The patients studied who received prescribed active treatments reported decrease in their pain at 4 to 8 weeks after the pain began. However, in many of those who did not have active therapy, the pain still decreased over time (8 weeks or longer). It would appear that the active therapy program achieved a more rapid resolution of symptoms in the early weeks after the whiplash injury. So therapy helps people get better quicker, and many people still get better without therapy, but it takes longer.

A recent study by Swedish researchers (M. Rosenfeld, *et al.*, *Spine*, 2000) evaluated 97 patients with a whiplash injury. The study evaluated early active mobilization versus a standard treatment protocol and the importance of early versus delayed onset of treatment after the injury. The results showed active treatment (manual therapy, McKenzie's principles, active exercises) reduced the pain more than standard treatment (initial rest, soft cervical collar, gradual self-mobilization), and early active treatment (within the first four days) was superior than delayed treatment.

When presented with a patient in acute pain, physicians usually choose to prescribe active treatments that include medications, therapies, manipulations and injections. If any patient's pain and suffering can be reduced over a shorter interval with treatment than without, the physician is certainly justified in ordering treatments.

Drug Therapy

Medications prescribed for treatment of whiplash-associated conditions include:

1. **Analgesics or painkillers.** Narcotic or opioid medicines are examples in this category prescribed to try to reduce pain.

2. **Muscle relaxants.** This type can reduce muscle spasms common after whiplash injuries.

3. **Anti-inflammatories.** Since inflammation often accompanies acute trauma, this type of medicine may be helpful in reducing swelling, inflammation, and pain. However, acute inflammation following trauma is beneficial to some degree since it leads to healing. The inflammatory response "clears the way" for the healing cascade. Using anti-inflammatory medicines like NSAIDs or steroids may blunt the inflammatory-healing responses, so the prescribing doctor should monitor for any delayed healing responses if considering these medicines.

There have been no specific studies of drug therapy for pain, spasm and inflammation after whiplash injury. In its review, the Quebec Task Force (*Spine*, 1995) found no studies addressing the benefits of drug therapies in the treatment of whiplash-associated disorders. Patients report decreased pain with these medicines, but studies haven't distinguished the pain relief from medicines from that of natural tissue healing and resolution.

When a patient reports decreased pain with prescribed medicines, this reinforces the treating physician's belief that the medicine is beneficial. The lack of scientific literature on pain medicines for whiplash injuries does not mean the medicines are not helpful. Rather it means the specific scientific study has not been done yet.

There have been no specific studies of drug therapy for pain, spasm and inflammation after whiplash injury.

Much clinical information is available that supports the effective use of medicines in treatment of pain from various conditions, including arthritis, tendinitis, headaches, neuropathy, cancer, and many more. It is not realistic to have encompassing scientific studies published on every possible condition that causes pain. Physicians are permitted to use clinical inference and conclude that medicines that help pain for some painful conditions will help for other painful conditions.

The prescribing physician must weigh potential benefits and risks for any medicine used in treating pain, whatever the cause. In the case of whiplash injuries, if prescribed medicines provide pain relief that would otherwise not have happened, and no serious side effects result from the medicines, the treatments may be deemed clinically effective. It is up to the individual doctor and patient to formulate strategies for which medicines to use and assess whether they are working.

Therapy Treatments

A wide variety of therapy treatments may be prescribed and include:

1. **Adjustments and manipulations.** Chiropractors and osteopathic physicians are trained to perform manipulations and adjustments to mobilize joints, improve range of motion, relax muscles, and reduce pain.

2. **Physical modalities.** Heat/cold treatments, electric stimulation, whirlpool, and ultrasound are examples of modalities that may help decrease pain. Treatments may be prescribed once a day to a few times a week to start, depending on the individual patient's condition.

3. **Manual therapy.** These include techniques to mobilize and restore injured tissues. One type of specialized spine therapy is called McKenzie's program.

4. **Exercises.** These include postural, stretching, strengthening, conditioning, and aquatic exercises.

5. **Acupuncture.** This ancient Chinese practice uses small needles to pierce body areas for therapeutic purposes, mainly to reduce pain.

6. **Cervical traction.** If cervical disc problems are present, this treatment may help relieve pressure and irritation of nerve roots.

As mentioned earlier, the combined data on these treatments support that early active intervention is better than passive "treatment" (*e.g.*, rest, over-the-counter medicines, heating pad) in reducing pain and expediting recovery from the whiplash injuries.

Injections

The use of injected medicines into specific body areas can reduce pain and improve recovery, as supported by a number of studies. In whiplash injuries, different types of injections that may help include:

1. **Trigger point injections.** A local anesthetic often combined with a steroid medicine is injected into a muscle area to reduce painful muscle spasms.

2. **Facet injections.** A mixture of local anesthetic and steroid is injected into these specific vertebral joints to block pain.

3. **Nerve blocks and epidurals.** Nerve root or disc problems may respond to specific injections into the spinal canal areas. A mixture of anesthetic and cortisone is often used.

4. **Prolotherapy.** A mixture of local anesthetic and a proliferative agent such as dextrose is injected into weakened, damaged ligaments to promote thickening and strengthening.

For acute whiplash related injuries, initial treatments I usually prescribe include drug therapy (pain medicines, muscle relaxants, and anti-inflammatories), pain management therapies (bioelectric, hot packs), manual therapies, and active stretching and range of motion exercises. I advise patients on nutritional strategies to promote healing (*e.g.*, glucosamine, chondroitin, MSM, magnesium). Smokers are advised to stop smoking to increase the body's ability to heal.

If the symptoms persist, I search for their cause, and try to design treatment strategies to eliminate the problems.

If the patient is improving within a week from the injury, I'll advance the therapy to more aggressive manual work and hands-on techniques which include McKenzie's techniques and other exercises. The patient is instructed on a progressive home program, and medicines are decreased, used only as needed, or discontinued.

If the symptoms persist, I search for their cause, and try to design treatment strategies to eliminate the problems. Different medicines, specialized injections, additional therapies, and other treatments may be tried.

When Injury Symptoms Don't Go Away

Healing is the expected outcome for most with acute injuries. Indeed, most people heal from whiplash injuries. The vast majority of authors who have studied the natural history of whiplash injuries have found that 82%–94% recover without residual permanent disability (Dr. Galasco *et al.*, review article in *Journal of Musculoskeletal Medicine*, 2000). Most recover, but not all.

The same percentages above can be interpreted that 6%–18% of those injured will have a residual permanent disability, such as severe pain interfering with functional abilities. Also, those who are classified as "recovered without residual disability" are not all symptom-free. In one study (Drs. Gargan and Bannister, 1990), up to 48% still had pain described as a "nuisance" in their daily activities. People who are reported "healed" are still hurting. Even if they are working, or have not been determined to have a disability from the whiplash injuries, they still have persistent pain.

If we pull back the curtain on the disparity between reported healing and persistence of pain, we discover the reasons:

1. **Not everyone heals the same from similar injuries.**

In the 18th Century, a German physicist, Johann Karl F. Gauss described the normal curve of distribution, known as a Gaussian curve. A Gaussian curve is a classic bell-shaped curve that shows the distribution, or range of "normal." Anything that has a normal value has a range of normal values, not just one single normal value. This is termed the normal variation and can be plotted out to reveal a typical Gaussian curve. Most of the normal values cluster together, forming the deep part of the bell. Some normal values are lower or higher than the "majority," and form the rims of the bell.

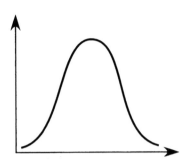

GAUSSIAN CURVE

Gaussian curves look the same whether plotting the normal human glucose levels, the incubation period of chickens, the size of duck feet, the height of adult giraffes, the weight of acorns, and the healing patterns of injured humans. If we could artificially create identical injuries in a group of humans, there would be predictable variations in the healing patterns.

Different factors are involved, including genetics, nutrition, regular exercise, stress level, quality of sleep, and exposure to potentially toxic substances, that affect each person's ability to heal. Some heal normally "faster," most heal normally "regular," and some heal normally "slower," consistent with normal variations in healing. Some who heal normally slower may have lingering problems or complications from the trauma. Those who heal abnormally for whatever reason will also be at risk for ongoing problems.

2. **Even with healing, one can still hurt.**

Healing is not synonymous with absence of pain or complete resolution of all symptoms. When soft tissues are injured, the body forms scar tissue to repair and "heal" the damage. Fibrin, the main component of the scar tissue, is formed as the "putty" for the damaged areas. Most of the fibrin that forms the scar tissue is already laid down by three weeks. Fibrin can be molded and reoriented into a flexible strong small scar with early active mobilization treatments.

 Healing is not synonymous with absence of pain or complete resolution of all symptoms.

If the window of opportunity to mold the fibrin is missed, the healed scar may turn into a large, inflexible, restrictive one. As we will see later in this book, this type of scar formation can cause chronic pain.

If patients are instructed to rest and wear a soft cervical collar immediately after the accident, they may be at increased risk for persistent stiffness, restriction of mobility, and pain in the injured areas.

Even though the healing phase is complete (*i.e.*, tissues repaired, scars formed), pain is still present. But the body does not sense anything wrong, nor is it signaled to reactivate the healing cascade. Like Stealth fighters, the persistent pain is eluding the body's radar, and all appears well to the healing command centers.

3. **Pain is different for everyone.**

The International Association for the Study of Pain (IASP) defines pain as an unpleasant sensory or emotional experience associated with actual or potential tissue damage (Merskey and Bogduk, 1994). This definition states pain can be present whether or not there is tissue damage. It also reflects how pain is always subjective and unpleasant, by definition.

Pain is difficult to measure, standardize or reproduce because its perception is influenced by multiple factors such as personal beliefs, education, culture differences, learned experiences, and genetics. But we know pain exists even if we can't measure it. All of us know about pain, but all of us perceive pain differently, uniquely.

No two patients are alike in how pain affects them, even if they were both in the same car involved in a rear-end collision. One patient may be hardly bothered by the pain, whereas another patient may be bedridden from it, even though neither may have any ongoing tissue damage or inflammation. Regardless of their functional status, if patients complain to me of persistent pain, I believe them.

Risk Factors for Chronicity

Innumerable variables and factors are involved in each whiplash trauma, and some of these are more apt to increase a person's risk for developing chronic symptoms. From the myriad of possibilities, research and experience can allow us to isolate some of the risk factors for predicting chronic complications. These risk factors include:

1. History of headaches or neck problems prior to the whiplash trauma

2. Surprised at time of crash, *e.g.,* an unexpected rear-end collision

3. Struck vehicle stationary when hit

4. Head turned or looking up at the time of the crash

5. Immediate headache and neck pain following the crash

6. Neurological symptoms resulting from the injury, *e.g.,* dizziness, unsteady gait, visual problems, and tinnitus (ringing in the ears)

Try as we may, doctors are not able to accurately and consistently predict which individuals are going to have chronic problems after a whiplash. We can identify risk factors for those more likely to get injured, those more likely to be severely injured, and those more likely to suffer chronic complications, but someone with no risk factors may still develop chronic problems, and someone with all the risk factors may not be injured at all.

Fibromyalgia As A Cause of Persistent Pain

Despite our best medical efforts to guide patients with acute whiplash injuries to a path of full recovery, chronic pain problems still develop. As if lacking an inner compass, the body's neuromuscular systems frequently drifts toward turbulent, irreversible changes that cause chronic pain.

I see numerous patients with chronic pain following injuries. They describe persistent pain despite various appropriate tests and treatments. The most common condition I diagnose in these people is fibromyalgia. Fibromyalgia is a common condition whose most common cause is trauma, such as whiplash trauma.

In 1996, Dr. Buskila *et al.,* published a study in the *Journal of Rheumatology* called "Increased Rates of Fibromyalgia Following Cervical Spine Injury." He examined 161 injured patients, 102 with neck injuries and 59 with leg fractures. Of the 102 with neck injuries, 67 of them had whiplash trauma. None of the subjects had chronic pain prior to the injury. He examined the patients immediately after the injury, and followed them over time.

His results confirmed what many specialists, including myself, have been noticing in our clinical practices: fibromyalgia is a common complication of neck trauma. In fact, Dr. Buskila found that fibromyalgia developed in nearly 22% of those with neck injuries versus about 2% of those with leg fractures (the control patients). Fibromyalgia was 13 times more frequent following neck injury than following lower extremity injury. This scientific study confirms that whiplash trauma can cause fibromyalgia, and does so frequently (about 22% of the time). Fibromyalgia is a complication of trauma. In the next chapter, we will learn more about how this complicated condition arises.

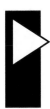 ## If You Want To Know More

1. Bogduk N. *Whiplash: why pay for what does not work?* J Musculoskel Pain 2000; 8: 29–53.

2. Buskila D, Neumann L, Vaisberg G, et al. *Increased rates of fibromyalgia following cervical spine injury. A controlled study of 161 cases of traumatic injury.* Arthritis Rheum 1997; 40: 446–52.

3. Galasko CSB, Murray PA, Pitcher M. *Prevalence and long-term disability following whiplash-associated disorder.* J Musculoskel Pain 2000; 8: 15–27.

4. Gargan MF, Bannister GC. *Long-term prognosis of soft-tissue injuries of the neck.* J Bone Joint Surg Br 1990; 72: 901–3.

5. Hendriksen IJ, Holewijn M. *Degenerative changes of the spine of fighter pilots of the Royal Netherlands Air Force (RNLAF).* Aviat Space Environ Med 1999; 70:1057–63.

6. Maimaris C, Barnes MR, Allen MJ. *"Whiplash injuries" of the neck, a retrospective study.* Injury 1988; 19: 393–6.

7. Merskey H, Bogduk N, eds. *Classification of chronic pain: descriptions of chronic pain syndromes and definitions of pain terms.* 2nd ed. IASP Press 1994.

8. Norris SH, Watt I. *The prognosis of neck injuries resulting from rear-end vehicle collisions.* J Bone Joint Surg Br 1983; 65: 608–11.

9. Pellegrino MJ. *From whiplash to fibromyalgia.* N. Canton OH: ORC Publishing, 2002.

10. Pellegrino MJ. *Post-traumatic fibromyalgia: a medical perspective.* Columbus OH: Anadem Publishing, 1996.

11. Rosenfeld M, Gunnarsson R, Borenstein P. *Early intervention in whiplash-associated disorders: a comparison of two treatment protocols.* Spine 2000; 25: 1782–7.

Fibromyalgia As A Complication Of Injuries

"The pain started after the car accident, and it has never gone away. Before the accident I was perfectly healthy, and now I hurt all over and nothing has helped."

This is a typical story I hear from patients who have chronic pain after a whiplash injury. Some of the treatments may have helped reduce the pain, but it didn't disappear. Many times, the pain is localized at first to the neck, shoulders and upper back areas, but over time, other areas of the body begin to hurt just as bad. Eventually, the person may say the classic 4 word sentence that practically epitomizes fibromyalgia: "I hurt all over."

Fibromyalgia caused by trauma is called post-traumatic fibromyalgia (PTF). Trauma to the body causes tissue damage. Whereas healing is the expected outcome for trauma, it doesn't always happen and PTF can develop. PTF does not occur immediately after an injury; it takes time to evolve and fully develop the characteristic tender points in distinct locations.

Just as trauma other than motor vehicle accidents can cause whiplash-type injuries, trauma other than whiplash-related ones can lead to PTF. Lifting injuries, falls, work injuries, sports injuries, and repetitive-type injuries are examples of other kinds of non-whiplash trauma.

The medical literature has numerous examples of persistent pain following trauma. Since fibromyalgia criteria were established by the American College of Rheumatology study published in 1990, various articles have appeared in the medical literature about PTF. Dr. Romano wrote in 1990 about patients with PTF who continued to require treatment for their condition years after settlement of litigation. In 1992 Dr. Greenfield published a paper describing reactive fibromyalgia syndrome in patients who report trauma as a precipitating event. Dr. Waylonis published a paper entitled "Post-traumatic Fibromyalgia, A Long Term Follow-Up" in 1994 that described a follow-up of 176 patients with PTF. Dr. Wolfe wrote a paper, "Post-traumatic Fibromyalgia: A Case Report Narrated by the Patient" in 1994. Dr. Buskila's 1997 study previously mentioned showed a higher rate (about 22%) of fibromyalgia following trauma to the cervical spine.

A study by Dr. Whalen (*Journal of Musculoskeletal Pain*, 2001) showed a remarkably high prevalence of over 90% of patients reporting at least one traumatic event prior to the onset of fibromyalgia symptoms. More and more researchers seem to be reporting on the importance of physical trauma as a factor in the development of fibromyalgia.

The medical literature and individual practitioners' experiences are revealing that many patients seen who are diagnosed with fibromyalgia have had some type of trauma that caused their conditions.

Among doctors in private practice, many (including me) have reported over half of fibromyalgia patients attribute the onset of their symptoms to a traumatic event. In my own private practice, about 65% of patients report a traumatic injury as the cause of their fibromyalgia.

The medical literature and individual practitioners' experiences are revealing that many patients seen who are diagnosed with fibromyalgia have had some type of trauma that caused their conditions. At a recent fibromyalgia convention (FAME 2000, California), 5 fibromyalgia panels experts, including me, opined that trauma can cause fibromyalgia. Whiplash injuries are the most common type of trauma that causes PTF.

Diagnosing PTF

Not all doctors believe in the existence of PTF. They may believe fibromyalgia is present, but trauma cannot cause it. Dr. Wolfe, a well-known fibromyalgia researcher, proposed that the term "post-traumatic fibromyalgia" be eliminated altogether (Vancouver Fibromyalgia Consensus Group, *J Rheumatology* 1996). Two years earlier though, he authored a paper entitled "Post-traumatic Fibromyalgia, A Case Report Narrated by the Patient." In a recent editorial, he wrote that few useful scientific data exist regarding fibromyalgia and trauma, and we should await more research that absolutely proves this causality relationship.

Yet the "absolute proof" standards are too strict to be useful in everyday clinical practices and common clinical diagnoses. As mentioned above, it is very difficult, if not impossible, to design research studies that will meet the standards of "absolute 100% proof." In the case of trauma and fibromyalgia, we physicians can use our astute clinical observations and current useful scientific data to recognize that trauma is a cause of fibromyalgia, more probably than not.

Trauma-related fibromyalgia, or PTF, is a specific medical condition that exists regardless of individual physician's beliefs or opinions. This diagnosis is never assumed before a patient is seen, or from the patient's history alone. In order for a physician to diagnose PTF, information from the overall clinical evaluation needs to be analyzed. This evaluation includes the patient's history and physical exam, supplemented by any diagnostic testing and review of any previous medical records. The final diagnosis of PTF is made if the total clinical picture "fits."

PTF can be diagnosed if these features are present:

1. No previous pain complaints before the trauma similar to those experienced since the trauma. That is, the person didn't already have a pre-existing fibromyalgia diagnosis or fibromyalgia-like symptoms before the trauma.

2. History of a trauma that led to the pain.

3. Pain resulting from the trauma that has persisted ever since the trauma. I call this the "unbroken chain of pain."

4. Widespread pain persisting for at least 6 months after the injury, well beyond the usual soft tissue healing time.

5. The presence of characteristic painful tender points as defined by the American College of Rheumatology criteria; *i.e.*, at least 11 of 18 positive tender points. If consistent reproducible tender points are present only in an injured region and not widespread, a subset of fibromyalgia, post-traumatic regional fibromyalgia may be considered.

A person can be diagnosed with PTF after one evaluation with an experienced physician. The physician does not have to order specific tests first, or reevaluate the patient over time, to conclude PTF is present. The tender points are the key findings on exam, but muscle spasms and trigger points may be helpful to the physician to clarify the diagnosis. The physician's exam will provide clues if something other than fibromyalgia (*e.g.*, inflammation, neurological disorder) or in addition to fibromyalgia is present.

Conditions in addition to PTF are often present. As previously discussed they can include, but are not limited to, post-concussive syndrome, disc disease, facet dysfunction, and reflex sympathetic dystrophy.

After the initial diagnosis of PTF, the patient may visit the physician for subsequent evaluations to review the condition and effects of any treatment. Re-demonstrating the initial tender points upon follow-up examination is a reliable and supportive physical finding of PTF. The exam abnormalities are expected to persist over time in PTF, and the physician can confirm this expectation upon re-evaluation at a later date.

The ability to diagnose PTF is not dependent upon the person being seen immediately after the trauma. PTF takes time to develop, and once it does, it leaves telltale puzzle clues. If the pieces of the puzzle fit and form the "big picture," a diagnosis of PTF can be made. The next chapter will explore the mechanisms by which PTF develops.

Mechanisms Of PTF

There is a difference between cause and mechanism. The cause is WHY something developed. Trauma is the cause of PTF. The mechanism is HOW something developed, or the pathological events that led to the problem. If you fall on the ground and break your hip, trauma is the cause of the broken hip (WHY you have a hip fracture). The pathological mechanism of injury (the HOW) is that high amounts of compressive forces (momentum) impacted the hip and resulted in a fracture.

Many times it is difficult to determine if an abnormal research finding is part of the cause or the mechanism of fibromyalgia. Changes occur after fibromyalgia has developed, so an abnormality can be one of the consequences of fibromyalgia. It's like asking the famous question, "What came first, the chicken or the egg?"

Injury Pain Mechanisms

Damage to body tissues from an injury can occur from muscle strains, ligament sprains, disc tear or herniation, joint impaction, direct nerve trauma, swelling and inflammation. A combination of injuries activates the normal pain cascades from multiple locations, bombarding the spinal cord and brain with pain signals. Dr. R. Munglani recently published a good review article on the neurobiologic mechanisms that can occur with whiplash injuries (*Journal of Musculoskeletal Pain*, 2000). His descriptions help explain how some people develop chronic pain and others do not.

The road to PTF travels first through acute pain, and then chronic pain. PTF does not happen immediately after the accident. It takes time to fully evolve. Presently, we have no way to determine which injured people will get PTF and which ones will heal and not develop chronic pain. Complete healing without residual pain is attempted in all with injuries, and expected in most. If chronic pain persists several months after an injury, complete healing is not likely to occur, and the risk for getting PTF increases.

The neurobiological mechanisms that lead to fibromyalgia after an injury are similar to what we've previously discussed. Let's review them again. Nerve injuries, tissue inflammation, soft tissue damage and scarring activate the nociceptors and signal pain. Localized injuries to the muscle components (spindles, intrafusal fibers, calcium pumps) can create biochemical, hormonal, and red blood cell changes that interfere with cells' ability to receive oxygen, glucose, and other nutrients. Blood flow, energy formation, and bioelectrical harmony are all disrupted. In those who ultimately develop PTF, the nociceptors probably remain "faulty" and continue to signal pain. Like faulty electrical short-circuits, the nociceptors continue to release pain-producing neurotransmitters.

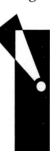

Presently, we have no way to determine which injured people will get PTF and which ones will heal and not develop chronic pain.

Hypersensitization of the nociceptors also occurs, so they respond more dramatically to any stimulation (called allodynia). The nerves cannot "turn off" these continuous painful signals and undergo profound functional changes. Pain arises spontaneously from the nerves causing the person to hurt "for no obvious reason." Instead of waiting to be signaled from outside sources such as trauma, pressure, touch, or temperature changes, the nerves signal spontaneous pain without any outside help.

Furthermore, permanent nerve changes cause outside sensory signals to be misinterpreted as pain. Instead of feeling ordinary touch, movement, or pressure, one feels painful touch, throbbing movement, and stabbing pressure. This exaggerated painful interpretation of ordinarily non-painful sensations is known as allodynia.

Autonomic Nerves Changes

The autonomic nerves are small diameter nerves that interconnect the major nerves with various tissues such as blood vessels, bones, muscles, glands and other organs. They regulate different body functions including sweating, digestion, pain responses, heart rate, blood pressure and more.

Dr. Clauw performed tilt-table testing on patients with fibromyalgia to investigate the autonomic nerve function and found abnormalities. The test subject had blood pressure, pulse and EKG monitored when lying flat and when tilted upward. One-fourth of those with fibromyalgia had an abnormal drop in blood pressure and increase in heart rate. These findings were felt to indicate a dysfunctional autonomic nervous system impairing the body's normal response to stress (in this case, gravity acting on the body). The most affected autonomic nerves are the ones known as the sympathetic nerves.

People with fibromyalgia, including PTF, often have symptoms attributed to a dysfunctional sympathetic nervous system. These symptoms include complaints of burning pain, swelling, rapid heart rate, hot flashes, cold hands and feet, anxiety, fatigue, poor sleep, irritable bowel syndrome, migraine headaches, and aggravation of symptoms with weather changes or increased stress.

There are several ways that whiplash trauma can lead to dysfunctional autonomic nerves, especially the sympathetic nerves:

1. **Hypersensitization.** Like the nociceptors and nerves described above, the sympathetic nerves can undergo physical and functional changes that cause them to be more sensitized to pain signals, or any sensory signals. They become extremely sensitized to any neurotransmitters circulating in the bloodstream (Dr. Devor, 1991). Sprouting of these sympathetic nerves onto any injured nerve enables the sympathetics to "hitch a ride" on other nerves. Whenever the other nerve is activated, the hitched sympathetics also get activated and cause exaggerated sensory symptoms (Dr. McLachlan, 1993).

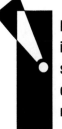

People with fibromyalgia, including PTF, often have symptoms attributed to a dysfunctional sympathetic nervous system.

2. **Direct trauma to the sympathetic nerves.** The cervical intervertebral discs have sympathetic nerve fibers in the front part. These nerve fibers can be injured with whiplash trauma to the discs (Dr. Munglani). As previously described in Chapter 2, major chains of sympathetic nerves are located in front of the cervical spine, and they can be stretched or damaged with neck trauma during the whiplash.

3. **Continuous stimulation from other sources.** The sympathetic nerves are obligated to do as they are told. If an outside source signals these nerves to fire, then fire away they must do. Following a whiplash trauma, different peripheral sources may continuously signal the sympathetic nerves to fire. These sources include muscle spasms, tissue swelling or congestion, soft tissue scars, painful facet joints, intervertebral disc problems, nerve root or plexus irritation and other areas (Dr. Munglani).

Spinal Cord Changes

At the spinal cord level, changes occur which propagate the fibromyalgia mechanisms. Spinal cord nerves are bombarded with continuous stimulation from the peripheral nerves, causing a progressive increase in electrical signals sent up to the brain. This phenomenon is called "wind-up," and is the neurological mechanism for amplification of pain. Wind-up leads to central sensitization where different sensory signals, not just pain, gets amplified and sent to the brain. The spinal cord is no longer able to normally sort out and filter these sensory signals.

Another key change in the spinal cord level is increased formation of a neurotransmitter called substance P (Dr. Russell). Substance P's primary role is to transmit pain signals at the spinal cord level and enhance the spinal cord's responsiveness to detecting pain. Persistent pain signals bombarding the spinal cord enhance substance P's production and it reaches abnormally high concentrations.

Excessive substance P begins to migrate up and down the spinal cord, away from the initial location of the pain signals. As a result, multiple levels of the spinal cord start responding to substance P. The spinal cord nerves at these levels become hypersensitized to pain and send pain signals to the brain. Thus, the pain "spreads" to different locations at the spinal cord level, and the person starts to report pain in other body locations, even areas that may not have been injured.

Glia Cells And Pain

Glia cells are part of the nervous system. There are several types, *e.g.,* microglia, astrocytes and oligodendrocytes found abundantly within the nerves of the spinal cord and brain. For a long time, they were thought to maintain and support the neurons, but not actually transmit nerve signals. Pain signals were felt to be a process that only neurons could transmit.

Glia cells probably play an important role in the overall function of the nervous system, including transmission of pain. Recent work by Dr. Linda Watkins (2001) supports the importance of glia cells in the transmission and perpetuation of pain signals. She found that glia cells, normally quiet, can become activated in response to specific triggers such as trauma or infection. Activated glia cells can release a number of pain generating chemicals, including substance P.

The glia cell malfunctioning can create a pathological pain state, causing persistent release of pain neurotransmitters and hypersensitization of the neurons. Since the glia cells are connected to all the nerves of the spinal cord and brain, they may be able to signal long distance malfunctions, *i.e.,* cause pain to spread from one body location to another by activating more distantly connected glia cells. Ultimately, the pain can become widespread and the person complains of hurting all over.

Regional To Generalized Pain

Dr. Bennett and others have described the phenomenon where pain spreads over time from a regional area to a more generalized area. A common example in whiplash trauma is where initial pain in the neck only evolves into generalized widespread pain over time. The injured neck area hurts, as expected, at first. Other areas such as the low back, hips, arms and legs may not hurt at all, and were never injured.

The neurobiological mechanism for this clinical migration of pain probably lies in the "rewiring" process that the nervous system undergoes in response to chemical, hormonal, and structural changes brought about by the trauma.

Yet over time, ranging from weeks to a few years, the patients report pain that seems to spread to these previously uninjured areas, often causing pain just as severe as the originally injured neck areas. Serial clinical exams on these patients reveal the correlation of regional painful areas at first (regional fibromyalgia), then widespread painful tender points that meet the ACR defined criteria for fibromyalgia.

The neurobiological mechanism for this clinical migration of pain probably lies in the "rewiring" process that the nervous system undergoes in response to chemical, hormonal, and structural changes brought about by the trauma. Neurons and glia cells probably reorganize and become dysfunctional. Too much substance P and other chemicals and neurohormones are produced and cause further changes in the spinal cord. The spillage of excessive substance P into other levels of the cord beyond the level(s) representing the injured tissues leads to cord changes. As a result, these previously "normal" levels of the spinal cord start signaling pain.

Like ancient Rome, all "roads" (nerves) lead to the brain. Whether the pain signals started at the neck, low back, foot, or finger, they all must travel the roads through the cervical spinal cord and into the brain. At first the brain might be able to distinguish the exact origin of the pain signals, but eventually a potpourri of sustained, amplified signals clouds the neurobiological picture.

Brain Changes

Central sensitization occurs in the brain as well as the spinal cord. The pain centers of the brain, the limbic system and the cerebral cortex, are continuously fed those amplified pain signals from the spinal cord. Previously innocuous sensations are being sent with pain signals attached (allodynia) which further feed the vulnerable central nervous system and permanently alters the way the information is handled.

Ultimately, the person who develops PTF reports constant, severe and widespread pain that cannot be ignored. The pain is spontaneous, occurring without any "provoking" factors. The pain also occurs with previously "normal" sensory signals such as touch, weather changes, air conditioning draft, movement, and more. Emotional components become "attached" to pain, including depression, anxiety, anger, hopelessness, and helplessness, which can further amplify the pain.

PTF Cascade Summary

To summarize, fibromyalgia from trauma results from changes in the pain pathways. It may start off as a peripheral irritant, but eventually it becomes a self-perpetuating process that affects the entire pathway from the nociceptors to the brain. Spontaneous pain is generated and amplified, and ordinary sensory input is interpreted as painful. Ongoing peripheral input feeds a sensitized and vulnerable central nervous system, giving rise to chronically painful PTF.

In my experience, PTF is the most common cause of chronic pain after whiplash trauma.

Not everyone with a whiplash injury has chronic pain, and not everyone with chronic pain after a whiplash has PTF. In my experience, PTF is the most common cause of chronic pain after whiplash trauma. Amplified pains are not everyday aches and pains. They are severe functionally limiting pains that cannot be ignored.

Persistent Triggers

Ongoing peripheral input that feeds into the centrally sensitized "fibromyalgia pain cascade" comes from different injured tissues. These areas are known as "triggers" or "pain generators" and can occur wherever there is residual damage or instability from injury. A number of pain generators exist and include:

1. **Muscle triggers.** Ongoing muscle spasms and restrictive muscle scars are examples of persistent triggers that can exist in muscles. Muscle bundles may go into protective spasms whenever there is inflammation or potential irritation in the region. For example, someone with a low back disc herniation may have spasms in the low back muscles as an involuntary attempt to protect, or guard from movements of the back. Any back movement could cause further damage or inflammation from the already damaged disc.

   In PTF, muscles have a double whammy effect on the pain-generating cascade. The injury itself caused muscle damage and persistent localized spasms, causing ongoing pain signals.

But the muscles may be forced to work harder because other tissues (*e.g.*, discs, facets, ligaments) were permanently damaged and cannot do their jobs of stabilizing the spine. Hence, the muscles tighten and spasm up to assist in the stabilization, and more persistent pain signals are sent...the double whammy effect.

Large amounts of restrictive scar tissue that formed in response to the muscle damage may impede blood flow and cause pain from lack of oxygen or nutrients. Or the scar may adhere to sensitive nerves and trigger them to fire pain signals.

2. **Facet joint dysfunctions.** Australian researcher Bogduk and his colleagues have demonstrated how the cervical facet joints especially are a major trigger of chronic pain. The facet joints may be unstable because the capsular ligaments were damaged or overstretched from the whiplash. Loose ligaments cannot hold the joints together as tightly as needed to stabilize them, and any "extra" movement in the facet joints triggers pain. The facet joints may be too restricted or tight, leading to instability. Muscle spasms can tighten or restrict the facet joints, causing pain from immobility.

3. **Intervertebral discs.** These areas can become chronic pain generators if the whiplash trauma caused tears or defects in the disc's annular ligament. Dr. Bogduk's work noted up to 50% of chronic whiplash patients have problems with these discs.

4. **Nerve injuries.** Direct injuries to nerves can result in chronic pain generation, as opposed to indirectly signaling chronic pain through normal uninjured nerves. Nerve roots, brachial plexus, and sympathetic nerves can all be bruised, stretched or damaged from the whiplash trauma and never heal properly, causing chronic pain signals.

All of the above sources can feed into the sensitized central nervous system (spinal cord and brain) and maintain, aggravate, and permanently worsen the PTF's chronic pain state.

Who Is Predisposed?

Presently, there is no way to predict who will get PTF after a whiplash trauma. In a group of people with whiplash trauma, we can say about 22% will get PTF over time (Dr. Buskila's study), but we cannot say which 22% will get it, or whether any one individual will get PTF after a whiplash. We know of risk factors that increase the likelihood of developing PTF after a whiplash, and I anticipate that additional research over time will shed more light on who is most predisposed.

In a group of people with whiplash trauma, we can say about 22% will get PTF over time, but we cannot say which 22% will get it, or whether any one individual will get PTF after a whiplash.

Based on what is currently known, I believe a number of risk factors exist that make one more vulnerable to getting PTF if a whiplash trauma occurs. People can have all of the risk factors and not get PTF, or have none of them and get PTF after a whiplash event, so an exact science does not exist for making predictions. We try to make the best educated medical guesses based on current clinical and research experiences.

The following are risk factors I consider in determining why certain people develop PTF after a whiplash injury:

1. **Genetics.** As mentioned in the last chapter, fibromyalgia can be inherited. Many people may inherit a vulnerability to fibromyalgia, even if they didn't have this condition at the

time of the whiplash. A specific genetic make-up that predisposes one to fibromyalgia is lurking inside the body, and the trauma unleashes the neurobiological cascade that causes PTF to develop. The predisposed state may be one that facilitates central sensitization if given the chance. Whiplash injuries provide the chance. People without fibromyalgia who have relatives with fibromyalgia, especially a parent or sibling, are more at risk for PTF in the event of an injury.

2. **Previous injuries.** Injuries can create "pain memories" that hurt for awhile, but then become masked or latent, especially if healing occurred. Later on in life, another severe injury may send signals up the previously traveled pain pathways and readily "unmask" the latent pain memories. The compounded effect leads to chronic pain that doesn't go away.

I've seen many patients who report previous injuries that healed. They may have had a prior whiplash injury or may have had treatments for the pain, but the pain eventually went away with no obvious residuals. These were not minor injuries like a shoulder sprain from throwing a baseball or a hamstring pull, but rather more severe injuries such as a fracture, previous whiplash, or back trauma. A subsequent whiplash may have an "advantage" to causing PTF because it can dust off the cobwebs of the unused pathways and quickly establish a chronic pain cycle.

Some people can have several previous whiplash injuries with no problems, and then the fourth whiplash causes PTF. Obviously, something unique happened the fourth time that triggered the irreversible PTF cascade.

3. **Preexisting cervical spinal stenosis.** Some people with fibromyalgia also have cervical spinal stenosis, a condition where the base of the skull and the top of the spinal canal are too narrow, causing pressure on the spinal cord and neurological symptoms. This problem can be inherited or can develop from disc and arthritic disease of the cervical spine. Dr. Pettersson (1995) showed that persons who sustained a whiplash injury were more likely to develop chronic pain problems if there was pre-existing narrowing of the cervical spinal canal.

Anyone without fibromyalgia and with pre-existing cervical spinal stenosis is at risk for PTF in the event of whiplash trauma. Neck injuries of normal necks can lead to PTF, so neck injuries of abnormal necks would be expected to lead to a higher incidence of PTF.

4. **Cigarette smokers.** Based on my experience, injured cigarette smokers heal slower and more incompletely than injured non-smokers. Much has been reported on the risks of cigarette smoking, and those who continue to smoke after a whiplash trauma are probably more at risk for developing PTF.

5. **Nutritional deficiencies.** Proper healing after trauma requires proper nourishment, including lots of protein which provide the body's building blocks. Those who are malnourished for whatever reason, such as medical ailments, dieting, poor dietary habits, or excessive alcohol drinking may be more at risk for developing PTF after a whiplash trauma.

6. **Medical profile characteristics.** Some characteristics seem to increase the risks of PTF. Women are more at risk than men, older persons more so than younger persons, taller people with longer necks more so than shorter short-necked people. As you may recall,

these factors make one more at risk for a whiplash injury in the event of a motor vehicle accident. By logical deduction, these same factors make one more at risk for PTF after a whiplash injury.

PTF is a common endpoint of different possible pathways. A person can have some or many risk factors, and be involved in a whiplash collision causing mild to severe injuries. Different tissues can become persistent pain generators, and peripheral and central nervous system changes can result. If everything happens just "right," PTF develops. Given the numerous factors involved, one who gets PTF is actually getting the "luck of the draw."

The person with PTF does not feel lucky at all. He or she has chronic severe pain and needs our medical help.

Treatment Of PTF

Just like in nontraumatic fibromyalgia, no one single treatment eliminates the symptoms of PTF. Currently there is no cure for this disorder. However, various treatments can help those with PTF even if the condition is not cured. Each person's treatment program needs to be individualized,

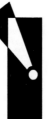

Just like in nontraumatic fibro-myalgia, no one single treatment eliminates the symptoms of PTF.

and what works for some may not work for others. Hopefully each patient will find some treatment that helps to deal with the chronic pain.

We've reviewed in detail already the various treatments for fibromyalgia. The treatments for PTF are really the same, since fibromyalgia is fibromyalgia regardless of the cause! Since some of you may be reading this section by itself (as a mini-book), I want to refer you to Section III to read about detailed treatments for fibromyalgia. For those of you who've read all the book so far, you can skip ahead, or enjoy a brief treatment review (if you've already forgotten the info due to Fibrofog!). I'll briefly review some aspects of PTF treatment here.

Treatment Goals

Six main treatment goals can be identified for each person with PTF:

1. **Decrease pain.** The ideal goal is to eliminate pain altogether, but this rarely happens because PTF has no known cure at this time. Many treatments can reduce the pain, however, even if it is still present. Sometimes a remission occurs where the pain is hardly noticed although painful tender points are still palpable on exam.

2. **Improve function.** The ability to perform everyday activities such as dressing oneself, driving, moving about, and eating is the basis for "quality of life" issues. If pain interferes with basic daily activities, the patient with PTF usually reports a poorer quality of life. Pain can interfere with work abilities, especially if the job requires a lot of reaching, bending, or lifting. Optimizing job functions is an important treatment goal.

3. **Promote healing of any residual injuries.** If residual damage to tissues is still present and contributing to pain, instability, ongoing irritation or inflammation, then treatments to promote healing of this damage should help.

4. **Prevent worsening or complications.** If residual damage to tissues is present and cannot be healed, then the goal becomes avoiding further damage or complications.

5. **Decrease the risk of re-injury or flare-up.** If one's PTF is chronic and permanent, then a goal is to keep it at a stable baseline, or a level where the pain can be successfully managed. A stable baseline free from annoying flare-ups may sound boring, but is exactly what is hoped for.

6. **Find a successful home program to control symptoms.** This goal is the ultimate prize. One hopes the therapy program works, and learns to do the program on his/her own to maintain a stable baseline.

In PTF various types of treatments are prescribed in order to achieve as many individual treatment goals as possible. Some treatments may work better than others, and usually the combination of all the different treatments can lead to overall improvement.

Education

No matter what the cause of fibromyalgia, I believe education is the most important treatment. In PTF, the patients already know the cause of the pain: whiplash trauma (or whatever trauma). They tell me that they never had previous pain complaints similar to those experienced since the trauma. They describe the "unbroken chain of pain" that started with the trauma and has been present ever since.

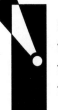

No matter what the cause of fibromyalgia, I believe education is the most important treatment.

I will confirm the diagnosis and discuss the mechanisms of how trauma led to the PTF, and why the symptoms persist. I'll review treatment goals. Having an accurate diagnosis helps validate patients' symptoms and give them closure. Once patients learn about PTF, they can begin to accept this condition and take better control of it.

Medications

Medications can be helpful in PTF. No magical pill exists, but many drugs can help reduce the pain. No one type of medicine works for everyone, and no one medicine causes 100% improvement. The patient and doctor need to experiment with different medicines, prescribed or over-the counter (OTC), to determine if any one or combination works well without bothersome side effects.

Therapeutic Injections

I frequently prescribe these injections for patients with PTF. Several types of injections can be done, depending on the particular pain-generating source.

1. **Trigger point injections.** For painful muscle spasms, these injections are commonly used. A local anesthetic and sometimes a cortisone medicine can be injected directly into the painful areas.

2. **Joint injections.** Injections into specific painful joints such as the knee, shoulder or facets may help if joint pain is a major problem. PTF can be aggravated by facet joint dysfunctions, shoulder tendinitis, knee inflammation, or other joint problems. Injections consist of a steroid

medicine mixed with some local anesthetic. Facet joint injections are common ones performed in those with PTF from a whiplash injury. A large percentage of these people will have persistent facet problems in the cervical and thoracic spinal areas.

3. **Nerve root blocks and epidural injections.** Whenever disc problems (*e.g.,.* herniated discs) or nerve root irritations (*e.g.,* radiculopathy) are present, these types of injections can be considered. Disc or nerve root problems will contribute to the ongoing PTF pain, so they need to be addressed as part of the overall treatment.

4. **Botox injections.** Studies on Botox injections have shown effectiveness for headaches and other pains caused by painful muscle spasms, thus these may help some with PTF.

5. **Prolotherapy.** The "prolo" in prolotherapy is short for "proliferate" because the injections stimulate growth or proliferation of tissue. This type of injection therapy is directed at weakened ligaments and tendons common in those with whiplash-induced PTF.

Typically, a dextrose (sugar) based anesthetic solution is injected into the injured ligament, tendon, or joint capsule areas. The body's injury-repair sequence is activated, and the areas injected behave as if a fresh injury has been caused. This controlled "injury recreation" activates the body's healing cascade which forms new soft tissues.

Combined studies by different researchers have shown that ligament and tendon size can increase by as much as 35 to 44% in areas treated by the injections, and hypermobile or loose facet joint capsular ligaments can be "tightened" and stabilized by prolotherapy. Seventy-five percent or more of patients who qualify for this treatment can improve (Vlad Djuric, MD, 2001)

These different injection therapies can help many with PTF. As with prescribed oral medicines, therapeutic injections can be considered on an individual basis as part of a multi-faceted treatment approach.

Physical Medicine Treatments

A physical medicine program is an important part of the overall PTF treatment program. It may also be called a physical therapy program or therapy program. It includes modalities such as heat, cold, massage, electric stimulation, or water therapy. Also included are exercises such as stretches, proper body mechanics, strengthening, stabilizing, conditioning, aerobics, and aquatics.

Manual therapy is helpful. A specific manual therapy program, the McKenzie program named after its founder, may help those with disc and spine problems present along with the PTF. Doctors need to determine what therapies ultimately work best for each patient.

Future Directions In Treatment Of PTF

What is expected in the future regarding whiplash injuries and PTF? As long as there are people who encounter momentum changes, there will be people who experience whiplash-type injuries. Some of these people will develop fibromyalgia as a chronic complication of their trauma.

We can't prevent qualified people from driving, and we can't strap everyone in a protective cage, race driver-style, when they drive. Somewhere in between, we need to find an effective compromise. A collaboration of physicians and engineers from multiple research centers (Crash Injury and Engineering Network) is working to rethink whiplash prevention and treatment strategies. Researchers are recognizing the devastation of auto accidents that is far greater than previously believed.

Instead of relying on crash dummies to understand crash dynamics, studies of human crash victims, precise measurements of damage to vehicles and recreations of the crashes are being documented. Test dummies that are crashed in the labs each day in no way act like humans in the real world. The physicians and engineers are changing the way they think and looking closer at safety standards and designs, and in medical treatments.

Engineers have learned certain safety features in the cars, such as airbags, seat belts, child safety seats, and headrests may not work effectively for different people or different types of collisions. For example, child safety seats that perform well in head-on crashes don't adequately protect babies from head injuries during a side collision. Seat belts that work well for younger drivers don't necessarily work well for elderly people. Airbags have caused fatal injuries in young children. Headrests need to be sturdy and properly fitted to the back of the neck.

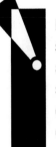

Engineers have learned certain safety features in the cars, such as airbags, seat belts, child safety seats, and headrests may not work effectively for different people or different types of collisions.

The team approach between doctors, researchers and engineers will hopefully produce a revolution in auto safety design that works for drivers and passengers of all shapes and ages. Redesigns and improvements in car interiors and crumple zones are already occurring. Legislative changes and modifications will likely continue to mandate safer vehicles.

Rethink Treatments

As we strive to minimize trauma to the human body, we need to rethink our acute treatment approaches when trauma occurs. As more research supports the advantage of early intervention with active mobilization and manual therapies (*e.g.,* the study by M. Rosenfeld, *et al.*), we should shift our focus from recommending rest and cervical collars to prompt interventions that include active manual therapy in acute whiplash injuries. Collaboration between emergency room/stat care physicians and manual clinicians may expedite the early interventions in the acutely injured patients. Doctors experienced in managing acute injuries and recognizing early signs of complications should be involved at the onset.

Treatment strategies that reduce inflammation and minimize further damage to tissues are important. Early nutritional strategies to help the repair process make sense as part of the treatment. Injection strategies such as prolotherapy will probably play a greater future role in reducing symptoms and helping tissues to heal.

The sooner the injured patient can be effectively treated, the less likely acute and chronic complications will occur. This is the hallmark of trauma medicine. As we refine the trauma interventions for whiplash related injuries, I anticipate less people will end up getting PTF.

If You Want To Know More

1. Aprill C, Dwyer A, Bogduk N. *Cervical zygapophyseal joint pain patterns. II: a clinical evaluation.* Spine 1990; 15: 458–61.

2. Bennett RM. *Emerging concepts in the neurobiology of chronic pain: evidence of abnormal sensory processing in fibromyalgia.* Mayo Clin Proc. 1999; 74: 385–98.

3. Buskila D, Neumann L, Vaisberg G, et al. *Increased rates of fibromyalgia following cervical spine injury. A controlled study of 161 cases of traumatic injury.* Arthritis Rheum 1997; 40: 446–52.

4. Devor M. *Neuropathic pain and injured nerve: peripheral mechanisms.* Br Med Bull 1991; 47: 619–30.

5. Greenfield S, Fitzcharles MA, Esdaile JM. *Reactive fibromyalgia syndrome.* Arthritis Rheum 1992; 35: 678–81.

6. McLachlan E. *Symposium on autonomic neuroeffector mechanisms.* J Auton Nerv Syst 1993; 45: 245–6.

7. Munglani R. *Neurobiological mechanisms underlying chronic whiplash associated pain: the peripheral maintenance of central sensitization.* World Congress on Whiplash-Associated Disorders in Vancouver, British Columbia, Canada, Feb 1999. J Musculoskel Pain 2000; 8: 169–78.

8. Pellegrino MJ. *From whiplash to fibromyalgia.* N. Canton OH: ORC Publishing, 2002.

9. Pellegrino MJ. *Understanding post-traumatic fibromyalgia: a medical perspective.* Columbus OH: Anadem Publishing, 1996.

10. Pettersson K, Karrholm J, Toolanen G, et al. *Decreased width of the spinal canal in patients with chronic symptoms after whiplash injury.* Spine 1995; 20: 1664–7.

11. Petzke F, Clauw DJ. *Sympathetic nervous system function in fibromyalgia.* Curr Rheumatol Rep 2000; 2: 116–23.

12. Romano TJ. *Clinical experiences with post-traumatic fibromyalgia syndrome.* WV Med J 1990; 86: 198–202.

13. Rosenfeld M, Gunnarsson R, Borenstein P. *Early intervention in whiplash-associated disorders: a comparison of two treatment protocols.* Spine 2000; 25(14): 1782–7.

14. Watkins LR, Milligan ED, Maier SF. *Glial activation: a driving force for pathological pain.* Trends Neurosci 2001; 24: 450–5.

15. Waylonis GW, Perkins RH. *Post-traumatic fibromyalgia. A long-term follow-up.* Am J Phys Med Rehabil 1994; 73: 403–12.

16. Wolfe F. *Post-traumatic fibromyalgia: a case report narrated by the patient.* Arthritis Care Res 1994; 7: 161–5.

17. Wolfe F. *The fibromyalgia syndrome: a consensus report of fibromyalgia and disability.* J Rheumatol 1996; 23: 534–9.

Legal Aspects Of Post-Traumatic Fibromyalgia As A Result Of Personal Injury

This chapter provides information on legal issues of post-traumatic fibromyalgia (PTF). The information is based on an interview with an experienced attorney, Nicholas E. Phillips, Esq. I am not an attorney, and I am not giving legal advice. However, educating people about PTF invariably involves educating them about medical and legal aspects because the two can be linked.

In my experience, very few people with PTF are involved in litigation, and a very small percentage of my time as a fibromyalgia specialist is spent addressing medical-legal issues of my patients. But issues arise, questions are asked, and information is requested. I always recommend patients seek advice of an attorney for any legal questions they may have.

I appreciate attorney Phillips' helpful and detailed information that comprises this chapter, and for those who seek this type of information, I hope you find it helpful.

What You Can Do If You Get Fibromyalgia From An Injury

By Nicholas E. Phillips, Esq.

Personal Snapshot

Nicholas E. Phillips, Esq. practices with Phillips, Mille & Costabile Co., L.P.A. in two locations in Northeast Ohio. Mr. Phillips has been trying personal injury cases for 30 years and has represented many clients with fibromyalgia. This firm includes six attorneys and provides a variety of legal services. Mr. Phillips heads the litigation department and is experienced in personal injury cases. One of only 100 Certified Civil Trial Advocates in Ohio, Mr. Phillips is also a member of both the Association of Trial Lawyers of America and the Ohio Academy of Trial Lawyers. The firm's website is http://www.pmlawyers.com; the e-mail address is pmstaff@pmlawyers.com, and the telephone numbers are (440) 243-2800 and (440) 460-4600.

Are you beginning to experience the symptoms of fibromyalgia as the result of an injury or is your fibromyalgia worsening because of an injury? If so, you may be entitled to compensation.

When you can identify the onset of fibromyalgia as the direct result of someone else's negligence you can attempt to recover compensation under that person's liability insurance policy. This is often the situation when you have been involved in an auto accident or other incident in which you are injured because of another's fault.

Can fibromyalgia be the direct result of an accident? It is often difficult to prove. And insurance companies are not going to compensate you without persuasive evidence, so it is wise to consult with an attorney if you think you have been injured by someone else's negligence.

The earlier you start to gather documentation of your injury the more likely you are to succeed.

You need to contact an attorney because you will deal with an insurance adjuster soon after the accident, and if you talk with an adjuster unprepared you could reduce your eventual recovery. Fibromyalgia is a difficult condition to discuss with insurance adjusters because most of them are unfamiliar with the condition. You should know exactly what to say to an adjuster before you discuss your case. Be prepared!

If you have just now begun to feel the effects of fibromyalgia from an accident which occurred some time ago, it's still important to contact an attorney to see what legal options you may have.

There is a significant amount of effort required in obtaining sufficient medical confirmation that you have fibromyalgia and that it is the direct result of the accident. The earlier you start to gather documentation of your injury the more likely you are to succeed. It is extremely important to document the body parts that are affected by the accident and may later lead to fibromyalgia. Again, the place to begin is with the first medical records following the accident.

How To Select An Attorney

Selecting an attorney in a post-traumatic (PTF) claim is similar to selecting an attorney for any other type of case. You will want an attorney who has experience trying cases, and more specifically, one who tries personal injury cases.

Personal injury attorneys are divided into two groups: defense attorneys who represent insurance companies and defend them and their insureds against claims such as yours and plaintiff's attorneys who represent people like you who have a claim.

Plaintiff's attorneys take cases like yours and file suits against the person at fault. They generally are compensated by charging a share of the amount of money recovered in a lawsuit. In other words, they usually don't charge you unless they're successful. However, you may be required to pay out-of-pocket expenses.

Many of the plaintiff's attorneys belong to the Association of Trial lawyers of America—ATLA www.atla.org. ATLA has local chapters in many locations so you may want to contact them. Also, your local bar association can recommend attorneys who handle your type of case.

The tried-and-true method for identifying an attorney to represent you is to talk to friends about their experience with attorneys. Any acquaintance who is familiar with the legal profession in your area would be a good person to talk with for a recommendation.

One resource you should check is a local fibromyalgia support group. Members often share information about doctors and lawyers who are knowledgeable about fibromyalgia, and you can easily tap into that source of information.

Before you actually retain an attorney to represent you it is helpful to sit down with him or her and ask a few questions. Since you probably already know at least something about fibromyalgia, you should be able to evaluate the attorney's understanding of the condition and how it is related to the accident. It is extremely important that you are well prepared with as much information about your accident as possible before you talk to an attorney, even for the first time. Bring a copy of the police report and medical reports.

There is still some controversy whether fibromyalgia can be caused by or worsened by trauma, and it is important to address this issue to determine your attorney's position on this issue. It is also appropriate to ask the prospective attorney whether he or she has handled any fibromyalgia cases before. If so, find out how successful your case would be based upon your medical history in relation to the attorney's other cases.

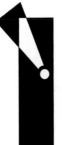

It is extremely important that you are well prepared with as much information about your accident as possible before you talk to an attorney, even for the first time.

If you're not satisfied with your attorney's level of knowledge or commitment to learning about fibromyalgia—and to your cause—it's best to select another attorney. You should be confident you are being well represented before you enter into an agreement for someone to prosecute your case.

Representation & Fee Agreement

One of the key issues for engaging an attorney to represent you in a personal injury case is the fee. You will be asked to sign a contingent fee contract which is a contract with the attorney to represent you. Be sure to read the contract thoroughly and make sure you understand it completely. Ask your attorney about any part of the agreement you don't understand. This will help avoid unpleasant surprises later on in your relationship.

Generally speaking, attorneys in litigation will charge somewhere between 33% to 40% and higher depending upon the difficulty of the case and at what stage the case is going to be resolved. The common fee is 33% if the case is settled before litigation, and it is not uncommon for fees to go up to 40% if the case is filed for litigation and there may be a few extra percentage points if the case actually goes to litigation.

With regards to your legal fees for claims made either through Social Security or Workers' Compensation or any another federal or state program, there may be regulations by that agency that set the level of fees. These cases will be discussed later.

In addition to your legal fees, there are costs of litigation. First there are court costs which are generated by the court and are charged to the parties, rather than the lawyers. Then there are case expenses. These include the costs of depositions (basically statements made under oath), preparation time for experts, video depositions, expert witness fees and preparation of any evidence that will be presented such as enlargements of photographs and other similar expenses. These costs are normally taken out of the recovery, either from the settlement or jury verdict.

Typically, legal fees are taken off the top of any award, and the costs are taken out of the client's share. So, it's something to look at when working with an attorney to ask these questions. Just make sure you understand where the dollars are going to be coming from. Often your attorney will pay these expenses during the course of the case and then recoup them out of your recovery.

You should be aware that even though the funds are being advanced by the firm during litigation, it is actually your money that is being spent, so you should keep track of it. Perhaps you would want a monthly statement of expenses. Remember that if you do not win, you still must pay these expenses.

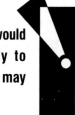

Any kind of accident that would cause the human body to suffer trauma is one that may cause fibromyalgia.

Again, make sure you understand the fee agreement, and once you sign it, make sure you obtain and keep a copy of it.

It is also a good idea to maintain a "shadow file" which will include all of the documents that the lawyer sends to you. The bottom line: keep your own records of every document in the case so that you have personal knowledge and some measure of control over what's going on. As with your health: be an active participant in the legal process. You will be surprised at how much better you will feel about the whole legal process if you do your part.

What Accidents Are The Basis For A Claim?

Any kind of accident that would cause the human body to suffer trauma is one that may cause fibromyalgia. The most usual cause is an auto accident where the patient is exposed to high G forces which cause the pulling and tearing of muscle and other connective tissues. Falls of any kind can also result in localized areas of fibromyalgia. This issue is explained in greater detail in the parts of this book dealing directly with medical issues.

What Types Of Insurance Are Involved In These Cases?

1. Private Liability Insurance

As we discussed in the section on retaining an attorney you will most likely be dealing with private liability insurance—regular auto insurance—in making a claim for fibromyalgia. The most common scenario involves making a claim against the insurer of the driver who caused the accident resulting in, or worsening, fibromyalgia. The person who caused the accident is known as the tortfeasor.

If you are the passenger in an auto that is struck you may make a claim against the automobile insurance of the auto you are riding in. Depending on the type of policy and state's laws, you can also make a claim against your own auto insurer for medical payment coverage, underinsured or uninsured motorist coverage, personal hospitalization coverage, and the medical payments coverage of other parties, such as the owner of land where an accident occurred.

2. Workers' Compensation

You may have a basis for making a claim under Workers' Compensation if your injury occurred while you are engaged in your work. Of course this applies if you are actually at your workplace and are injured in some way. Also, depending on the situation, you may be able to make a claim if you are in an auto accident while traveling to work from home, during work, or returning home from work.

Workers' Compensation claims are handled in what is known as an administrative proceeding with an agency of the state, in some states called the Industrial Commission. This is not a court, but in some ways performs the function of a court because the agency determines whether you are entitled to compensation for your injury. As part of the process of making a claim, you will be examined by a physician who will report to the agency about your ability to work.

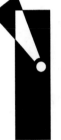

There are a myriad of factors that influence the outcome of a Workers' Compensation claim. There are different categories of disability, and depending on the evidence and the medical examination, the agency will rule on the extent of your disability, if any. Categories include temporary or permanent, partial or total. Rehabilitation from your injury is another factor.

The most common scenario involves making a claim against the insurer of the driver that caused the accident resulting in, or worsening, fibromyalgia.

Another consideration is the work you have been engaged in and whether you can continue that work or some other kind. In some instances you are entitled to certain restrictions on your duties which your employer must follow. Also, you can be asked to undergo rehabilitation to help you maximize your physical capabilities to be able to return to work.

If your injury involved a work-related automobile accident, you may be able to make a claim against a private insurance company as well as for workers' compensation. If you are successful in your claim against the private insurance company, whether you need to reimburse Workers' Compensation for your award varies by state, and you may need a lawyer to let you know your obligation in that regard.

3. Medicare

Medicare is another consideration when an accident brings the onset or worsens fibromyalgia. Depending on the situation, Medicare may pay for all of the medical treatment needed for a patient. If you are simultaneously bringing an action against a private insurance company and receive compensation in a trial or a settlement, federal law gives Medicare a statutory right to be reimbursed for the amount you collect. There are specific reporting rules for this situation that should be discussed with an attorney before signing any settlement. Medicare will usually share in the cost of pursuing the claim and will reduce its claim for reimbursement.

4. Other Insurance

Some states provide insurance coverage by case law, and this is known as insurance coverage "by operation of law." This might create a right to file a claim against an insurance company that is not readily apparent to you. For example, in Ohio there are certain circumstances where a person may file a claim with his or her employer's commercial automobile insurance company, and the possibility exists that additional funds can be collected under the employer's underinsured motorist provisions. Coverage by operation of law varies from state to state, so you should ask your attorney about this and any other special circumstances that may provide you a basis for making a claim.

Making A Claim

Once you have retained an attorney, and he or she is satisfied that you have a basis for recovering for PTF, your attorney can proceed with the legal process. Initially your attorney will file a claim with the adjuster of the insurance company of the individual who caused the accident. In an auto accident situation, this is the other driver.

Typically, the function of the insurance adjuster is to look for information (evidence) concerning the medical bills and perhaps the medical records. Fibromyalgia is a condition which insurance adjusters are very reluctant to recognize at all. If it is determined that you do have fibromyalgia, the adjuster may be even more reluctant to agree that your fibromyalgia is accident-related or the result of some type of trauma. Therefore it is important that your attorney understands what fibromyalgia is and how it needs to be proven within the insurance process.

The Best Way To Resolve Your Case

The best way to make sure your case is resolved if you have PTF is to retain an attorney as soon as possible who definitely knows about fibromyalgia. Assemble your medical evidence early in the claim process. Present your claim thoroughly and forcefully to the adjuster—the person who must be convinced of the legitimacy of your claim—and give this person some hard evidence to support your claim. If there is enough medical evidence in your file, you are going to make it easier for the adjuster to settle your case.

Present your claim thoroughly and forcefully to the adjuster.

Fibromyalgia presents a difficult set of circumstances for achieving just and full compensation. If the case is settled too soon, the full extent of the disease may not be accounted for in a settlement. On the other hand, if you wait too long to file a claim you may be outside the period of time in which a lawsuit must be filed.

Generally, it is best if the case is not settled until the patient has completed treatment for fibromyalgia—meaning that there is no further treatment because the disease has plateaued. Or it may be settled once the physician can reasonably predict what will be the end stage of this condition.

It is important to remember the competing interests (settling the claim as quickly as possible against the possibility of losing the right to make a claim if you wait too long) to get as complete a picture as possible of the extent of your disease. Many times fibromyalgia is difficult to diagnose by doctors who aren't familiar with this condition. You may have to go to several doctors before you find one who recognizes the condition. So the sooner you see a doctor who understands fibromyalgia the better off you will be. Getting the medical information as concrete as possible will drive the resolution of the case.

Be aware that statistics show that over 90% of personal injury claims will be settled before trial begins. Do your part to help avoid the costly and time-consuming process of going to trial. Adequate evidence is the key determinant to a just result of your case.

Evidence You Need For A Successful Claim

You need to do your part in making a successful claim. That means you need to supply your attorney with medical records from a physician who understands fibromyalgia and is familiar with diagnosing it. Doctors need to know that what they write in their medical records about a patient will be used in negotiations with insurance companies and possibly used in court.

If a patient comes in soon after an accident and the doctor doing the examination believes the patient has fibromyalgia, the doctor will identify any abnormal findings as part of the medical record (*e.g.*, positive tender points). The identification of tender points is objective evidence of fibromyalgia. Ultimately, beyond having the medical records that reflect the findings, doctors may likely be required to provide a written narrative report. This report provides a medical opinion of not only what the condition is, but most importantly, that there is a cause-and-effect relationship between the condition and the accident, if one does exist.

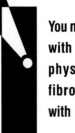

You need to supply your attorney with medical records from a physician who understands fibromyalgia and is familiar with diagnosing it.

Finally, it is very important that in the written opinion, the doctor provides a prognosis of the patient and the likely future course of the condition. If you are doing well with fibromyalgia, you may plateau, but if there is an injury, your fibromyalgia may escalate, and then reach another plateau. And then it may escalate again. The doctor has to be able to explain this in the report. The emphasis is to be armed with solid medical evidence early enough so that the case can be settled without resorting to the time-consuming and expensive process of litigation.

Objective Tests

In other parts of this book the kinds of objective tests doctors use to confirm a diagnosis of fibromyalgia are explained. We will just briefly touch on this point here because it is important to have a knowledgeable doctor who is familiar with fibromyalgia.

One of the main objective tests is examination for tender points. The legal importance of tender points is that a doctor can record and map them out on the human body and report these as being "objective findings." Subjective reports of pain and discomfort have very little weight when they come from an individual who is trying to recover money in a claims process. The claims process is set up to rely heavily upon objective findings.

Tender points in fibromyalgia are the main objective findings. A record of the results of this test needs to be made whenever a doctor does an examination and finds the tender points. Other tests done by specialists such as physiatrists or rheumatologists are helpful as well.

Your physician may not be the only one who will examine you if you are making a claim and initiating litigation. Once the case is going to be litigated, in most jurisdictions (but not all), the insurance company is entitled to have the claimant examined by a doctor of its choice. Defense attorneys refer to this as an independent medical examination, and they call these doctors defense experts.

In the independent medical examination, the doctor may see the patients for 20 minutes, provide no treatment, and write a report saying that there is no fibromyalgia and no injury related to the accident. The insurance companies' defense attorneys get to choose any doctors they want, and those doctors may know little or nothing about fibromyalgia. Or if they know something about it, they may not believe that trauma can induce or worsen fibromyalgia.

If you are applying for Social Security disability or if you are applying for Workers' Compensation benefits or any other type of disability payment related to fibromyalgia, you can anticipate being ordered to see a government-appointed physician for an examination.

Before undergoing such a medical examination you should talk with your attorney about what is the purpose and goal of such an examination. You should be prepared to make sure you explain your condition to the examining physician so that regardless of the neutrality of the examination, the report will at least have your statements. Once you have retained an attorney, you may be able to bring someone from the law office to the examination or you may be able to tape what is said during the examination so there is no mistake about what is said.

Time Limits On Your Claim

You should be aware that in all states the administrative process with the insurance company does not suspend or terminate the need to file a lawsuit against the wrongdoer. The lawsuit must be commenced before the statute of limitations (time within which a lawsuit must be filed) of your state has expired. You need to check with your attorney to find out what the statute of limitations period is in your state. For example, if the statute of limitations is two years you cannot file your suit after that period of time has elapsed from the date of your accident, with some specific exceptions. After the statute of limitations passes, you lose all rights to your claim and the matter is closed.

There are other administrative proceedings which you can be involved with—generally with governmental agencies. We've already talked about Workers' Compensation. There are other agencies such as the one dealing with unemployment benefits; in some states it is known as the Bureau of Employment Services. There are a variety of governmental agencies which may relate to some aspect of your case depending on your particular situation.

You should be aware that in all states the administrative process with the insurance company does not suspend or terminate the need to file a lawsuit against the wrongdoer.

Each agency has its own limitations period that require claims to be filed within a certain amount of time. Some of these administrative procedures can have deadlines less than one year duration so you have to be very careful in protecting your rights in filing an administrative claim at the state or federal level. The proceedings before any of these agencies usually does not extend the statute of limitations for filing a lawsuit in court.

The fact that litigation needs to be initiated where there's no basis for suspending the statute of limitations is very important. If you are involved in dealing with an insurance carrier and the insurance adjuster continues to exchange letters and requests information past the statute of limitations period, the insurance carrier is no longer responsible for paying the claim at all and your claim may be entirely lost because you failed to file a suit within the statutory period.

In the situation where the driver who caused the accident has no insurance, you may have to become involved in the administrative process in filing a claim against your own insurance company under the uninsured motorist coverage. Your policy must be read very carefully to determine whether or not there's a limitation period in that as well. The policy may require you to sue your own insurance company.

Many insurance policies do include arbitration clauses requiring that arbitration be pursued with the insurance company rather than going into litigation. Also, some insurance policies require that a lawsuit be filed in a period less than the time specified in the statute of limitations. There are a number of pitfalls that have to do with the period for filing your claim when you're dealing with the administrative process and also thinking of going into litigation. Again, your attorney can guide you through these issues.

Going To Court

Do you want to go through the difficult process of a trial? You should consult with your attorney about the probability of winning your claim. Also be aware that the possibility of settling continues even though you are going to court. This possibility runs parallel with the trial and is an option at any point before final resolution in the court. Usually a case takes anywhere from one to three years to be resolved.

As the medical profession becomes more enlightened about fibromyalgia, more courts will recognize it as the basis for a legitimate claim. In Ohio the courts and The Ohio Bureau of Workers' Compensation both recognize fibromyalgia.

Whether or not the court is going to rule that a particular person has fibromyalgia and whether or not the court will allow evidence to be presented on this subject and allow the jury to consider a claim on this basis depends upon the strength of the medical evidence that comes in. That is why it is of the utmost importance to have a physician who understands fibromyalgia and how fibromyalgia is related to trauma. There are few, if any, courts that would not permit an argument to be made and evidence presented that a patient is suffering from fibromyalgia.

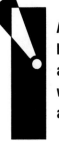

As the medical profession becomes more enlightened about fibromyalgia, more courts will recognize it as the basis for a legitimate claim.

A lawsuit is initiated by filing a complaint in the name of the plaintiff, who would be the victim suffering injury in an automobile or other kind of accident. In many states if the plaintiff is married and/or has children, he or she could include his or her spouse and children in the lawsuit. The legal theory for including the spouse and children is that because of the injury to the victim, the family members are also injured because the victim cannot interact with them in the same way as before the accident. Their loss is characterized as the loss of the victim's services to them.

The complaint must be filed with the clerk of the local court within the statute of limitations in order for it to be valid. After the suit is filed, the defendant has to be located and served a copy of the complaint. Once this is accomplished, litigation in most situations can take anywhere from one to three years.

In the litigation process, it can be expected that if someone has fibromyalgia or any other medical condition, the defendant's lawyers will request all medical records to determine whether or not the condition is fibromyalgia or a pre-existing condition or whether it was something that manifested itself immediately or shortly after the trauma of the accident. Be prepared to sign authorizations so you can have your medical providers deposed (or questioned before trial by the opposing counsel) about your medical records.

While the privacy of your medical records is protected by federal and most state laws, you impliedly waive most of your rights to medical privilege for the purpose of trial when you engage in litigation with the objective of recovering compensation for your fibromyalgia.

Discovery

Filing a suit starts the process which includes discovery. Discovery means that the attorney representing the insurance company attempts to find out anything he or she can find out about your medical condition. This includes all present and past medical records. Depending upon how aggressive the defendants are, they may try to discover all of your medical records. This is their right to attempt to obtain all of your medical records; however, they may not be entitled to all of your medical records.

Your attorney—the plaintiff's attorney—would resist each discovery request on an individual basis if what the defendants are looking for is too remote or not related at all to this particular case.

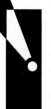

You have to work with your attorney to assess the potential for recovering for fibromyalgia in your case.

For example, if a female plaintiff had a hysterectomy at an earlier time and she is now claiming fibromyalgia primarily in the upper shoulders, then an argument should be made that the hysterectomy information should not be discoverable by the defendants since it is not related to the fibromyalgia claim. There would have to be a cause-and-effect connection or nexus between the medical records sought and the claim in order to allow the records to be discovered.

Litigation goes through the discovery phase, then through a preliminary hearing phase. The pre-trial conferences are held and ultimately the case is set for trial for the jury to hear all of the evidence. The pre-trial phase of litigation involves meeting with the judge and discussing issues which might arise during the trial. The most important aspect of these meetings is to try to settle the case so it doesn't have to go to trial. This is a very important part of the legal process since most cases are settled. You have to work with your attorney to assess the potential for recovering for fibromyalgia in your case.

Litigation requires that your doctor appear in court, either live or by videotape trial deposition. When the doctor actually appears in court, you will have to pay for the doctor's time, and this issue must be addressed by you and your attorneys.

The Trial

The trial itself consists of jury selection, which can take time if the attorneys question each of the jurors to determine how the jury will respond to the testimony and to determine their attitudes towards victims of fibromyalgia. Attorneys are entitled to a fixed number of challenges to jurors whom they think will be unlikely to respond favorably to their side of the case. Once the jury is selected, the trial can begin with an attorney from each side making an opening statement to the jury. This statement is designed to outline the position of each side for the jury to give them a way to place the testimony in the context of the entire case. After the opening statement, the plaintiff's attorney—your attorney—calls witnesses to the stand and asks them questions which are designed to establish the onset or worsening of fibromyalgia as the direct result of the accident. This usually consists of medical expert testimony or accident expert testimony. The defendant's attorney has the opportunity to cross-examine your witnesses to try to demonstrate the weaknesses in their testimony.

As the plaintiff, your attorney has the responsibility to establish your case for fibromyalgia by a preponderance of the evidence. This is referred to as having the burden of proof. After you have called your last witness, the judge is often requested by the defendant to make a ruling on whether you have provided enough evidence to meet your burden of proof. If you haven't, the case can end at that point and you receive no compensation.

The defense presents its case next. The attorney presents witnesses who provide testimony contrary to the testimony of your witnesses, and your attorney questions each of the defense witnesses to challenge their statements. At the conclusion of the defendant's case, each attorney is allowed to give a closing statement to the jury which sums up the testimony for each side.

The final step before the jury deliberates is important: this is when the judge explains to the jury the law which they are supposed to apply to the facts. Each attorney can submit jury instructions to the judge with the law stated the way each attorney recommends; however, the judge makes the final determination of how the law should be explained to the jury. Finally, the jury deliberates and makes its own decision. If you lose the case or are unhappy with the amount of recovery, you are entitled to file an appeal.

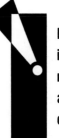

Making a successful personal injury claim for fibromyalgia requires you to be very formal and literal in your presentation of evidence.

Your Award Of Damages

If you win the case, you are awarded damages. Since there is usually an insurance company involved, this company usually pays the amount awarded by the jury, unless there is an appeal of the verdict. If there is a settlement instead of a jury verdict, the insurance company will pay the amount agreed upon by the attorneys.

Usually, a lump sum check is given. If it is a significant amount, there may be some benefit in having the insurance company provide you with what is called a structured settlement, which would essentially have the insurance carrier purchase an annuity. If that is going to be the case, what you want to do is to value the case at its full value and use the full value to be paid into the annuity.

In some instances when you win a case, the defense may appeal the verdict. If the verdict is very large, expect the defense to appeal the verdict. The higher the jury verdict, the more likely the insurance company will appeal the judgment. Appeals tend to delay ultimate recovery for another one to two years, depending on the individual case. If your award withstands appeal, you will receive your payment when all the appeals are exhausted. Sometimes, however, the appellate court will send the case back to the trial court for a second trial.

The judge can, in very rare cases, change the award that a jury gives. But the jury verdict carries a tremendous amount of weight and unless there is either misconduct or a gross misapplication of the evidence to the verdict, judges are generally not going to change the award.

Do not forget that throughout the course of litigation the possibility of settlement continues to exist and "runs parallel" with the court proceedings.

A Final Word

Making a successful personal injury claim for fibromyalgia requires you to be very formal and literal in your presentation of evidence. At your very first visit to the hospital or doctor after an accident, plan for the possibility of eventually going to trial. There is still the perception that fibromyalgia is a subjective condition with no objective criteria for its existence. You need to overcome this perception with well-presented solid evidence.

The material in this chapter is for informational purposes only and is not intended to substitute for the advice of an attorney. Every case is different, and you should contact an attorney experienced in these types of cases to do a thorough evaluation of your claim and to represent you.

ADDENDUM

Examples Of Verdicts Rendered In Personal Injury Cases Of PTF

1. In Dallas, Texas, a woman was stopped at a stop sign when another driver drove into the back of her car. The injured woman claimed a cervical strain and fibromyalgia. She asserted the driver who hit her was driving negligently by not keeping assured clear distance and not keeping a proper lookout. This woman was awarded $2,400 for fibromyalgia and two children who were her passengers also received awards.

2. In a similar case in northern Ohio, a woman began to suffer from fibromyalgia after she injured her back, shoulder, wrist, ankle and both knees when the car in which she was a passenger was hit in the back by another driver. The woman claimed that the driver did not: control his car; keep assured clear distance; or keep a proper lookout and that the driver was intoxicated and left the scene of the accident. The injured woman was awarded $5,000.

3. A woman was awarded $10,000 for her PTF and chronic fatigue syndrome after her car was hit in the back by a bus. In this accident the woman also suffered significant injuries to her arm and hand and bruised her collarbone, foot, and knees. She claimed that the other driver was negligent in failing to keep assured clear distance and did not keep a proper lookout.

4. In a 1999 Washington state case, a woman aggravated her fibromyalgia along with injuring her back as the result of a chain reaction rear-end collision. After claiming the other motorist was negligent, the woman received an award of $25,450.

5. A woman from the state of Washington started to suffer from fibromyalgia primarily in the cervical and lumbar spinal areas as the result of a collision at an intersection. She claimed the other driver drove through a red light after she entered the intersection, while the other driver asserted that woman failed to yield the right of way. The injured woman prevailed and was awarded $38,042.

6. A 51 year-old man slipped on a grape on the floor of a grocery store in Missouri and began suffering from fibromyalgia which disabled him. His problems arose from injuring the soft tissue around his cervical spine and developing a tumor in his right hip for which he needed hip replacement surgery. Failure to keep the store safe or to warn about the unsafe condition

was the basis for the injured man's claim, and the store responded by claiming that the man did not properly look at the condition of the floor. The injured man was awarded $75,000. The award was reduced by 25% because the injured man was himself negligent to some degree.

7. A man started to suffer general weakness and pain from fibromyalgia after he slipped on a ladder to a ferry boat while he was carrying a bag of sand as part of his job. He claimed his employer was negligent in allowing him to carry the sand bag in violation of state labor codes which require that an individual's hands must be free when climbing up or down a ladder. The injured man was awarded $2,370,000 in this 1996 Washington state case.

8. A woman was injured in a number of auto accidents and brought this case for the 2 most recent accidents from which fibromyalgia evolved. The appeals court in Canada affirmed a total award of $334,961, of which $175,000 was for potential loss of future earnings. The court said: " The injuries she sustained in the fourth and fifth accidents were superimposed on her weakened back. An award of damages should compensate her for the increased discomfort she has and will experience as a consequence of these accidents."

9. A cervical strain suffered in a broadside auto accident resulted in the development of fibromyalgia in an Ohio woman. In this accident which occurred in a parking lot, the woman claimed that the driver who hit her car was negligent, and the parties settled for $2,500 after the driver admitted liability.

If You Want To Know More

1. Pellegrino MJ. *From whiplash to fibromyalgia*. N. Canton OH: ORC Publishing, 2002.

2. Pellegrino MJ. *Understanding post-traumatic fibromyalgia: a medical perspective*. Columbus OH: Anadem Publishing, 1996.

Controversial? Says Who!?

As I've mentioned several times already, some doctors declare their beliefs that fibromyalgia doesn't exist and, most certainly, trauma could not possibly cause fibromyalgia, even if fibromyalgia did exist! Yet these same doctors are never heard to utter opinions that migraine headaches, depression, irritable bowel syndrome and other conditions do not exist. We know less about some of these conditions than we do about fibromyalgia, so why aren't these doctors voicing opinions about other less understood conditions? Why are they reluctant to believe in fibromyalgia?

Anti-Fibromyalgia Bias

Perhaps some physicians have a strong bias against acknowledging fibromyalgia. Physicians, like everyone else, base their opinions on their education, experiences, and biases. If a physician never learned about fibromyalgia during medical school, or was told by an instructor the condition did not exist, he or she may conclude, with conviction, there is no such thing as post-traumatic fibromyalgia (PTF). These doctors will point to the absence of absolute proof, the "hard evidence," to bolster their expert opinion.

As long as there are doctors willing to voice their opinions, there will be those who say fibromyalgia doesn't exist or trauma cannot cause fibromyalgia. I have never understood how a doctor who adamantly denies the existence of a condition, and therefore has never "seen" it or diagnosed it, feels qualified to say it doesn't exist. I would not ask a medical colleague for a knowledgeable opinion on a condition if I knew that person never made the diagnosis. I would assume that "no experience" with a particular condition means "no expertise" about the condition.

A Third Model For Chronic Pain

Some physicians have a misconception that chronic pain cannot exist unless a detectable tissue lesion is present and, if pain is reported, it must be solely psychological in nature. This belief is akin to saying the victim is responsible for the pain, rather than the whiplash trauma. Blaming patients for their symptoms is not what Hippocrates seemed to have in mind when he wrote about the care of patients nearly 2500 years ago.

Dr. Yunus has proposed the medical community embrace a third model to explain chronic pain that is different from the traditional dual model: structural/anatomic pathology versus psychological explanation. He proposes a neuroendocrine dysfunction/central sensitivity model as a third way to correctly explain a condition like fibromyalgia.

Fibromyalgia does not have structural changes in joints like degenerative arthritis. Nor does it have microscopic or usual lab changes of an anatomic pathological disease. Yet many abnormalities are found in fibromyalgia by specific biochemical and hormonal testing, EEG studies, or functional imaging of the brain. These dynamic and dysfunctional abnormalities do not fit neatly into either the anatomic model or the psychological model, but define a unique "new" model. I hope doctors will be open minded in accepting this new manner of thinking about fibromyalgia.

Trauma Bias

There exists a bias among many physicians that trauma implies liability, which means potential lawsuits. The mere implication of "trauma" being involved in a medical diagnosis pushes sensitive medico-legal buttons in many. The actual appearance of the word "trauma" in a diagnosis such as whiplash trauma or PTF may be too difficult for some to accept, so the diagnosis is avoided.

Unfortunately, these medico-legal perceptions can carryover into the actual practice of medicine. Many physicians choose not to get involved in the treatment of patients with work-related injuries or motor vehicle accident injuries. They may feel threatened or uncomfortable with treating someone who may have an attorney because of trauma issues. I don't think we should let our perceptions of the legal system ever influence how we practice medicine.

Our country has laws governing liability issues related to trauma, so sometimes patients find themselves involved in litigation matters. Patients have legal rights, and their attorneys, not their doctors, can advise them of these rights. We doctors should practice medicine on patients who seek our help, regardless of whether they've had an injury. The medical diagnosis of PTF is independent of any medico-legal activity the patient may be involved in.

Interestingly, an article published in the *New England Journal of Medicine* (2000) tried to imply that litigation interfered with recovery. In reality, only a very small percentage of patients with PTF are involved in litigation. Studies have shown the pain in PTF persists whether or not any financial settlement is awarded (Dr. Romano, Dr. Waylonis).

Research studies performed in environments that are "hostile" to the whiplash-injured patient, *e.g.*, countries with "no-fault" systems, no insurance benefits, or disapproval of medical treatments, must be interpreted with caution as the negative biases can cause the results to be misleading.

People with whiplash injuries and ongoing problems living in a "hostile" environment may choose not to seek treatment, may not be medically acknowledged if they seek help, or may be denied treatments by the insurance company. The "whiplash ship" is sailing the seas looking for a friendly harbor to dock, but none exists. Yet the harbor masters (insurance companies, governments) are proclaiming that the coast is clear, and no whiplash problem exists!

It is unfortunate that the insurance industry and other special interest groups seem eager to perpetuate a myth that most people are faking their injuries and that whiplash trauma is not serious enough to cause chronic pain. The medical condition of PTF needs to be managed by medical doctors, and not by governments or insurance companies. The doctor appreciates the actual human patient who has real medical problems. The true malingerer is rare, and only a small percentage of those with fibromyalgia are ever awarded disability benefits or financial settlements.

The vast majority of people with fibromyalgia are truthful and reliable. They are seeking help for their chronic pain and want to improve their quality of life. A few may ultimately be forced to seek financial relief options, such as applying for disability benefits because of the severity of their condition, which prevents them from sustaining employment.

Many people with PTF have not had any treatments despite the chronic pain and functional impairment. They are not seeking "secondary gains" or some type of reward for their pain such as therapies, money, or an excuse not to work. If you ask these people, they will tell you there is no "reward" to having a condition that causes severe pain for the rest of their lives.

Consensus View

Sometimes the well-ingrained perceptions among scientists and physicians hinder the ability to be open-minded and see ideas from a different perspective. This "consensus" view can be wrong because science is not determined by consensus. Galileo was judged to be wrong by his peers for his view that the earth rotated around the sun. The consensus opinion against Galileo resulted in his imprisonment. Today, we know he was right.

In 1983, two doctors, Dr. Barry Marshall and Dr. Robin Warren, said bacteria caused stomach ulcers and the ulcers should be treated with antibiotics. They were ridiculed by their gastroenterologist peers because the consensus at that time was that ulcers were caused by stress and poor diet and the treatment was acid-neutralizing drugs. Today, a bacteria called *Helicobacter pylori* is recognized as the major cause of stomach ulcers, and is treated with antibiotics.

Consensus is not science, and neither is the belief that something cannot exist unless absolute proof is available. Physicians who treat PTF could use the same rigorous absolute proof standard to support their conclusions as attempted by those who do not believe in PTF. Just as one doctor may say there is no absolute proof that says whiplash trauma causes fibromyalgia, another doctor can say there is no absolute proof that says whiplash trauma does NOT cause fibromyalgia.

We are allowed to accept the notion that trauma from whiplash injury causes severe injuries, and some injured patients get fibromyalgia because no other explanation accounts for the observations, experiences, and scientific studies we've accumulated to date. We are not abandoning scientific standards, rather we are accepting the evidence we have as the most reasonable explanation.

Ultimately we are trying to help the patients do as well as they can. Because at the end of each day, when the courtrooms are quiet, and when all the scientists, medical experts, and authorities have gone to bed, the patients still have pain and need our help.

I've learned from patients that they are most concerned about what's going to happen to them and what can they do to help their condition. Patients do not care about the attempts by disbelieving doctors to create "controversies" regarding whiplash related fibromyalgia. The patients already know their trauma was the cause of their fibromyalgia. They want their doctors to help them make the best recovery possible and restore as much ability as possible, not to tell them that some think their condition is "controversial."

Personal Snapshot—Ongoing Controversies

by Mark J. Pellegrino, M.D.

I have my opinions about the so-called "controversies" regarding fibromyalgia. Being the diplomat I am(!), I will summarize some of the current controversial points in a Point-Counterpoint fashion.

Point	Counterpoint
No obvious pathology in fibromyalgia	We know a lot about the pathophysiology and have objective tender point abnormalities
Therapy does not cure fibromyalgia	Treatments can heal fibromyalgia even if there is no cure
Treatments are costly	What is the price of improving the quality of life?
No proof that trauma causes fibromyalgia	Much evidence that trauma causes fibromyalgia. No proof that trauma DOESN'T cause fibromyalgia
Legal system too involved in fibromyalgia	This country has laws regarding trauma and liability
Labeling people with fibromyalgia has gotten out of control	Fibromyalgia is a legitimate, valid medical diagnosis
It is a syndrome, not a disease	It is a disease of pain perception
We should limit treatments of fibromyalgia	We should teach home programs and personal responsibility
A few people use most of the care	Some require more treatments to achieve a better outcome
Fibromyalgia is over diagnosed	Fibromyalgia is undertreated
There should be no disability awards for fibromyalgia	Each person's situation is unique and decisions regarding disability should be individualized
Illness magnified by medical model of care	Illness helped by chronic pain approaches

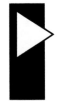

If You Want To Know More

1. Bernikow P. *Missing links*. FM Frontiers 2001; 9: 11–9.

2. Cassidy JD, Carroll LJ, Côté P, et al. *Effect of eliminating compensation for pain and suffering on the outcome of insurance claims for whiplash injury*. N Engl J Med 2000; 342: 1179–86.

3. Ewald PW. *Plague time. How stealth infections cause cancer, heart disease, and other deadly ailments*. Simon & Schuster, 2000.

4. Pellegrino MJ. *From whiplash to fibromyalgia*. N. Canton OH: ORC Publishing, 2002.

5. Romano TJ. *Clinical experiences with post-traumatic fibromyalgia syndrome*. WV Med J. 1990; 86: 198–202.

6. Waylonis GW, Perkins RH. *Post-traumatic fibromyalgia, a long term follow-up*. Am J Phys Med Rehabil 1994; 72: 403–12.

7. Wolfe F. *The fibromyalgia syndrome: a consensus report of fibromyalgia and disability*. J Rheumatol 1996; 23: 534–9.

8. Wolfe F. *For example is not evidence: fibromyalgia and the law*. J Rheumatol 2000; 27: 1115–6.

9. Yunus MB, Bennett RM, Romano TJ, et al. *Fibromyalgia consensus report: additional comments*. J Clin Rheumatol 1997; 3: 324–7.

SECTION VI—HANDLING FIBROMYALGIA'S UNIQUE SITUATIONS

You've already read about prescribed and self-directed strategies for managing fibromyalgia. In this section, I will focus on some unique situations we encounter with fibromyalgia, and hopefully you can pick up some tips on how to handle them. This section has new information combined with information you've already read; I've done this to reinforce what you've learned and to apply the information to specific, unique situations. Some of the chapters in this section may not apply to you, so you can browse past them if you wish (or skip them if you don't want to browse past!). You should not be offended when you get to Chapter 39, OK? Don't be making fun of the stick diagrams in Chapter 39. (I said "stick" not "sick.")

The Fibromyalgia Homemaker

An example of a personalized answering machine message of a fibromyalgia homemaker:

"I can't come to the phone right now. In fact, I can't move from the couch because I hurt all over. If I reach for the phone, it would hurt my arm, so I'm just lying here instead. My ears are fine, though, so feel free to talk away when you hear the beep."

Whoever invented fibromyalgia never had to vacuum! Homemaking chores can be a difficult challenge for someone with fibromyalgia. I always ask my patients if their fibromyalgia interferes with activities in the house and they almost always tell me "yes" (even the men!). The bending, reaching, lifting and pulling required of these tasks causes increased pain and often leads to painful flare-ups. The fibromyalgia homemaker is faced with the dilemma of wanting to have a clean home, but not having the physical abilities to complete these routine tasks without pain. What does the homemaker do?

Options To Consider:

1. **Stop doing housework altogether.** Yes, just go on strike! See if the work gets done by others. Watch as nothing gets done and your house becomes a health hazard! You can't stop everything, but daily or weekly tasks can be analyzed to determined if they can be done less frequently. Consider a rotating system where different parts of the house are cleaned on different days and not all at once. Instead of doing one heavy task in one day, spread it out into several mini-tasks over the course of a week. Your whole house may not be perfectly clean all the time, but parts of your house are perfect every day!

2. **Have someone else do it, with you supervising.** This is a good way to teach responsibility to your children (or your spouse, the biggest kid of all). The shared housework concept divides the responsibilities among the entire family, and you do the share of tasks that you can comfortably handle. The heavier tasks (vacuuming, carrying laundry loads) should be delegated to other family members. You supervise—and be sure to look busy at all times!

3. **Pay someone else to do it, if you can afford it.** Try to have the paid person come weekly or every other week to do the major cleaning, scrubbing and vacuuming. You can do the minor "touch-up" work in between visits. Bribe your kids to work cheap!

4. **Modify the way you are doing particular tasks.** This allows you to continue doing the homemaking, but do it in a way that is kinder to your muscles. Since homemaking chores are done with your body in unusual and awkward positions that aggravate your fibromyalgia, proper attention must be paid to fibronomics.

Four Rules of Fibronomics:

1. **Arms stay home.**

2. **Unload the back.**

3. **Support always welcome.**

4. **Be naturally shifty.**

Probably a combination of these options works best for each homemaker. New strategies can be learned and used successfully.

Below is list of usual homemaking tasks that individuals with fibromyalgia have difficulty performing:

- Running the vacuum cleaner
- Doing dishes
- Ironing
- Dusting
- Scrubbing
- Laundry
- Washing windows
- Getting objects in and out of high or low cupboards
- Lifting or moving heavy objects or furniture
- Prolonged writing
- Yard work of any type
- Dog walking

Sometimes unusual projects cause flare-ups. For example, one patient described how she spent several hours decorating cakes for her boy's basketball team and had severe pain in her shoulders and arms. Another woman had a flare-up in her back when she was lifting heavy bird seed bags into the trunk of her car. Both ordinary and unusual homemaking tasks and projects can cause flare-ups, so you must be constantly on guard to try to prevent them. Wear your mental seat belt and follow fibronomics.

The following pages are devoted to showing you some strategies and homemaking fibronomics to apply to usual tasks.

1. **Problem:** Vacuuming is Housework Enemy Number 1. It can aggravate pain in the back, shoulders and arms because your arms are reaching out to push and pull the heavy vacuum, and you are bending forward while pushing, which puts stress on the back.

Solutions:

a. Obtain a lightweight vacuum cleaner to minimize the load on the arms and back.

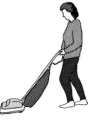

b. Hold the vacuum cleaner by holding arms down against the side and lightly holding the vacuum handle but not squeezing hard. The handle of the vacuum cleaner rests against the upper thigh and hip area. Walk forward with back maintaining a normal curvature to push the vacuum cleaner forward, and then backing up, squeeze the handle harder and pull the vacuum backwards with steady force. Repeat these steps to cover different areas of the carpet. Be sure that the arm does not reach out away from the body, but that the whole body moves forward along with the arms.

2. **Problem**: Standing at the sink washing dishes hurts your lower back because you have to lean forward.

   Solutions:

   a. Alternate leg on a stool or inside sink cupboard to unload the back and decrease the pain.

   b. Use disposable paper plates, paper cups, and paper cereal bowls. (Don't hurt your back throwing them away!)

   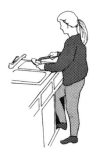

   c. Do a few dishes at a time, do something else, then do more dishes. The alternating method helps reduce prolonged back strain.

   d. If the sink is too short for your height, place a large plastic dishpan on the counter top and wash dishes in this.

   e. Use one of those sponges that have dish detergent in the handle. You can rinse and wash dishes easier.

   f. Cook and eat from same dish. Use a microwave bowl to cook and then eat out of it. If you're eating alone, just eat out of the pan.

   g. If cooking for your family, serve from the stove so you don't have extra serving dishes and spoons to wash.

   h. If using a dishwasher, have family members load their own dishes, and assign the job of unloading clean dishes to children or spouse.

3. **Problem:** Ironing. Bending forward increases back strain and repetitive arm reaching hurts.

   Solutions:

   a. Alternate leg on a foot stool to unload the back.

   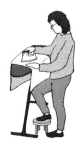

   b. Avoid overextending the arm; keep the elbow bent and the iron as close to the body as possible.

   c. Use a drive-through dry cleaning service.

   d. Buy fabrics that don't need ironing.

   e. Wash clothes at home; hang dry so you don't have to use dryer. Take them to the cleaners for pressing.

4. **Problem:** Dusting. The major problems with dusting are reaching for the tops of shelves and bending to reach difficult low areas of furniture.

   Solutions:

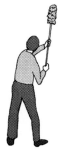

   a. Use a longer handled dust mop to allow the equipment, not your arm, to reach the spots.

   b. Use a hair dryer to blow dust off.

   c. Store all knickknacks in glass-enclosed shelving.

5. **Problem:** Scrubbing. Scrubbing the floor, furniture or countertops is an invitation to a flare-up. You bend and reach and you hurt!

   Solutions:

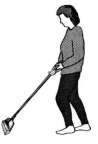

   a. Use a long-handled mop when scrubbing the floor. Take advantage of any cleaning solvent that will perform the chemical scrubbing for you, so all you have to do is wipe up.

   b. Use an electrical device that does the scrubbing for you.

   c. Hire someone to clean your floors yearly.

6. **Problem:** Doing laundry. There are various components to laundry that cause problems, including gathering up dirty clothes, carrying them up and down stairs, and loading and unloading the washer and dryer.

   Solutions:

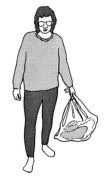

   a. Use dry cleaning services whenever possible, especially the drive-through or pick-up and delivery service.

   b. Instead of using the laundry basket to carry clothes up and down steps, place the clothes in a mesh laundry bag and throw them down the steps. Drag them up the steps behind you.

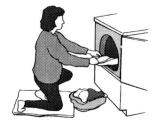

   c. Dryers that have front openings are preferred. You can get closer to the opening to pull out the clothes, making it easier on your low back and arms.

   d. Do one or two loads at a time; wash enough clothes for two or three days, instead of a week.

   e. Use an assistance device (a reacher/grabber device) to reach into the washer or dryer and avoid bending over.

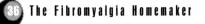

7. **Problem:** Washing windows. Another enemy of housekeepers and almost everybody else! Reaching, straining the back, wiping; it hurts me to write this, and I don't do windows!

   Solutions:

   a. Use a long-handled window cleaner with a squeegee to clean the outside windows so you can observe proper fibronomics.

   b. Don't try to do all your windows in one day; wash only one window every other day.

   c. Hire window cleaners once a year.

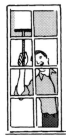

8. **Problem:** Getting objects in and out of high cupboards. The reaching and lifting can hurt your shoulders and back.

   Solutions:

   a. Use footstools or kitchen step ladders so you can practice fibronomics when getting objects out of cupboards.

   b. Store your everyday pots and pans in the most accessible cupboards; the rarely used and heavy cooking items can go in the higher cupboards or less accessible locations.

   c. Store all cooking utensils in a basket on your kitchen counter so they are always accessible.

   d. Use a reaching device.

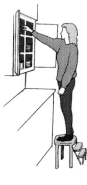

9. **Problem:** Lifting or moving heavy objects or furniture. Every once in a while, we decide it's easier to move something ourselves and we usually will pay the price.

   Solutions:

   a. Do not buy heavy objects unless they can be placed in a permanent resting spot, and I do mean permanent, forever, always, OK?

   b. Do NOT lift heavy objects; leave them where they are as long as they are not bothering anything.

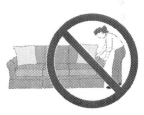

10. **Problem:** Prolonged writing. This might include bill paying or writing letters. Also, frequent typing on computer keyboards can increase neck and shoulder pains.

   Solutions:

   a. Instead of paying bills all at one time, designate two nights a week for the task.

   b. Use marker pens or pens with a medium point to minimize the amount of pressing required.

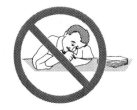

c. Reduce the total number of checks to be written by consolidating loans or using automatic deductions. Some banks offer online bill paying services that might save you time and effort.

d. Write or type a "master" letter and photocopies for your different friends, adding personal tidbits to the individual's copy.

11. **Problem:** Yard work. This can be especially challenging since many patients with fibromyalgia love being outdoors and working on the flowers, garden, or lawn. Rather than giving this up completely, I encourage patients to find ways to enjoy some aspects of yard work without doing work that is too strenuous or painful.

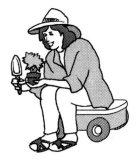

Solutions:

a. Buy a garden seat and cart to allow sitting and other proper fibronomic techniques.

b. Don't be a yard warrior. Break up large tasks into a series of smaller tasks and spread them over a longer period of time. Cut the front grass one night, the back the next, and do the trimming on a third night instead of doing it all in one day.

c. Hire a lawn service for heavy duty tasks, like spring clean-up, edging, or mulching. You do what you enjoy.

12. **Problem:** Walking the dog and the dog jerks on the leash, causing your arms, shoulders and back to hurt. Walking the dog is exercise for both you and the dog, however.

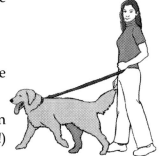

Solutions:

a. Use an extendable leash which will significantly reduce the torque and force on your arm.

b. Obedience school for your dog (heck, you are in "Fibromyalgia Obedience School" if you're reading this book!)

c. Train your dog to use a treadmill! I have a patient who actually did this. Now the dog gets a lot of exercise but not my patient!

Grocery Shopping With Fibromyalgia

Grocery shopping can be a dreaded activity with fibromyalgia. The fibromyalgia homemaker should prepare some shopping strategies. One of the first steps is to choose a time to arrive at the store when no one else wants to shop. It is that simple! During early morning or late evening, most stores are not crowded. Determine the peak shopping hours at your favorite stores and avoid those times. Those times are usually during the lunch hour, after school and work, and Saturday. It is easier to pick a small store that does not have miles of parking lots to cross just to get to the front door. Thus, the

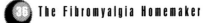

super store is usually out. Even if they have a better selection and price, what good is that if you are exhausted even before you get into the store!

Remember where you park your car. Park in the same section all the time if you can.

A shopping list is a must. To make your shopping fast and easy, prepare a master list of all of the products that you will use and purchase. Then, in your mind, go through the store and write down the items in the order that the aisles are arranged in the store. You've made your grocery map from your master list. Check this "master map" before you leave home, and when you arrive at the store you will be organized and can shop fairly quickly with a minimal amount of walking. Conserving your energy is important so you can get those newly purchased groceries into your car!

So you park close, get to the store quickly, avoid any long lines, and keep a list. What other strategies can be helpful to get your groceries into your home? Consider these tips:

1. When you enter the grocery store, look for those small plastic baskets you can carry, and put one in the bottom of the shopping cart basket. Thus you only have to bend and lift one time at the checkout to place the items on the counter, and your grocery cart is easier to unload.

2. Buy smaller amounts of groceries. Beware of quantity. It is better to make two or three trips a week than to buy jumbo sizes of laundry detergents, cereal boxes, and milk containers that are too heavy to handle on a daily basis.

3. Ask for help to get your groceries into the car. The bagger can pack them lightly and in paper bags so they are easier to handle.

4. Keep small laundry baskets in the trunk of your car. These baskets can keep grocery bags upright and prevent them from sliding to the back of the trunk where it is hard to reach. Keep a reacher/grabber (an assisting device) in the trunk to get items you can't reach.

5. Once you arrive home, take the bags containing items that need refrigeration inside; you can unpack the rest at a later time. Or bring the bags into the house and put them away later. Or have a family member or friend carry the bags into the house. You might even pay someone to go out and get your groceries in the first place!

Conquering Cooking

Getting groceries is a challenge, but cooking is a true adventure. The fibromyalgia homemaker may have chosen to not work outside the home, but still have difficulty finding time, energy, or physical stamina to prepare meals. You can cook and not feel guilty in spite of your fibromyalgia.

Prepare meals that can be done quickly and do not require extensive physical labor. Choose recipes that you can rely on when you are tired and operating on very low energy reserves, and prepare meals with ingredients that you have on hand. Avoid meals that require standing for long periods of time to cut vegetables or standing with arms extended over a kitchen counter.

You can keep it simple. Adding items to the meal directly increases the time needed for preparation, serving, and cleaning up. Try to use foods that are already prepared such as salads in a bag, cole slaw, macaroni, and bean salad. Use paper plates, napkins, salad bowls or whatever you can throw away.

Choose meals that can be prepared the night before. Salads, desserts, and vegetables can be prepared early and refrigerated overnight. Make sure you have all of the ingredients as nothing is more frustrating than making a mad dash to the store when you are trying to prepare a meal.

Any job can be made easier if it can be broken down into smaller tasks. Divide and conquer is a good plan. If you've picked a meal that is "fibro-friendly," gathered the necessary ingredients, prepared some items the night before, all you need to do is divide and delegate the work. If you are preparing the meal for yourself, you can take it one step at a time and rest in between. Prepare your salad, sit, eat, take a short rest, and then progress to the next item. Clean-up can always be done the next day. If you are preparing for others, divide the task so that each person has a job. Remember, clean-up tasks are to be delegated as well.

Make sure your body is in the best possible position while you are in the kitchen to help avoid increased pain.

Examples Of Fibronomic Applications In The Kitchen:

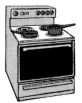

1. Use disposables to save time. Paper towels, paper plates, paper napkins, paper cups, etc.

2. Use reacher/grabbers and long-handled items.

3. Avoid hanging things over the stove or places where you have to lean or reach.

4. Use the front burners on the stove; less reaching is involved.

5. Store items in mid-range; avoid using the top or bottom shelves. If you must use high shelving, use a step-ladder. Use a plastic basket on each shelf so you can pull it out and search through it.

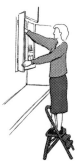

6. Store items in the same place every day (remember, we have fibrofog).

7. Wash dishes a few at a time. Use a sponge with soap in the handle. Place a container on top of the sink and wash.

8. Sit down to clean up spills on the floor. Or use the Ann Evans Bath Towel Method (A.B.T.) to clean up spills. Stand on a towel and use the foot to wipe up the spill!

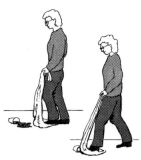

9. Buy a refrigerator with the freezer on the bottom. The fridge will be at a more comfortable height, and the lesser-used freezer will be out of the way. Don't forget to put a magnetic notepad (your Fibrominder!) on the refrigerator.

Get The Kids Involved

Your kids make great helpers in the house (cheap too … usually!). Don't forget to get them involved. Older kids can take out the trash or run errands for you (if they drive). Meal preparation responsibilities can be divided up. Younger children can help set the table and assist mom and dad in other chores.

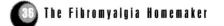

Delegate responsibilities and try to make it "fun." If you find out how to get your kids to work for fun, please write me and tell me what you are doing!

Before doing any type of housework, both physical and mental preparations are necessary. Pretend that you are about to perform an event in the Homemaker Olympics and you are representing your fibromyalgia. In order to make the best representation, you should make certain that adequate time is allowed for warm-up exercises that include stretching and flexibility. Emphasis is placed on the muscles that are going to be used most, and stretching should be done just prior to the event. Mentally visualize how you will perform from start to finish, seeing yourself cross the finish line free from flare-up. Psyche yourself up and tell yourself that you will do the best you can and that you anticipate no surprises.

Hopefully, you will be successful in all your homemaking events and win a lot of gold medals. Who knows, you may even be inducted into the Fibromyalgia Homemaker's Hall of Fame where each recipient is honored with a bronze dust pan!

If You Want To Know More

1. Pellegrino MJ. *Inside fibromyalgia*. Columbus OH: Anadem Publishing, 2001.

2. Pellegrino MJ, Evans AM. *The fibromyalgia chef*. Columbus OH: Anadem Publishing, 1997.

The Fibromyalgia Worker

Many of my patients are faced with a major dilemma: their fibromyalgia interferes with their jobs. The fibromyalgia person who is the sole breadwinner of the family can be in an extremely stressful financial situation if the job cannot be performed properly. Post-traumatic fibromyalgia (PTF) due to work injuries is being seen more frequently. There may be a single trauma such as a back strain from lifting, or it may be a cumulative trauma that appears over time from continuous performance of specific job activities. Acute injuries and repetitive trauma can worsen pre-existing fibromyalgia. Whether the fibromyalgia was actually caused by work injuries, or whether the work is aggravating the pre-existing fibromyalgia, the worker has to make changes in the way he or she approaches work to minimize pain and functional impairment.

Job Considerations

Individuals with fibromyalgia must consider various factors when looking for a job, or when trying to modify an existing job. First, one must develop a realistic outlook for the type of job that he or she would qualify for from a physical standpoint. Since individuals with fibromyalgia have a difficult time performing activities that require reaching, overhead use of the arms, bending and heavy lifting, certain high risk jobs would not be considered realistic. Even jobs that involve little or no lifting may not be tolerated if a lot of reaching or repetition is involved.

Examples of high risk jobs involving a lot of reaching and overhead use of the arms include assembly line jobs, dry-walling, hair styling, secretarial, computer programming, transcription, carpentry, and bricklaying. These types of jobs are more demanding on the neck, shoulders and upper back. I have seen a number of women hair stylists and school bus drivers who gradually developed fibromyalgia over the years. Some of them had to give up their jobs because of the pain. Examples of jobs that require a lot of bending and heavy lifting include construction work, welding, truck driving, and being a mover. These jobs are more demanding on the low back. You need to know the risk factors and risky jobs and try to avoid them as much as possible when looking for a job.

Job hunting is difficult enough, even without fibromyalgia. *Know your strengths and weaknesses, and know that, in spite of fibromyalgia, you can be a reliable, dependable, efficient and intelligent worker who would be an asset to any company.* Research the companies and fields that particularly interest you and take advantage of any professional guidance that might be available through various schools, career centers, and reference books. Let your natural ability to be organized, concise and "perfect" help you in developing a professional resume and plan.

Explore the type of hours available at any prospective job. Part-time, flexible hours might suit you best compared to a full-time job. Swing shifts and strictly night jobs are more difficult due to the disruption they cause to the already impaired sleep pattern. Even persons who work permanent night shifts never develop the quality of sleep of persons who work the day shift, so keep this in mind and seek stable daytime hours if you can.

Health insurance is certainly an important issue. Persons with fibromyalgia require periodic medical attention ranging from seeing the doctor, taking medication, participating in therapies, to taking time off work altogether. A job that provides adequate health insurance and acceptable sick time is certainly a plus.

Checklist To Think About When Considering A New Job:

HOURS:
- ❏ What type of shift?
- ❏ How many hours over 40?
- ❏ Flexible schedule?
- ❏ Commute time?
- ❏ Part time vs. full time?
- ❏ Can you make up missed time on weekend?

BUILDING:
- ❏ Can you park close?
- ❏ Stairs, elevator?
- ❏ Climate, cold, damp, basement?
- ❏ Furniture, ergonomic?

PHYSICAL:
- ❏ Standing too much?
- ❏ Sitting too much?
- ❏ Can you pace your work?

WORK LOAD:
- ❏ Can you rotate tasks?
- ❏ Are deadlines critical?
- ❏ Are others depending on your work before they can finish theirs?
- ❏ How much pressure?
- ❏ How much politics?
- ❏ Work quotas?

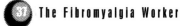

WORK ENVIRONMENT:

- ❏ Lighting?
- ❏ Heating?
- ❏ Cooling?
- ❏ Drafts?
- ❏ Quiet?
- ❏ Disruptions?
- ❏ Phones?

INSURANCE:

- ❏ Is it adequate?
- ❏ Long term paid medical leave?
- ❏ Pharmacy plan?

Should You Reveal Fibromyalgia?

A frequently asked question is whether an individual should reveal his or her fibromyalgia to a potential employer. I always advise my patients not to volunteer any information regarding their health, specifically as it relates to fibromyalgia, because chances are a potential employer will not know what the condition is and will consider it something negative. The Americans with Disabilities Act, otherwise known as ADA, protects people who have disabilities from job discrimination. A potential employer is not supposed to ask about any medical condition, either on the application or during the interview, according to the ADA. However, the employer can perform medical testing on a newly hired employee to make sure the employee is medically able to perform the job.

I understand that both the potential employer and potential employee have specific interests and concerns. The employer does not want to hire someone who may have a pre-existing medical condition which will worsen once the individual begins a new job, thus costing the employer. From this standpoint, any medical information about the employee might be harmful to him or her, particularly if the employer were to assume that fibromyalgia, because it causes pain, would mean that the employee would not be able to perform a particular job. Of course, the potential employee wants to be honest and not hide anything, but why should you volunteer information that could cost you a job? I feel the potential employee should receive the benefit of the doubt.

By law, this question should never come up before a job is offered, but if it does, you need to answer in the manner in which you are most comfortable. If you choose to reveal your fibromyalgia, it should be done in a manner that focuses on your abilities, not your inabilities. I would try to convince the employer that you have a good understanding of your condition and know your limitations. Point out that you are capable of handling the job, and that you consider yourself a responsible, reliable and efficient individual who would be an asset to the company. An honest and confident approach is probably your best long-term strategy, even though this approach could still scare away some potential employers. But don't offer anything about your fibromyalgia unless you have to. If you are hired, you may be asked to undergo a medical evaluation to assure you are medically fit for a particular job.

Once an individual finds a job, what can be done to prevent fibromyalgia from developing or flaring up? Preventive measures focus on stopping the problem from ever developing in the first place, or in the case of the fibromyalgia worker, preventing flare-ups from occurring. Maintain a regular stretching and exercise program to reduce the chance of injury. A worker should approach his or her job in the same way a trained athlete approaches a sporting event. Prior to attempting any sport, the athlete will perform warm-up exercises, especially those that include stretching. The fibromyalgia worker must also perform warm-up stretching exercises prior to performing the daily event. The stretching exercises will improve flexibility and circulation, decrease the tendon tightness, and decrease the chance of stretch and tear injuries.

Pay attention to increased pain and early symptoms of a flare-up. The company doctor or nurse should be notified. Contact your personal physician, if available. Over-the-counter pain medications, modalities (heat, ice or muscle creams) and work restrictions can be part of the initial treatment. If the flare-up worsens or a new problem develops in spite of what you do, further medical evaluation by your own physician will be necessary. The earlier a flare-up or injury is treated, the better the chance of resolving the problem.

Ongoing training and education involves periodically analyzing your work site and recognizing and correcting any ergonomic or fibronomic hazards. Work positions, power tools, ergonomic chair, telephone headset, or other adaptive equipment may be helpful. Working with your company's safety committee to review any injury trends or identify any patterns that can be further analyzed and remedied, if possible, is part of the ongoing follow-up needs.

Reasonable Accommodations

The employee, the employer and the doctor can work together to create a safe, pain-free workplace. The Americans with Disabilities Act requires employers to provide equal employment opportunities for people who are able to do the job, but who are limited by physical disabilities. The employee has a right to reasonable accommodations provided by the employer to help overcome any physical limitations.

Examples of reasonable accommodations for fibromyalgia workers (and all workers) in an assembly line setting might include:

1. Rotating jobs to minimize the chance of flare-ups rather than performing a single job all the time

2. Rearranging work stations and providing ergonomic tools to optimize proper body mechanics and use of the rules of fibronomics

3. Providing rubber mats where prolonged standing is required

4. Allowing frequent breaks during the work day

5. Allowing scheduled time for stretching exercises

6. Forming an education and prevention committee

Examples of reasonable accommodations for a clerical worker might include an ergonomic chair, a phone headset, a couch in the break room to lie down, and allowing frequent stretch breaks at the workstation.

In general, patients of mine who work in small business or professional offices report that their employers are very understanding and cooperative. From patients who work in larger corporations, I frequently hear that an employer is not as receptive and responsive to some of the individual issues. Know what your legal rights are under ADA and work with your union representative or legal advisor if necessary.

The fibromyalgia worker's personal physician has an important role in helping the worker preserve gainful employment. Flare-ups of fibromyalgia occurring at work need to be evaluated by the physician and treated aggressively. Most of the time, a flare-up is related to a temporary situation that can be successfully treated. The person can resume a normal baseline and return to regular job duties.

Part of the treatment approach of a fibromyalgia worker who is experiencing a flare-up is the need to consider work restrictions. These can range anywhere from complete time off work to limiting certain activities.

The Family Medical Leave Act (FMLA) was passed to allow workers to take time off work when they (or family members) are incapacitated and require medical treatment for a serious health condition. An employee who takes an FMLA leave is assured that his or her job will remain available once the medical condition has disappeared or stabilized. A health care provider must certify a FMLA leave. I complete FMLA forms for my patients when necessary.

On the FMLA form, fibromyalgia is defined as a serious health condition under Category 4: Chronic Conditions Requiring Treatment. This chronic condition requires periodic visits for treatment, continues over an extended period of time and may cause episodic incapacity (flare-ups that make the person unable to work). I describe the medical facts supporting the diagnosis of fibromyalgia and the need for FMLA certification and would indicate if the condition is incapacitating or can cause intermittent inability to work a full schedule. I usually state that fibromyalgia is a condition that may unpredictably flare-up from time to time resulting in impairment of work ability and may require a time off work on a temporary basis. I describe the health services needed, such as medications, therapies, or injections, and explain the justifications for a leave from work. A leave from work may be brief—one or two days—or may require a few months. The patients and I work together to keep time off work to a minimum and prioritize returning to work and staying there as much as possible.

If the patient is able to continue working, work restrictions may be necessary. Examples of work restrictions specific to a patient with fibromyalgia include:

1. Not working more than eight hours a day, five days a week; specifically, no overtime or weekends

2. Working part-time hours, working day hours only, or working flexible hours

3. Avoiding temperature changes (no exposure to cold or damp weather)

4. No direct air-conditioning drafts

5. No repetitive reaching or overhead use of the arms

6. No repetitive bending or leaning forward

7. No sitting, standing, or walking for a long period of time without altering positions

In addition to work restrictions, a prescription for specific adaptive devices may be necessary. This could include:

1. Phones with headsets to minimize the reaching and bending required to manually hold the phone

2. An ergonomic chair

3. A modified typing station that includes a drop keyboard, wrist bars, and arm rests

4. A back brace to be worn at work only

Many times I will place absolute restrictions on patients in terms of weight lifting (no lifting more than 20 pounds frequently and 50 pounds occasionally). If a person is experiencing a flare-up, I may temporarily place more restrictions depending on the individual situation. If the flare-up resolves and the person returns to baseline state, the restrictions can be removed. I prescribe rest often as part of a treatment program. If repeated flare-ups are occurring within a certain job description, it may be necessary to place permanent restrictions on the worker.

Up Close Patient Snapshot

by Mark J. Pellegrino, M.D.

Denise (age 43) is a patient of mine who has fibromyalgia. Her occupation is a Fitness Instructor and Coordinator at a local health club. One would never guess that "exercising" regularly as part of the job could aggravate fibromyalgia over time, but that's what's happening with Denise. In the past several years she has been having more neck and back pain despite remaining very active and following a superb stretching program.

We checked X-rays on her neck and back and found a lot of cervical and lumbar arthritis, more than expected for her age. This arthritis and worsening of her fibromyalgia are both causing her increased pain and increased difficulty performing her daily job duties.

Her job requires her to teach three aerobic classes a day (1 hour each), do a kid's stretching program (30 minutes), teach 1 senior citizen's arthritis aquatic class (1 hour) and do administrative work the rest of the time. She had been doing this job for over fifteen years, and until about five years ago, she has taught as many as 5 aerobic classes a day. As a teenager, Denise was active in gymnastics and dancing.

We discussed accumulative and repetitive trauma as the major mechanisms of her increased pain and arthritis changes. The gymnastics and dancing probably "started" the initial low grade trauma, and over the years the repetitive and sustained occupation trauma from her aerobic teaching (increased gravity on the spine, increased tendon and muscle forces) aggravated and worsened the pain to the point where work changes needed to be made.

For Denise we decided on a program of medicines, supplements, and physical therapy to try to reduce the pain to a lower, more stable baseline. We also tried to "lighten" her workload. She gave up her more intensive aerobic classes, took on another stretching class and one more aquatics class, as well as doing more personal training with members one-on-one. By reducing the weightbearing and repetitive forces (no aerobic, substituting "no gravity" aquatics), Denise was able to successfully modify her job to decrease the aggravating risks. She was fortunate that her job was flexible enough (no pun intended!) to allow her to make these changes and remain productive and employed with less pain. Plus, it didn't hurt that she's in charge of the Fitness Programs!

continued on next page...

Quite often a person can be off work, obtain therapy and treatment, and feel pretty good. But if no attempt is made to alter the job situation, it is not surprising that when returning to work, another flare-up occurs. The flare-up may occur within days or may take months. Long-term strategies are vital in helping a fibromyalgia worker sustain gainful employment.

Most patients will indicate that their pain level is less when they are not working. When a person returns to work, the pain baseline creeps up. Hopefully, it stabilizes at a level that enables one to continue working at a comfortable baseline.

I frequently write letters to patients' employers on their behalf to explain what fibromyalgia is and how it causes muscle pain and interferes with certain activities. I will indicate restrictions, but at the same time focus on what the person is able to do. Employers who are receptive to open communication between patient, doctor, and employer usually make every effort to facilitate effective strategies at the work site.

The fibromyalgia worker is responsible for continuing his or her regular home program even though he or she may be working full time. If this home program is not maintained, the work pain baseline will probably creep up even higher and be very easily triggered into a flare-up or recurrent flare-up.

If various treatments such as modifying the physical stresses at work, rearranging the workstation, placing work restrictions, prescribing rest, or completing a physical therapy or occupational therapy program do not help the fibromyalgia worker maintain a regular job, a different job altogether needs to be considered. Vocational counselors can help persons find different jobs that allow for medical restrictions, retrain for new skills, or pursue educational programs for entirely new careers. There are vocational bureaus at the state level that offer qualified vocational counselors.

Disability

It is my experience that the majority of fibromyalgia workers are motivated and determined to maintain their jobs, but issues of disability may need to be pursued. I think that total disability should be rare in fibromyalgia, and despite all the problems, there should be something that the individual should be able to do. However, the economy is not always receptive to a worker with various restrictions due to a medical condition, and all factors have to be considered when determining whether total, partial or no disability applies to a person with fibromyalgia. The patient and doctor need to work together to reach these difficult decisions.

I believe in maximizing one's abilities despite his or her medical condition. In an ideal situation, there will always be some type of job an individual with fibromyalgia could perform despite the pain. Individuals with pain who are gainfully employed will think less about pain. I recognize a big difference between the ideal situation and the real world, and I certainly work with each individual's situation to try for the best possible quality of life.

I'm often asked how I can continue a hectic full time schedule with my fibromyalgia. I remind them that everyone's fibromyalgia is different. My job is a sedentary one. I'm supposed to be using my brain mainly. I am able to shift my body positions to avoid strains. I can control my hours to allow rest times. Sure, I get flare-ups like everyone else, and I deal with them when they happen. I hope I can continue to work for a long time. I always think ahead, but I take one day at a time.

Disability Paradox

I frequently see patients who have "dual" objectives. On one hand, these patients indicate they want to improve their fibromyalgia condition, but on the other hand, they are also seeking disability. These objectives are actually conflicting, hence my term: disability paradox.

To improve one's condition is to focus on ability, or what can be done to help a person become more functional. The Latin word "habile" in rehabilitation means "to make able again." It is difficult to improve one's abilities if disability issues are requiring the lack of abilities to be spotlighted.

To become "disabled," one must convince the disability organization of an inability to perform certain functions required to maintain any type of employment and that these impairments are expected to persist over time and not improve. The very nature of the disability process requires patients to "prove" they are not able to function, which is in direct conflict with rehabilitation treatment philosophy. Hence, a disability paradox exists when someone is seeking both treatment and disability.

Treatment may help a patient feel better, but a disability award provides income. Which do you think takes priority? Whether the patient seeking disability is consciously aware of it or not, the overriding priority is to "win" a disability award and not risk "losing" one by feeling better with treatment.

Based on my experiences with the disability paradox, I find it very difficult for patients to report to me ANY improvement with any treatments as long as the disability status is pending. No matter what I prescribe or try, practically everyone who is pursuing disability will indicate that the treatment didn't help or made very little difference. I don't think it is cost-effective anymore to try new treatments on these patients, so I now recommend that any new fibromyalgia treatment be deferred until AFTER a disability decision is made.

Long-term follow-up studies on patients with fibromyalgia who have been rendered disabled or awarded a legal settlement have shown that the majority of them continued to be bothered by fibromyalgia and then seek medical treatment for this condition. In surveys, people with fibromyalgia rank their condition as more disabling than individuals with rheumatoid arthritis, heart disease, lung disease, and other chronic disorders. There is no question that the debilitating effect of fibromyalgia persists even if the jobs are stopped, stresses are relieved, life-styles are altered, or disability is awarded. The next chapter will address disability issues with fibromyalgia.

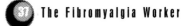

Hazardous Occupations With Fibromyalgia

I have created a list of hazardous occupations for someone with fibromyalgia. The hazard is designed to have a double meaning to indicate unique problems we have with fibromyalgia. They are supposed to be cleverly humorous, so if you don't laugh, they're probably too clever!

OCCUPATION	HAZARD
Railroad Conductor	Lose "train" of thought
Fireworks Distributor	Spontaneous flare-up
Ship Captain	Continuous fog
Plumber	Troublesome leaks
Shirt Starcher (day shift)	Excessive morning stiffness
Window Installer	Too many "panes"
Dog Trainer	May not "heel"
Proctologist	No "end" in sight

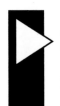

If You Want To Know More

1. Pellegrino MJ. *Inside fibromyalgia*. Columbus: OH: Anadem Publishing, 2001.

2. Romano TJ. *Clinical experiences with post-traumatic fibromyalgia syndrome.* WV Med J 1990; 86: 192–202.

3. Waylonis GW, Perkins RH. *Post-traumatic fibromyalgia, a long term follow-up.* Am J Phys Med 1994; 72: 403–12.

Disability Claims For Fibromyalgia

Disability issues may arise with some individuals with debilitating fibromyalgia. My experience is that fewer than 5% of fibromyalgia patients receive a permanent disability award. Patients do not want to become disabled from fibromyalgia or any condition. They all want to be better. If everything has been tried and the patient is still doing poorly and not functioning well, the disability route may need to be considered.

The ultimate decision regarding disability rests with "organizations" which review the applications and determine if the disability criteria are being met. Sometimes it seems as if the disability criteria are as complicated as fibromyalgia itself! My patients frequently ask me questions regarding the disability process and if an attorney is necessary. I am not an attorney, so I am not knowledgeable on specific legal issues regarding disability. I can provide medical advice and information if fibromyalgia is severe, chronic or functionally limiting for a given patient of mine, but sometimes an attorney who specializes in disability may be helpful when pursuing disability.

This chapter was written by two attorneys who are very knowledgeable in disability and fibromyalgia: Paul Kimsey, Esq., and Edward A. Doskey, Esq. I appreciate their helpful information and I hope you find this chapter helps answer any questions you have regarding disability claims.

What You Can Do If Fibromyalgia Prevents You From Working

By Paul Kimsey, Esq. and Edward Doskey, Esq.

Personal Snapshot

Paul Kimsey, Esq., is managing partner of Kimsey Law Group in Tampa, Florida. The firm's practice areas include personal injury, employment law, workers' compensation and insurance law. Mr. Kimsey focuses his practice on disability insurance claims, including ERISA cases. He is a member of the Academy of Florida Trial Lawyers, the Florida Bar Association and American Bar Association. Mr. Kimsey serves on the board of the Tampa Bay Trial Lawyers Association and on the Ethics Committee.

Edward Doskey, Esq., is the Director of the firm's Disability Insurance Litigation Division. He is a graduate of the Boston College School of Law and a member of the Academy of Florida Trial Lawyers Association and Tampa Bay Trial Lawyers Association. Mr. Doskey is also a member of the Employment Law and Workers' Compensation sections of the Florida Bar. For more information see the firm's website at http://ProtectingYourRights.com. The firm's e-mail address is info@kimseylaw.com, or contact them by telephone at (813) 265-9292.

If you have fibromyalgia (or suspect that you do) and it is interfering with your ability to work, you may be eligible for disability income. Disability income is compensation to replace the income you would earn if you were still able to work.

Types Of Coverage

If you begin experiencing difficulty with your work because of fibromyalgia, an attorney can help you determine your legal options. Generally, your options fall into the following categories:

1. You may be covered by a disability plan through your employer, particularly if you work for a large company. A plan like this is called an ERISA disability plan. ERISA stands for Employee Retirement Income Security Act, and if you make a claim under such a plan, it will be governed by federal law.

2. You may be covered by an individual disability insurance policy, for which you would be paying premiums.

3. A third possibility is that you may be able to obtain benefits under Social Security if you qualify.

4. If you are injured on the job, you may also be able to make a claim under Workers' Compensation, which is provided under state law.

Knowing what your options are is only the beginning of the process. Understanding how the legal process works under each of these types of "insurance" is essential. You need an attorney to help you navigate through the process and to help you make a successful claim.

How To Select An Attorney

You will have the best results with an attorney who has experience in representing individuals such as yourself in making disability income claims and, of course, is familiar with fibromyalgia.

How do you identify the ideal attorney? Word of mouth is still an effective way. Your local fibromyalgia association can be a good resource for suggesting an attorney, and you may also contact your local bar association for a referral.

Internet & Yellow Pages

The Yellow Pages and the Internet can be helpful in finding an attorney to assist you, but don't be frustrated by some initial difficulty using these methods because attorneys may not be listed under the categories you are familiar with, such as disability law.

Most Yellow Pages now have a separate listing under legal specialties and many attorneys have advertisements that state what types of law they practice. The categories you should look for are: disability insurance; employee benefits; government administrative law; and Social Security disability. Remember that ERISA plans and Social Security are quite different, and you need to engage an attorney who specializes in the exact type of situation in which you are involved.

You can also look at legal directory websites on the Internet. Two directories that are helpful are www.Findlaw.com and www.Martindale.com. Under Findlaw go to the section for Public & Consumer

Resources, click on Find a Lawyer and go to Browse by Practice Area. On the bottom of that section click on More Practice Areas. In that list you can click on Employment Law—Employee, Insurance Law, Administrative Law and perhaps Workers' Compensation if you think your fibromyalgia is the result of a work-related accident or condition.

In Martindale, good places to start are Employee Benefits, Insurance or Administrative Law (or if you are contemplating Workers' Compensation, go under that heading). You might also want to look at your state or local bar association website. Also, you can check with www.Google.com as well as other popular search engines. Try several variations of terms such as disability income or disability lawyers.

ERISA Disability Plans

When you first think about making a claim for your inability to work because of fibromyalgia, contact your human resources department to see if you are covered by a disability plan through your employer. A disability plan is considered an employee benefit and is usually handled by a payroll deduction. When an employee becomes unable to work, the plan usually provides the employee anywhere from 50% to 70% of income minus setoffs such as Social Security or Workers' Compensation.

There are two types of disability income compensation under ERISA plans: short term (usually for about six months) and long-term beyond that initial time period. This is a very important issue and needs to be addressed with your attorney at the earliest possible time. Although I have described the typical plan, every plan is different. It is important to get a copy of the plan from the Plan Administrator and read it carefully.

How To Get Started

You should start thinking about making a disability claim when your physical condition begins to interfere with your work. When you think you are having difficulty doing your work because of fibromyalgia symptoms, make an appointment with an attorney who can help plan the steps you will take to pursue your claim. Your doctor or specialist will be able to provide findings to confirm your fibromyalgia and the effect it has on your ability to work.

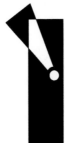

You should start thinking about making a disability claim when your physical condition begins to interfere with your work.

When you are making a claim for disability, the issue is whether your fibromyalgia prevents you from doing your job—not what caused your fibromyalgia. It doesn't make any difference whether your fibromyalgia was caused by trauma (unless you are claiming Workers' Compensation—discussed later in this chapter) or if the origin of your fibromyalgia is unknown. That's one less issue you need to prove to recover under your insurance.

Medical Report

If your doctor determines that you are disabled because of fibromyalgia, it is important to obtain this finding in written form so an initial claim can be made. As you know, there is some controversy about the ability to objectively diagnose fibromyalgia, and this issue becomes important when your claim is made under an insurance plan.

Your attorney can help you provide the medical information that insurance companies consider when deciding to allow or deny a claim. It may be advisable to consult a physician who focuses his or her practice on diagnosing and treating fibromyalgia. That doctor may be able to provide you a more objective diagnosis of fibromyalgia than a practitioner who is not familiar with diagnosing fibromyalgia. Additionally, a fibromyalgia specialist may also garner more credibility from the insurance company and the court.

A Knowledgeable Doctor

The more knowledgeable the physician is with fibromyalgia and its effect on the ability to work, the greater the likelihood of success in making a claim under a disability plan. This is important because insurance companies often contend that even though a doctor finds a patient disabled by fibromyalgia, such a diagnosis is not supported by an objective medical test.

Indeed, there is an objective medical test known as the tender point test, and if you truly have fibromyalgia this test should reflect that diagnosis and be used to document your claim. There are ways the doctor conducts the tender point test that help to ensure its objectivity.

The more knowledgeable the physician is with fibromyalgia and its effect on the ability to work, the greater the likelihood of success in making a claim under a disability plan.

If representatives of the insurance company still contend you do not have fibromyalgia, your attorney will put the burden on them to demonstrate on some objective basis that you do not have fibromyalgia. This is an impossible task, and this type of challenge to the company should strengthen your position.

By building a strong file with evidence of your disability—early in the process—you will be more persuasive and in most cases be much better prepared than the insurance company. Your attorney will help you assemble this kind of medical documentation. By proceeding with your claim *without* the best evidence, you may be jeopardizing your claim.

The Claims Process

Once you have retained an attorney and have gathered evidence of disability, you can proceed by notifying the human resources office at your company. They may refer you to the insurance company to file your claim and begin what is known in the law as the administrative process.

You should be aware that under many plans there are actually two levels of disability payments. The first is short-term disability and the second is long-term disability. Insurance companies often use a different basis to decide whether to award disability income for each of these categories.

Occupational Testing

When you make a claim, the insurance company may require you to be tested using a functional capacity evaluation (FCE). This is a half-day test that is supposed to be an objective measurement of your ability to perform work duties. It tests whether you can make basic movements that would be part of your job.

Often an individual with fibromyalgia is able to complete the FCE; however, this does not mean the person is not disabled by fibromyalgia. In most instances the day following completion of the FCE, the person is unable to do anything. The stress of performing the test can cause the person to have to stay in bed all day. Therefore, you can pass an FCE but still be disabled from fibromyalgia. The FCE by itself is not an appropriate test for determining whether fibromyalgia is disabling, and you need to rely on your attorney to make that argument.

In the ERISA context, the carrier's representatives may agree that you have passed the FCE and that they have identified various jobs in your geographic area that the test shows you can perform. Therefore, you're not disabled and they are not going to award you benefits.

You may want to have your own vocational evaluation tests done, depending on the situation. Your attorney or doctor can suggest other tests that more accurately reflect your actual capacity to do your job. You can often provide test results that refute the FCE and give your claim more validity.

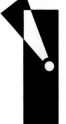

Often an individual with fibromyalgia is able to complete the FCE; however, this does not mean the person is not disabled by fibromyalgia.

Short-Term & Long-Term Disability Benefits

For short-term disability, the test is usually whether you can do the material duties of your own occupation. This is known as the "own occ" test. If the company determines that you cannot do the duties of your own job, you should receive short-term disability benefits. These short-term disability benefits usually last for six months, but it depends on your plan. The most important thing to do is to get and read you plan with your attorney. Under this "own occ" standard, if you do a job that is more than sedentary, such as standing on your feet all day or lifting, you will probably have a greater likelihood of having your short-term disability claim allowed.

Once the two years elapse, the definition of "disability" usually changes. The insurance company asks: "Can you perform the material duties of any occupation?" It is often a lot more difficult to show that you are incapable of performing any type of work than to show that you cannot perform the work that you did before suffering symptoms of fibromyalgia.

If the insurance company denies the claim, you have a right to an ERISA appeal—still within the administrative process. There may be one or two appeals. Your attorney will be helpful in giving you the best chance of prevailing at any of these appeals. It is important to provide as much documentation in as persuasive a way as possible to succeed on your claim.

Unfortunately, many individuals who are claiming disability fail to understand that even if they make a successful claim for the short-term disability, they may not be successful for the long-term income. Often they retain an attorney only after being denied long-term disability. An employee disabled by fibromyalgia would be in a much stronger position if he or she were represented by counsel at the outset and disability rights were preserved with a view to obtaining long-term disability income.

When the employee receives a letter that says the administrative process was exhausted, many employees do not realize they have already concluded the most important part of the claims process.

Into The Courts

If your claim is denied at every step during the administrative process, you can appeal this final ruling to federal court, since ERISA is governed by federal law. Depending upon the wording of the ERISA plan, the court may be able to rule in your favor only if it finds that the ruling at the administrative level was "arbitrary and capricious."

As with any disability income claim, you will be in a much stronger position if you retain an attorney as soon as you believe you have a basis for a claim.

This means the court does not look at all the evidence and consider if you are, indeed, disabled. The court will often consider **only** the information contained within the claims file. The court will not substitute its judgment for that of the insurance company. The court merely looks at the decision of the insurance company and determines if it had some reasonable basis for denying the claim.

The bottom line is that it is difficult to overturn an ERISA administrative decision once it gets to the point of being reviewed by a court.

Key Points To Remember

1. As soon as you begin considering whether to file a claim, you may want to retain an attorney to help you evaluate your situation and decide whether to make your claim.

2. Make sure your diagnosis is supported by accepted medical standards. This may mean arranging for an examination with a physical medicine (physiatrist) or rheumatologist. These specialists often have more experience with fibromyalgia than primary care physicians and know what tests accurately and objectively reflect your physical condition.

3. Explore with your attorney the options for evaluation of your capacity to perform your job. The FCE test may not accurately reflect your actual capacity to do your job. You can provide other test results that refute the FCE and give your claim more validity.

4. If your initial claim is denied, consider hiring a vocational expert during the ERISA administrative claim review process to help support your claim.

Individual Disability Insurance

Some individuals purchase disability insurance policies which are similar to any other individual insurance that you purchase for yourself. This type of insurance is different from company-funded plans governed by ERISA discussed above.

The purpose of disability insurance is to provide income when an individual cannot continue to work at his or her job because of some disability. For example, if a chiropractor has fibromyalgia and cannot do back adjustments, but can work as an administrator, he may be able to recover under disability insurance.

Seeking recovery is similar to any other type of insurance in that you make a claim under the policy. If your claim is denied, then your attorney can file a suit in state court against the insurance company. The legal basis for such a suit is called "breach of contract." One advantage to private insurance is that any appeal of a denial is not subject to the ERISA "arbitrary or capricious" standard of review.

As with any disability income claim, you will be in a much stronger position if you retain an attorney as soon as you believe you have a basis for a claim.

A Word About Workers' Compensation

As you consider your options in recovering for your inability to work because of fibromyalgia, you may be able to make a Workers' Compensation claim.

To recover Workers' Compensation benefits, you must show that your disabling fibromyalgia was the direct result of some injury or condition acquired because of an accident at work or because of your work environment.

For disability income you only need prove that your fibromyalgia is disabling which results in your inability to do your job. It doesn't matter whether your fibromyalgia resulted from a job-related cause or some other cause. This is an important distinction to be aware of.

Social Security

Before taking any action for a Social Security disability claim, you should consider contacting an attorney and also review the information provided directly by Social Security. For a detailed outline of Social Security disability benefits go to http://www.ssa.gov/pubs/10029.html.

Following is a brief outline of some of the key points on Social Security disability. When we talk about Social Security, we are usually talking about the Social Security Disability program (Title II). There is also the Supplemental Security Income (SSI) program (Title XVI), and this applies to people who are indigent. In general, to qualify as disabled under the SSD Program, the Social Security Disability Administration must determine that you are unable to do the work you did before and that you cannot adjust to other work because of your medical condition(s). For purposes of a condition like fibromyalgia which is not life threatening, your disability also must last or be expected to last for at least a year.

Eligibility depends on whether you have worked long enough and recently enough under Social Security. This is based on a points system and you can earn up to 4 points a year. Generally you need 20 credits earned in the last 10 years ending with the year you became disabled. However, younger workers may qualify with fewer credits.

Application

You can make a disability claim at your local Social Security office in person, by phone or in the mail. First you are checked for eligibility: age, employment, marital status, income and resources and Social Security disability coverage. Then the issue turns to medical eligibility, and to make this determination you are sent to a Disability Determination Service (DDS), which is a state agency, for evaluation of medical eligibility.

Many disabled claims are decided on the basis of the claimant's own medical sources. Therefore, it is important to get the best possible evidence of your fibromyalgia at this point. The Social Security Administration states that it places great value on the reports of the claimant's own physician because that doctor has the perspective of treating the patient over a period of time—something a single encounter with another doctor or hospital does not provide. The DDS may ask the treating physician for more information or enlist an independent medical or source.

Many disabled claims are decided on the basis of the claimant's own medical sources.

Your doctor will make a medical report which asks the following questions: What is wrong? When did it begin? How does it limit your activities? What have the medical tests shown? and What treatment has been provided?

They also are asked for information about your ability to do work-related activities, such as walking, sitting, lifting and carrying, and remembering instructions. A physician who is knowledgeable about fibromyalgia will be able to supply the appropriate information for you.

Speed Up Your Claim

It usually takes up to 60 to 90 days to process initial Social Security claims. This process can be shortened by providing certain documents when applying and providing the medical evidence that reflects a disability.

Documentation includes: the Social Security number and proof of age for each person applying for payments; names, addresses and phone numbers of doctors, hospitals, clinics and institutions that treated you, and dates of treatment; names of all medications you are taking; medical records from your doctor; laboratory and test results; summary of where you worked and the kind of work you did; a copy of your W-2 Form (Wage and Tax Statement) or, if you are self-employed, your federal tax return for the past year; and dates of prior marriages if your spouse is applying.

Even if all these documents are not available, Social Security suggests immediate filing and letting their office help develop the file. Your attorney should certainly be involved at this point and will assist you with documentation for your claim.

Disability Determination

The procedure for determining if a person qualifies for benefits is a step-by-step process involving five questions. They are:

1. Are you working? If an individual is not working, then go to the next step. If an individual is earning an average of more than $800 a month, the person is not considered disabled.

2. Is your condition "severe"? The person's condition must interfere with basic work-related activities for the claim to be considered. If it does not, there will be a finding of no disability. If it does, go to the next step.

3. Is your condition found in the list of disabling impairments? Social Security maintains a list of impairments for each of the major body systems that are so severe they automatically mean there is disability. If a condition is not on the list, the Social Security Administration has to decide if it is of equal severity to an impairment on the list. If it is, there is a finding of disability. If it is not, go to the next step.

4. Can you do the work you did previously? If a condition is severe, but not at the same or equal severity as an impairment on the list, then it must be determined whether it interferes

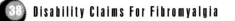

with the person's ability to do the work he or she did previously. If it does not, the claim will be denied. If it does, go to the next step.

5.   Can you do any other type of work? If a person cannot do the work he or she did in the past, it is determined whether the person is able to adjust to other work. Social Security considers the claimant's medical conditions, age, education, past work experience and any transferable skills he or she may have. If the person cannot adjust to other work, the claim will be approved. If the person can adjust, the claim will be denied.

If Your Claim Is Denied

If your claim is denied there is the right to an appeal. It is of utmost importance to have a lawyer represent you since there are time limits for appeals, and if you miss the deadline you will lose your rights and the opportunity to receive disability income.

If Your Claim Is Approved

If your claim is approved you should normally receive the first Social Security payment for the sixth full month after the date disability began and then for each month following the month benefits are due.

The amount of your monthly disability benefit is based on your lifetime average earnings covered by Social Security. You can get an estimate of your disability benefit by going to the link *Social Security Statement* (www.ssa.gov/mystatement/), which will display your earnings with an estimate of benefits. You can also get this information by calling or visiting your Social Security office. The form is also available on the Internet on *www.socialsecurity.gov* .

Your disability will be reviewed periodically by the Social Security Administration to determine if you are still disabled.

A Final Word

Obtaining disability benefits for fibromyalgia is more difficult than it is for more well-defined traditional medical problems. For this reason it is of utmost importance that you engage an attorney as soon as possible to protect your rights. There are many details of your case which may not seem important to you, but may be very important to the success of your case. Your attorney will present the most persuasive case to help you obtain benefits if you are disabled by fibromyalgia.

The material in this chapter is for informational purposes only and is not intended to substitute for the advice of an attorney. Every case is different, and you should contact an attorney experienced in these types of cases to do a thorough evaluation of your claim and to represent you.

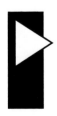

If You Want To Know More

1.   Americans with Disability Act (ADA). Public Law 101–336, enacted 7/26/90. www.doc.gov

2.   Family and Medical Leave Act (FMLA) Public law 103–3, enacted 2/05/93. www.doc.gov

Sex & Intimacy In Fibromyalgia

Chronic pain and illness can affect sex and intimacy in a relationship. Fibromyalgia and its chronic pain often intervene and introduce new fears, concerns, and anxieties into a relationship. Fibromyalgia affects everything else, so why shouldn't it cause some unique problems with sex and intimacy as well? The main problem is pain, and pain is the physiological equivalent of a cold shower!

Pain

Muscle pain can result in painful intercourse. People with fibromyalgia hurt all over and are more sensitive to pain. Muscles are particularly sensitive to pressure and squeezing, and these muscles usually "talk louder" during attempts at intimacy. Sometimes, no matter how careful or gentle you may be proceeding, each and every muscle that gets involved or is touched will scream out. This is a distraction, to say the least.

The muscles can hurt with any pressure or weight on them, and that makes it difficult to be on the bottom. Many women with fibromyalgia have pelvic pain due to the involvement of the pelvic and sacroiliac muscles as well as the low back muscles. This can cause pain during intercourse attempts. Men with fibromyalgia may have severe low back pain, particularly when the man is on top. Sometimes intimacy is moving along fairly smoothly, then suddenly a muscle develops a painful cramp right in the middle of intercourse.

Fatigue

Fatigue is also a problem. Energy is required to be sexually active, but there is very little energy at times with fibromyalgia. This physical fatigue makes it difficult to feel like moving your body at all, much less being sexually active. The mental fatigue is just as bad as it can result in decreased motivation and loss of libido.

The person with fibromyalgia may be going to bed several hours before the partner and be asleep by the time the partner gets ready for bed. It is difficult to have a successful sexual intimacy when one person is asleep! For persons in a deep sleep stage, this particular sleep stage is highly coveted for it is short-lived. I guarantee this deep sleep will be more desired than sex at 11:30 PM!

Associated Conditions

Irritable bowel syndrome can cause nausea, abdominal pains, and more bowel alertness than sexual alertness. Depression can cause additional loss of motivation, loss of interest, and loss of libido. Frequently, weight gain is a problem with fibromyalgia, and this can lead to further loss of interest due to low self-esteem or embarrassment.

Medicine Side Effects

The medications used to treat fibromyalgia can cause side effects that interfere with sexual abilities. Specific medicines, particularly those that increase the serotonin level, can decrease the sexual response. In women, this means decreased sexual desire, responsiveness, or inability to achieve orgasm. In men, there may be decreased libido or difficulty achieving erections. Other medicines can cause extreme sedation, which prevents sexual alertness. Some medicines cause nausea or gastrointestinal side effects, which shift the focus of attention to the bathroom rather than the bedroom.

Fibromyalgia does not physiologically interfere with the sexual function, however, even though there may be some problem because of the pain, fatigue, or treatments.

Benefits Of Sex

If you focus on the benefits of sex rather than the problems, you can reassure yourself that becoming intimate is good for you and your relationship. Think of sex as being therapeutic. It is a physical activity that increases the body's endorphins (natural pain killers). It improves blood flow, removes toxins from the cells, and boosts the immune system. The physical activity provides stretching, conditioning, and relaxation of the muscles. Plus, one tends to forget about pain during intimacy.

Strategies To Improve Sex And Intimacy

You need to be reassured that you are not hurting yourself by being intimate; rather you are helping both your fibromyalgia and the relationship. Your partner is also dealing with fears and anxieties about hurting you, so you both need to be reassured about the positive aspects of being intimate.

Open Communication

Open communication is the most important factor in dealing with sex and intimacy problems. Talk to each other and discuss what hurts and what helps, and attempt to overcome any fears and anxieties that are present. Frequently, couples tell me that they are not comfortable having conversations about sex and may find it embarrassing to speak freely at first. If a couple's relationship is already built on solid communication, talking about intimacy will be more comfortable. Begin discussion and communication gradually, then become more open in your sharing.

Re-discover The Romance

Intimacy does not mean sex alone or having sex at all. Men seem to be confused at times regarding this concept! I frequently hear women complaining that their husbands ignore them during the day, or don't bother to say two words to them, but then when they get into bed, they expect a switch to turn on and proceed with sexual activity. Intimacy does not happen in the bedroom only; it is something that occurs throughout the day.

Men need to learn that what they do during the day is the most important factor in whether or not they will be intimate (by man's definition) that night. Women must realize that they too need to be responsive to their mate throughout the day. Make sure you notice your significant other, compliment him or her, smile to send intimacy signals, and be a loving mate.

Touching, hand-holding, kissing, couples massage, and couples hot tub can be excellent forms of intimacy. Stroke gently and massage to rediscover touch, and make sure your significant other learns the definition of the word gentle. Educate your partner to not poke, squeeze, or slap playfully.

Take more time to get ready. Yes, I'm talking about foreplay; remember this? Sex or intimacy is natural and needs to be felt as such. The physical environment should have a comfortable room temperature without drafts. If you need more time and attention to get aroused, let your partner know. Remember that sexual activity will not damage fibromyalgia muscles, so have fun.

Find Comfortable Positions

Certain positions may be painful for the person with fibromyalgia. Examples of common positions that are painful include:

1. The missionary position. For the woman with fibromyalgia who has pain with any pressure on the muscles, being on the bottom can be very painful. Men with fibromyalgia who have particular low back problems may find this position too painful because it requires arching of the back. And how did the missionary position get its name? Supposedly, when missionaries came to America, they saw the native Americans copulating in all types of unusual positions. These missionaries apparently observed these native American practices, and trained the native Americans in a new "traditional European" sex position with the woman on the bottom. Apparently this training was done by actual demonstration. Being a missionary at that time must have really been a tough career!

2. Positions that involve arching the back, straightening the legs, twisting the spine.

3. Positions that involve an unsupported dangling leg, require supporting or holding up the weight with arms, or positions that require body weight on an arm or a leg.

Experiment with different positions and find out what will work for you. You need to redefine what is "traditional" for you. Lying on the side, positions with the knees bent, sitting positions, or positions where there is support of the back or neck usually work better for those who have fibromyalgia.

You need to follow your fibronomics during sexual activities as well. Remember to be naturally shifty, that is, don't be in one position too long as it can cause muscle cramps; rotate different positions just like you would rotate between sitting, standing, and walking. Remember that support is always welcome, whether it be a chair, a pillow, or your partner's arm, leg, or body. Train your partner to support your back or hips during sexual activity to minimize pain.

Specific Examples

I was debating whether or not to include diagrams in this chapter. I don't want this chapter to be censored! On the other hand, diagrams can be helpful in demonstrating specific types of information, in this case specific sexual positions that may be less painful and more pleasurable for you. I played it safe, however, and used stick people.

A. Lying on the side

1. Partners facing each other. Man and woman on their sides facing each other. The bottom arm of each partner is placed under the neck or under the armpit to minimize direct pressure on the arms. This position allows for pleasurable body contact without forcing the body to bear weight.

2. Partners in the same direction (overhead view). This position likewise avoids weight on the body and allows for rear entry vaginal intercourse with the knees and hips in a bent position that may be more comfortable.

B. Fibromyalgia partner on top

1. Man is on the bottom with knees straight or bent. His hands are holding and supporting her lower back. Woman is on top with knees bent, leaning forward with back in a natural position, arms forward providing some support.

2. Man on the bottom, woman sitting straight up with back naturally supporting itself. This position takes pressure off the lower back, and both the man and the woman can move with minimal strain on the back and pelvis.

C. Fibromyalgia person on the bottom

1. Woman on the bottom with knees bent. Man on top with arms supporting him. This position unloads the woman's back and pelvis and avoids weight pressure on the woman because the man is holding up his weight with his outstretched arms.

2. Woman on the bottom with knees bent and a large pillow supporting her upper back and neck, man on top. This position provides support to the woman's upper back and enables the couple to have more physical contact with upper body as the full weight of the male partner is disposed in this angle twist position. Closer intimacy is allowed.

3. Woman on the bottom with a pillow supporting the low back and hips, man on top. This position relieves the pressure on the woman's back and hip areas and allows more tolerance of her partner's weight. This position allows for maximum body contact between partners.

4. Woman on her back at edge of bed, knees bent, and legs supported by partner's upper body.

D. Sitting positions

1. Partners facing each other. Man sitting, woman on the top, chair for support. Partners' arms embrace each other for additional support. The floor can support the legs.

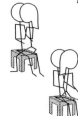

2. Partners facing the same direction.

Professional Counseling

Sometimes it may be necessary to work with a health professional who is experienced in treating problems related to sex and intimacy. As I've mentioned, it may be difficult to talk about intimate, personal problems to each other, or even to a doctor. Many physicians and health professionals are skilled and comfortable discussing sexual matters. They have expertise and training to provide valuable insight and recommendations. Counseling is a definite option. Don't be reluctant to see someone who might be able to help you.

Showing love is a mental and an emotional process, not just physical. If fibromyalgia has interfered with your total process of showing love, then you and your partner need to acknowledge this and make a commitment that the interference will only be temporary as you learn to redefine intimacy on your own new terms.

Your new terms can include oral sex, masturbation of each other, or other sexual activities if intercourse is too difficult or painful. It's okay to do other things and not have intercourse. An intimate relationship does not have to focus all on sex, so don't base a successful relationship on whether or not you have intercourse. But most importantly, don't let fibromyalgia rob you of the pleasure of enjoying each other.

New Moms (& Dads) With Fibromyalgia

Fibromyalgia affects mostly women, and many of them are first bothered by symptoms in their early reproductive years, so it is common for issues regarding pregnancy to surface. This entire chapter is devoted to mothers-to-be or new mothers who have fibromyalgia. New dads with fibromyalgia will also benefit from reading this chapter.

A frequent question is whether or not a woman should consider getting pregnant if she has fibromyalgia. From a medical perspective, there is no contraindication or unusual medical risk involved with fibromyalgia and pregnancy. Fibromyalgia has not been shown to cause infertility or increased miscarriages. Endometriosis frequently occurs with fibromyalgia and may cause problems with getting pregnant. Fibromyalgia has a hereditary component and could be passed on from parent to child, but this is not considered a dangerous medical risk or a reason to avoid pregnancy.

Another concern is whether or not the pregnancy will cause a significant flare-up for the pregnant woman, or perhaps aggravate the condition to a more severe level that persists after the pregnancy. I have treated many women for whom pregnancy has played a major role in the onset of fibromyalgia. A number of women in my practice have indicated that they were never bothered by any symptoms before pregnancy, but since then, they have had persistent muscle pains and have been diagnosed with fibromyalgia. Surprisingly though, I find that more women who develop fibromyalgia from pregnancy do so after their second pregnancy, not their first.

Another group of women have indicated that they had some pre-existing mild muscle pain, but pregnancy worsened their overall condition and led to fibromyalgia. A few individuals traced the onset of their initial low back problems and generalized fibromyalgia to their epidural procedure during delivery. Overall, a large number of women with pre-existing fibromyalgia state that their condition flared up during the pregnancy. In some, the condition became worse overall, but most have said their conditions returned to their previous stable baseline after the baby was born.

Because many people seem to have problems with increased pain, does that mean the hopeful mother-to-be should be advised not to consider pregnancy because of her fibromyalgia? Absolutely not! Despite the numerous reports, these same women will also tell you that the reward, a beautiful baby, was well worth any pain and suffering they had to endure. The benefit far outweighed the risk. Their advice to mothers or potential mothers with fibromyalgia is this: "Go ahead with it, you will be glad you did. I have no regrets and I would do the same thing all over again." (And many do!) I think that the more sophisticated one's knowledge, the better she will anticipate and deal with any increased pain during the whole process of making a new family member.

The woman with fibromyalgia must consider many issues when deciding whether or not to have a child. There may already be a strained marital relationship, which could be further strained by adding a child. The potential mother needs to know how much help the spouse and relatives are willing to give, especially if extra help is going to be needed because of fibromyalgia. Finances can be a big concern. Will the mother still be able to work and care for the baby? These issues and many more need to be carefully considered when making the decision.

Once the decision is made, the first thing that should be done, even before becoming pregnant, is to review all the medications related to fibromyalgia. Very few medications have been found to be completely safe during pregnancy; so as a rule of thumb, all prescription medicines should be reviewed with the primary care doctor for advice on whether or not they can be discontinued altogether. Some medicines can be completely stopped. Others have to be weaned gradually. Remember that medicine should be completely out of her system before the woman attempts to become pregnant (about a week after stopping medicines). If one waits until the pregnancy is confirmed, the fetus will already have been exposed to the medicine for a month. Vitamins and nutritional supplements also need to be reviewed with the doctor prior to actual pregnancy. Don't just stop medicines as some may need to be gradually weaned away from; check with your doctor first.

Very few medications have been found to be completely safe during pregnancy; so as a rule of thumb, all prescription medicines should be reviewed with the primary care doctor for advice on whether or not they can be discontinued altogether.

Fibromyalgia dads should review their medications as well prior to actual attempts to impregnate their partners. However, sperm cells are well protected from medication side effects, and the chance of causing a defective sperm that will affect the fetus at the time of conception is very remote.

If medications were a crucial part of the overall pain management, there may some increased pain once the body realizes the medicines are no longer in the system. However, there is also a readjustment phenomenon. The pain settles down again after it rebounded upward, and levels off to a more stable baseline, even though the baseline may be a little higher than the one achieved with medication. This is the time to take advantage of more natural measures to control pain, such as using moist heating pads, hot baths, ice packs, massage, or trying to get pregnant! Certain over-the-counter pain medications may be allowed during pregnancy. Check with your primary care physician.

A hopeful mother-to-be can take several measures to decrease the risk of fibromyalgia flare-up, whether or not medications were being used. Here are a few tips.

1. **Exercise.** Stay with a regular exercise program that includes stretching and conditioning exercises, with emphasis on the back. This is always easier said than done, but hopefully the mother-to-be will already be performing a regular exercise program. This program does not have to be time-consuming. Our studies have shown that 20 minutes of exercise 3 times a week will significantly improve overall conditioning and strength. Stretching exercises should be done daily, however, and the trick is to integrate an overall program into your lifestyle and then continue even after the baby is born.

2. **No smoking or exposure to secondhand smoke.** Nicotine decreases the blood flow to the muscles by constricting the arteries, which decreases the oxygen and increases the pain in the muscles. Cigarette smoke can also be harmful to the fetus. Frequent coughing can strain the back and cause exacerbation of the fibromyalgia.

3. **Follow fibronomics.** The mother-to-be needs to perfect the techniques of proper posture and body mechanics (and fibronomics). She will really need to call upon these skills once she has the baby.

4. **Get proper rest.** Proper rest resets the body's physiologic mechanism to help ward off injury, illness, and stress, and reduces the chance of a flare-up.

5. **Schedule time for yourself.** The mother-to-be should try to set aside at least an hour a day for her own private time. This is the time to relax, listen to music, read a book, work on a hobby, or enjoy recreational activities. This will help deal with physical and emotional stress.

Pregnancy Changes

What happens to the body during pregnancy as it relates to fibromyalgia? At the beginning of pregnancy, the body's hormones are undergoing rapid changes. The changes in the blood level concentration of various hormones such as estrogen and progesterone are necessary to enable the fetus to grow in a proper well-balanced environment and to prepare the mother for the birth. Surging hormonal changes in the first trimester can have opposite effects on the muscles of women with fibromyalgia. About half of my patients state that their muscles become more painful and they experience an overall aggravation of their fibromyalgia. In addition, many types of smells and various foods are not tolerated well, especially in the morning. These symptoms lead women to describe a feeling that they have the flu.

About half of the women, however, actually feel better from a fibromyalgia standpoint during the first trimester of pregnancy. This is somewhat surprising since, normally, any type of change in the body causes increased muscle pain. However, not all changes must be bad, since a good percentage of women actually feel better. The reason for this improvement is probably due to hormonal changes that cause positive psychological mood changes and decreased sensitivity of the muscle pain receptors. Your body physiologically tries to make you feel "happy" during pregnancy.

During the second trimester of pregnancy, the stress to the body slowly increases. As the fetus grows, the resulting protrusion shifts the body's center of gravity forward. In order to compensate for this shifting weight, the lumbar spine must curve backwards, and in doing so increases the swayback posture, also known as lumbar lordosis. This position creates unusual strain on the back muscles as they work harder to maintain a balanced erect posture, and the risk of back pain increases.

For every pound of extra weight in the front of the body, there are more than two pounds of extra force exerted on the low back to compensate; so there isn't an even trade-off. The back works harder. These muscles become stressed and are more likely to cause pain and fatigue. Also, the back is more vulnerable to injury and strain. This is true for overweight people as well.

Hormonal changes during pregnancy cause the back and pelvic ligaments to soften to enable easier stretching during delivery. However, this softening alters the structural balance of the back, increases the mechanical stress, and results in more back strain.

As the pregnancy progresses, the fibromyalgia mother-to-be becomes more at risk for increased generalized pain, especially in the low back area, and increased fatigue. It is important to continue the regular stretching and conditioning exercises during pregnancy, especially for the low back.

Towards the end of pregnancy all the muscles, especially the spinal muscles, are more strained. The physiologic weight gain during pregnancy has increased the energy demands and requirements on the muscles. The extra breast weight further destabilizes the upper spine and mid-back area and contributes to an unnatural strained positioning. The muscles are becoming overwhelmed and aren't "happy" anymore.

The majority of fibromyalgia women report increased muscle pain particularly in the low back towards the end of pregnancy. By then, all of the various factors have compounded to cause increased pain. It is difficult for the new mother-to-be to find comfortable positions or control her pain. I have had many of my patients participate in a supervised physical therapy program that includes heat and massage to the low back during the later stages of pregnancy. Also, trigger point injections have been helpful. This technique is not contraindicated during pregnancy, but the obstetrician and the fibromyalgia doctors need to carefully review this possible treatment method and indications for each individual patient.

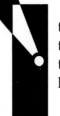

There is no evidence that natural childbirth vs. epidural vs. C-section makes any difference in terms of whether or not the woman will experience a flare-up of fibromyalgia back pain during childbirth.

Although late pregnancy may be a difficult time, it is almost the end. The mother can call upon all of her tricks and techniques to control the pain, with a little extra help from therapy or other medical treatments if needed, and hopefully keep the condition manageable.

After childbirth, additional factors can cause acute exacerbation of back pain or fibromyalgia symptoms. During labor and childbirth, sudden strenuous contractions pull on the back structures. If the labor is prolonged, the already vulnerable low back can sustain acute injury.

There is no evidence that natural childbirth vs. epidural vs. C-section makes any difference in terms of whether or not the woman will experience a flare-up of fibromyalgia back pain during childbirth. There are several patients in my practice who feel that the epidural itself was the cause of the fibromyalgia, first starting off as back pain, then generalizing. It is theoretically possible that there could be a "trauma" associated with the epidural, particularly difficult epidurals as my patients described, to result in a post-traumatic fibromyalgia. However, epidurals are generally safe and only rarely result in complications, and may be necessary and recommended for childbirth. I think the potential benefits of epidurals, such as decreased pain, far outweigh any potential risk concerning fibromyalgia.

Fibromyalgia mothers become fatigued easily during labor. However, there is no evidence of defective uterine contraction pattern unique to fibromyalgia mothers, nor has there been any evidence showing that fibromyalgia mothers should have more C-sections compared to vaginal deliveries.

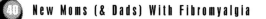

Post-Pregnancy Factors

Back pain may develop within hours after delivery, whether it was a vaginal delivery or a C-section. The abdominal and pelvic muscles which were stretched and weakened during the pregnancy and delivery are not able to balance the spine well, and painful muscle spasms can occur. After delivery, there is decreased mobility and activity as the new mother adjusts to the post-pregnancy changes and restores the body's energy supply. This is a risky time for flare-ups.

Back stretching and strengthening exercises should be started within a few days after delivery, with an attempt to resume the fibromyalgia home program as quickly as possible. Sometimes extra support is needed, such as a back brace or abdominal binder for a few weeks until the muscles can regain their strength and provide support. Larger breasted women who are nursing should wear a supportive bra so the extra breast weight does not further de-stabilize the spinal balance and increase neck, shoulder, or back pain.

By far the biggest challenge to the new mother's fibromyalgia is the newest member of the family, the infant! This lovable, irresistible little person who weighs less than ten pounds manages to get in strategic locations that are most challenging to the new mother's ability to maintain proper low back and body posture. Whether the baby is in a crib, on the floor, or nestled in a car seat, the new mother must bend, and bend frequently, to a level below her waist. Twisting and reaching go hand-in-hand with bending, and all three of these positions are hazardous to the vulnerable back and the fibromyalgia mother. Carrying the infant is also difficult, and the burden on the back increases as the child grows.

Both physical and emotional stress can cause a flare-up of pain. As we know, people under stress often tense their muscles, which causes spasms and pain. New mothers are certainly under a lot of stress due to the physical and emotional responsibilities of a newborn. Even though this type of stress may be considered good, the fibromyalgia muscles do not make a distinction.

By far the biggest challenge to the new mother's fibromyalgia is the newest member of the family, the infant!

An additional imposed stress on the new mother is sleep deprivation. Lack of sleep is synonymous with being a new mother! Increased pain and fatigue result.

Mothers who breastfeed their babies are at particular risk for sleep deprivation and this is a factor to consider when deciding whether or not you want to nurse your baby. Mothers who nurse will probably not get back on medications as quickly as mothers who choose to bottle feed. Most of my patients choose to bottle feed, particularly after the first pregnancy, because it causes fewer sleep problems and enables the partner to be more involved in the nighttime feedings.

Postpartum depression is also common and can lead to additional poor sleep, increased fatigue, and increased pain. Fibromyalgia women don't seem to be more prone to postpartum depression than their non-fibromyalgia counterparts, but I wouldn't be surprised if future research shows otherwise since people with fibromyalgia are more prone to clinical depression. Given all of these stresses, it is no wonder that a new mother is more vulnerable to pain. If all of these stresses overwhelm the muscles, acute flare-ups can occur.

How does the new mother decrease her risk for an acute injury or flare-up as she cares for her new baby? Here are a few tips.

1. **Resume your regular exercise program of stretching and conditioning exercises as soon as possible.** Start with 5 minutes of stretching twice a day for a week and then increase to 10 minutes twice a day the second week. During the third week and thereafter continue with 15 minutes a day. The second week after delivery, begin a regular exercise program which might first include casual walking for ten minutes 3 to 4 times a week, gradually progressing to at least 20 minutes 3 times a week. The trick is to integrate a regular exercise program into your new mother's lifestyle.

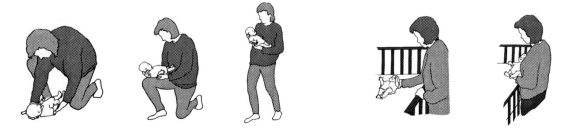

2. **Follow fibronomics** (Moms and Dads). Although it is impossible to avoid dangerous positions (bending, twisting, reaching, lifting), a new mother can learn to practice proper posture and body mechanics, specifically fibronomics, when lifting and carrying the child or engaging in other activities.

   To properly place the infant on the floor, or to pick the infant up from the floor, avoid bending at the waist; instead, bend at the legs and allow the legs to do the lifting while maintaining a natural back position. The one-knee lift technique allows you to bring your baby close to the body before completing the lift. Keep your elbows close to your sides.

   To properly carry the infant, always hold the child close to your own center of gravity, which is from the chest to the navel area. Keep your elbows at your side and avoid reaching out and lifting. To place in or pick up from the crib, first drop the crib side to the lowest position possible to minimize the bending required. Spread your legs apart and bend your knees slightly to lower your chest and the infant as much as possible. Keep back in neutral position. Slowly bend forward with the infant still held close to your chest and then slowly open the arms, keeping your elbows against your abdomen. Set your infant down in the crib and gently ease into the proper lying position. To adjust your baby's position once in the crib, try using a technique called the Golfer's Lift (see page 123).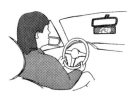

   To place the infant into the car seat, put your foot onto the car floor, and lean as close as possible to the car seat. Try to keep your elbows as close to the side as possible during the transfer into the car seat. Since baby's car seat has to go in back because of front seat air bags, it is hard to turn around and see the baby. Many new mothers say turning the neck causes pain to flare-up. A trick is to secure another mirror below the rear-view mirror to allow you to see into the middle of the back seat. You can glance in this mirror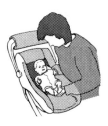

and monitor your baby without twisting your neck. As your child gets older (and heavier), take advantage of his or her developing motor skills to protect your back. Let your child crawl onto your lap instead of picking him up. Whenever possible, sit instead of stand to hold. Encourage your child to walk from point A to B instead of carrying her.

3. **Get proper rest.** Proper sleep resets the body's physiologic mechanisms. Avoid caffeine at night. You may take naps during the day as needed.

4. **Schedule your own time.** Try to set aside at least an hour a day that you consider your own private time. This is when you should achieve relaxation, and do other leisurely activities such as reading a book, listening to music, or working on a hobby.

5. **Pain relief can be obtained by various measures.** Check with your doctor to see what over-the-counter medications may be allowed. All of these medicines, except Tylenol, can help decrease both pain and any acute inflammation. (Tylenol decreases pain but does not help inflammation in a strained muscle.) Application of light heat or an ice pack can help decrease pain and spasms and increase blood flow. Sleeping medications should usually be avoided. A sleeping medicine may prevent the mother from hearing the infant cry or have side effects such as drowsiness, confusion, or impaired balance.

   If the new mother is not nursing, she should try to work out a call schedule with her husband to handle nighttime feedings so she can get a good night's sleep. Although a new mother with fibromyalgia may be at a higher risk for developing flare-ups or acute low back strain, she can learn how to prevent or minimize these consequences so they do not interfere with the wonderful task of having and raising a new baby.

6. **Consider taking longer than the usual six-week medical leave to recover.** Sometimes fibromyalgia delays recovery and you may need a few more weeks before you are ready to return to work.

Fibromyalgia Fathers

Fibromyalgia fathers certainly experience a lot of stress and anxiety during the wife's/partner's pregnancy. It is natural to have concerns about the well-being of the developing fetus and the mother's health, and these natural stresses can cause fibromyalgia flare-ups.

The fibromyalgia father needs to pay special attention to proper fibronomics just as the mother does. If the mother chooses to bottle feed, as my wife did, the fibromyalgia father should be involved in the bottle feeding. I took on feeding responsibilities particularly on weekends. I am not sure which was worse, my weekend night call duties feeding the baby, or my medical on-call duties! Truthfully, I didn't mind the night feeding call duties at all because I was happily fulfilling my duty as a new parent. I was able to psyche myself up for these upcoming weekend duties, and my wife and I worked out an arrangement so I could catch up on my sleep when I was "off duty." This helped me to minimize potential fibromyalgia flare-ups.

▶ If You Want To Know More

Pellegrino MJ. *Inside fibromyalgia*. Columbus OH: Anadem Publishing, 2001.

The Fibromyalgia Traveler

Vacation time should be relaxing and free from pain. Many of my patients complain that they have more pain or flare-ups from their vacations than other situations. One particular woman was surprised at the severity of her fibromyalgia flare-up, but when I asked exactly how she spent her vacation, she explained that she jetted to Europe, walked in five different countries in seven days, returned to the U.S. and flew across the country to California for a reunion with family members, many of whom she had not seen in years. She then returned home to help her daughter move to a college dormitory for the fall semester. My back started to hurt just listening!

Vacation time can be extremely stressful. Remember, fibromyalgia does not distinguish good stress from bad. They both hurt. There are many reasons why vacations cause paradoxical flare-ups of our fibromyalgia: happy stress, a hectic schedule, increased physical activities (walking, hauling luggage, etc.), and changes from our proper posture. In our eagerness to take our vacation, we often forget our necessary daily routine for controlling fibromyalgia. We must remember that we are bringing our fibromyalgia with us, and we have to make sure our fibromyalgia has a good time too! Vacations, like everything else, have to be planned in detail. We need to think of as much as possible ahead of time to anticipate potential problems and avoid surprises. Always try to plan a few days at home after the vacation, strictly to rest and recover before returning to work or whatever you do in the "real world." Getting home from vacation on Sunday night and returning to work Monday morning will only invite a prolonged fibromyalgia flare-up.

Decide What You Want To Do

So how does one prepare for vacation to include fibromyalgia? We can't fly to Europe and then see how it goes. Trying to decide what to do after you are already there is inviting stress, confusion, disagreements and, of course, pain.

Top Ten Vacation Activities to Avoid

1. Annual North Pole Expedition, Fort Yukon, Alaska

2. Cross-country Unicycling Tour: starting point, Plymouth, Indiana

3. Human Mannequin Contest, Los Angeles, California

4. Moose Hunting from Trees, Northern Canada

5. Family Triathlon Olympics, Steubenville, Ohio

6. Amateur Lumberjack Festival, Spokane, Washington

7. Drywallers' Fantasy Camp, Iowa City, Iowa

8. Backpacking with the Pack Backers, Green Bay, Wisconsin

9. Marathon Rock Climbing, Bryce Canyon National Park, Utah

10. Camping Stargazer's Reunion, Eureka, Nevada

First, decide on a suitable vacation spot for both you and your fibromyalgia. Locations with hot, dry climates are best. I haven't met anyone who has taken a vacation to Siberia. However, I have met a city employee with fibromyalgia who has traveled all over the world, including Antarctica, Indonesia, Uganda, Brazil, and Portugal! Another patient plans a local getaway where she checks into a local hotel for one week a year from Monday to Friday. No one stays there during the week so it is quiet and she has the pool to herself. There is no long drive, minimal packing and expense, and lots of rest and relaxation!

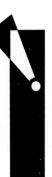

One way to avoid being overwhelmed by the big picture is to plan and organize (and write down) every detail of your trip as exactly as possible, and try to follow this agenda.

If you like to stay busy, pick locations that offer a variety of attractions or events involving sitting as well as standing. Theme parks can be difficult places because of all the required walking and standing in lines. Avoid locations that require sleeping on the ground (camping out in a tent!) or sleeping on an impossible bed (recliner cot in an RV, Aunt Mae's sofa, etc.). My idea of camping is fishing, hiking, and boating during the day, and at night staying in an air conditioned hotel with a king-sized bed (firm mattress) and my pillows from home. You're allowed to get away to some relaxing resort and do absolutely nothing.

Some people have a difficult time planning for a major vacation and this stress can increase pain even before the vacation starts. I've had several patients tell me they were so overwhelmed by everything that had to be done beforehand, that they chose not to take a vacation at all. Or they didn't want work to pile up while they were gone, so they never left!

One way to avoid being overwhelmed by the big picture is to plan and organize (and write down) every detail of your trip as exactly as possible, and try to follow this agenda. Take care of all your home activities such as paying the bills, doing the laundry and shopping. Prepare a list of various vacation packing duties and spread out these duties each day for two weeks before you actually leave on vacation. Arrange for coverage at work so you can minimize the dreaded work pile-up.

By planning each day and activity, you can keep your mind occupied and off the pain as much as possible. This also breaks down the very big stressful vacation into a series of small mini-events that are not as intimidating and seem possible to accomplish and enjoy. Organizing your vacation into a series of smaller events allows you to focus your attention and energy on smaller tasks that can be accomplished, whereas if you look at the whole vacation and what you are trying to accomplish, you may be overwhelmed and not feel that you have the energy or motivation to do it.

Taking Care Of Yourself

Since the majority of vacationers often spend several hours more on their feet during each vacation day than they would under non-vacation circumstances, we need to recognize the potential for aggravation of back, hip and leg symptoms. Carefully organize the vacation event so that you allow frequent breaks between walking, sitting and standing. It is a good idea to plan a rest day every third day for sitting and browsing only. Plan on watching a show, taking a seated sightseeing tour, or lounging at pool side. Planned rest breaks in a hectic schedule are very much appreciated by our muscles.

If you are traveling by car, make sure you allow plenty of extra time so you can give proper attention to your fibromyalgia. A good rule of thumb is to add 10 extra minutes per every hour of travel. Ideally, we should stop the car for every hour of driving and take a 2-minute stretching break and a 5-minute walking break before resuming the trip. Every 4 hours we should take a 5-minute stretching break, a 5-minute walking break and at least a 30-minute seated break (eating a meal in a restaurant).

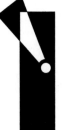

If you are bothered by a lot of neck pain and fatigue during prolonged driving, you would be a good candidate for wearing a soft cervical collar during your trip.

Watch your position and body mechanics while you are seated in the car. Don't turn your head in an awkward position to talk to someone for long periods of time. Likewise, if you are taking a nap, try not to lean on a pillow with your head tilted for a long period of time.

Many fibromyalgia patients are bothered by motion sickness, especially those who try to read while riding in the car. Some patients don't even attempt to take cruises because they have overwhelming motion sickness. An airplane ride is usually tolerated better except during prolonged turbulence. The apparent increased motion sickness probably relates to a hypersensitive vestibular system that overreacts to extra signals.

There are several strategies for minimizing motion sickness. If you are prone to developing motion sickness, your doctor may prescribe a pill or patch to use as needed. Avoid reading while riding in the car; be especially careful when looking at maps while riding. When it's necessary to look at a map, look at it for no more than 15 seconds at a time before shifting your focus to outside the car at moving scenery for 15 to 30 seconds; then look at the map again, no more than 15 seconds at a time. Breathing fresh air, getting out of the car and walking, and switching roles with the driver are all helpful in combating motion sickness.

Watch out for drafts; vacation time seems to be a drafty time! Avoid direct air conditioning drafts in the car or in the restaurant and have a light coat to keep your arms and neck covered if it is chilly or drafty in an area. Don't roll windows down, especially when driving on the freeway.

If you are bothered by a lot of neck pain and fatigue during prolonged driving, you would be a good candidate for wearing a soft cervical collar during your trip. A soft collar can help rest the neck muscles while supporting the head; it can be particularly effective while driving over bumpy areas where there are more demands and strains on neck muscles. I recommend that the collars not be worn more than 50% of the time while driving or riding, and no more than one hour at a time to prevent the neck muscles from getting stiff.

Help your fibromyalgia in any way you can while driving or riding in a car. Taking over-the-counter pain medications thirty minutes to an hour before an anticipated strenuous activity may help dampen the pain. Rubbing muscles with creams that generate either heat or cold can help. Bring along a tape player with earphones and play your favorite music or relaxation tape.

If you are traveling by airplane you need to maintain proper body mechanics and frequently reposition your body. An aisle seat is best so you can stretch out your legs and alternate positions, especially on long flights. Take your portable music player with you. If you hate flying like I do, practice your deep breathing exercises especially just before take-off. Bring your own comfortable pillow to increase the chance of getting some restful sleep during those transcontinental or transoceanic flights at night. Your doctor may be willing to prescribe a sleep modifier to use especially on the plane to help achieve good quality sleep. In planes with larger aisles, walk around frequently. If your budget permits, buy first class or business seats simply for the extra space. Watch out for those air blowers above you so they don't shoot cold air right onto your neck.

Luggage can cause special problems. If you are loading your own luggage into the trunk or carrying it around for long distances, you are particularly prone to developing increased pains in your neck, shoulder, back and arm muscles. Take less! Use luggage racks, carts, and wheels whenever you can. Don't sling straps over your shoulders as this will aggravate your trapezius and back muscles. The best way to transport luggage if you have fibromyalgia is to let someone else carry it for you. The next best way is to push a luggage rack on wheels in front of you. Pulling it behind you is harder. If you have to carry your own luggage, make sure that you switch arms frequently, take rest stops every hundred yards and actually set down your luggage, stretch your arms and massage your shoulders.

In addition to taking your own pillows, remember that many hotel air conditioners blow air directly on the bed, so be certain that you either block or redirect the air to avoid direct drafts. Have a VCR set up in your room so that you can play your favorite exercise video that you have remembered to bring. Always make sure that the hotel you will be staying in has a hot Jacuzzi so you have a relaxing, deep heat modality. Pack your bathing suit. If you like ice packs, bring some instant cold packs or a locking plastic bag to make your own.

Don't forget to take your medicines along, especially sleeping pills or medicines that you use only for flare-ups in case you need them. I have had patients call me from different states wondering if I could prescribe something because they forgot to bring their medicines. Never leave drugs in visible areas where they could be stolen.

There is no need to let fibromyalgia ruin a perfectly good time. Nor should you let it prevent you from taking a well-deserved vacation. Bon voyage!

Traveling By Car

Some of us may travel by car to vacation getaways, but most of us spend considerable time in our cars every day regardless if we are vacationing. Commuting to and from work, running errands, traveling, and repeated trips to our doctors (!) give us the opportunity to know our car very well. We should not buy a vehicle based on how it looks, but how functional it is for our fibromyalgia. If you have the opportunity to shop around, some important features of a car may help decrease your fibromyalgia pain, or help prevent it from being aggravated while you are traveling.

I think an important preventive feature is an adequate headrest. As you may know, whiplash injury commonly occurs after a rear-end collision and is one of the most common causes of post-traumatic fibromyalgia (PTF). A good headrest can help reduce the severity of a whiplash injury during a rear-end collision, although this has never been proven with studies. Headrests do not prevent whiplash injuries, nor do they help in head-on or side collisions.

When you are seated in the car, the headrest should rest just behind the middle of your head. When you move your head backwards, it should come against the headrest very quickly. Make certain that the headrest has strong supports even if it is raised into the upper position so it won't snap off in the event of a rear-end collision. Ask questions and do your research so you can make knowledgeable choices. Make sure you keep the headrest up whenever you are driving or riding.

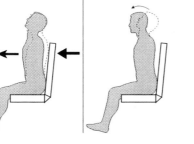
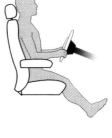

Another important feature is armrests. There should be armrests on both sides of us, whether we are drivers or passengers. Prolonged driving with unsupported arms is a major cause of fatigue in the arms and upper back area. Armrests on both sides enable us to unload the upper back muscle by supporting our arms while we maintain safe control of the steering wheel. Make sure the armrests have adequate padding so as not to put pressure over the bony elbows or nerves inside the elbow. I find my arms are most comfortably positioned when the steering wheel is held in the 4 o'clock and 8 o'clock spots.

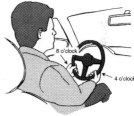

We need to adequately support our spine. Cars should have adjustable seats **and backs**. Power controls are better than manual devices, allowing you to make adjustments while you are driving. This feature not only enables us to find an individual comfortable position, but to adjust position while driving if needed. I have a favorite adjustment of my car seat, but I will change this position several times

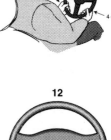

a week depending on whether my upper back or lower back is bothering me more. A more reclined position helps decrease my lower back pain. Each person needs to experiment in order to find the right balance of back/pelvic/leg angles. Keeping the seat as close to the steering wheel as possible helps prevent painful reaching to hold the wheel, and it also better positions feet and knees to unload the back.

If you move your seat too close to the steering wheel, you may have to disable your air bag to avoid air bag injury in case of a collision. Check with the law enforcement officials in your state before doing this. The highway patrol officials I've talked with tell me air bags save lives and disabling them could increase your risk of serious injury. Some cars are equipped with lumbar supports, which can be helpful if low back pain is a problem. Avoid very deep seats that you sink into, which make it difficult to get in and out. You may have a favorite lumbar roll or cushion that you can bring into your car for more comfortable seating while you are driving or traveling.

A good climate control system is mandatory in a car. Without an air conditioner, we must rely on open windows for air circulation during hot days, and this invites the humidity, dust, pollen and drafts which all can irritate our sensitive skin and muscles. If you can control the air, you can keep some control of your condition. Make sure that the heating and air conditioning units are functioning properly.

Car vents should be adjusted so as to redirect the cold air away from the body. Direct cold air hitting the skin can trigger reflexes that cause muscle spasms and flare-ups. Warm air from defrosters can cause nausea or stuffiness if it directly hits your face, especially for those of us who are sensitive to odors and fumes and have overactive nasal responses. Adjust the vents so air does not hit you directly. If some vents cannot be adjusted to redirect the air, they can be closed.

Mirrors are also important; make sure there are lots of them so you can scan the outside world without turning your head too far. When you are comfortable in the driver's seat, you should be able to glance into the rear view mirror and the side mirrors by moving your eyes mostly to see easily everything that is happening beside and behind us. When you turn your head to the left to see in your blind spot, be sure that your properly positioned headrest is not obstructing the view or causing you to strain your neck. Power mirrors let you make more adjustment choices and are worth the money.

Be sure your car has an automatic drive. No stick shifts or clutches allowed unless you want your right shoulder and left leg to fall off! One patient thought a stick shift would be good exercise for her arm; she quickly learned that it caused bad flare-ups instead. Let your car do as much work for you as possible.

Be careful about twisting and reaching for items that always manage to be just beyond a comfortable reach. I am talking about items that end up on the floor such as tapes, sunglasses, pens, or snow scrapers. One of my patients uses an assisting device called a reacher/grabber which she keeps in the front seat and uses to retrieve those impossible-to-reach items. This enables proper body mechanics. The reacher/grabber can also be used in the trunk to retrieve items and prevent risky bending.

In general, the bigger and roomier the vehicle, the easier it will be on fibromyalgia posture. We need to be able to easily step into the vehicle. It's better to climb up a little to get into the car; getting out will then be simple. If you have to drop down into your car seat, it will be hard for you to lift yourself up and out of the car. Let gravity work for you when you get out of your car, not when you get into your car.

▶ If You Want To Know More

Pellegrino MJ. *Inside fibromyalgia*. Columbus OH: Anadem Publishing, 2001.

Handling The Holidays

For many fibromyalgia patients, the worst time of the year is the holiday season, starting in late November and hitting full peak in December. Return visits for increased fibromyalgia pain and flare-ups are common. I actually see most of these patients in January because they are hurting after the holidays.

There are numerous reasons why fibromyalgia is so susceptible to flaring-up during the holiday season. The most prevalent reason is the increased stress at this time of the year.

The extra stresses are a problem for women especially since they are traditionally the ones responsible for preparing for the holidays. Extra duties of buying gifts, wrapping, cooking, baking, decorating, entertaining, and transporting various family members to and from school and related activities are superimposed on the everyday responsibilities—a good recipe for a fibromyalgia flare-up.

Various physical stresses during the holidays include:

1. The shopping required with prolonged standing, walking, and carrying.

2. The cookie baking and other cooking involved. Somehow the holiday pans are always on the highest shelves, and there seems to be some sort of relationship between the heavier the pan, the higher and the more out of reach it will be.

3. The holiday decorations, putting up lights, Christmas trees, and the hundreds of other items that get arranged throughout the house and yard to prepare for the holidays.

4. Increased job demands during the holidays, particularly with factory workers and retailers who may work many overtime hours.

5. Increased school and social activities demand more physical effort. This includes our children's school holiday plays and activities, all the holiday parties and get-togethers.

In addition to physical reasons, there is increased stress caused by weather changes. By now the weather is changing to cold and damp, particularly for those of us who live in the northern part of the country. There is less sunlight as the days get progressively shorter, and this combination disrupts our fibromyalgia baselines. Seasonal affective disorder (SAD) is a form of depression caused by lack of sunlight.

There are also plenty of mental stresses during the holiday season:

1. Family relations are often strained as everyone is experiencing a higher level of stress. Numerous family get-togethers, out-of-town visitors staying over, and other events that brings families together for lengthy periods of time may create both anticipated and unexpected stresses.

2. Depression is common during the holidays. Multiple factors are involved, but it seems that everywhere you go happy Christmas music and decorations abound, and everyone appears to be joyous and excited . . . but you hurt more.

3. Procrastination is a mental stress and can lead to an overwhelming sense that everything will not get done in time. I tell my family members to make sure they've bought my presents first . . . and then they can procrastinate!

4. Worries about finances abound at this time of year with extra holiday expenses, savings depletions, tax concerns, and more.

Another cause of feeling bad around the holidays is the change in our usual eating patterns. From Thanksgiving to New Years, many of us eat large quantities of refined sugar. We may eat out more and eat more fatty foods, gourmet foods, or unusual foods that are not a part of our routine diet. The altered eating and over-eating disrupts our usual gastrointestinal balance and may aggravate fibromyalgia by draining energy, aggravating irritable bowel symptoms, or simply causing us to not feel like ourselves.

Holidays happen at predictable times, so don't act surprised when they come, and don't assume you have no control over this situation. You can recognize potential stresses and take specific steps to decrease your risk of a flare-up.

Here are some tips for handling the holidays:

1. **Stress:** Don't forget to practice your stress management techniques. Recognize that the holidays are a difficult time of the year, but the higher stress level is temporary. One patient told me she got particularly upset because she literally lost all of her purchased Christmas gifts. She had so much stress and worry about getting all of the gifts that she simply forgot where she put them. I saw her in early January and I reassured her that the gifts would probably be found in some closet she never knew she had! I suggested to her that she create a special temporary space for the holidays. In this space, whether it be a closet or a corner of the room, she will have her gifts, gift wrap, and accessories needed to wrap the gifts. She can get bankers' boxes and label them and stack them neatly, and she knows that this is her temporary holiday special space.

   Weather changes may force you to revise your schedules suddenly, so don't worry if you don't get everything done. Be glad you got ANYTHING done. Make an extra effort to follow through with your exercise program.

2. **Shopping:** Start your shopping in July. Order your gifts from catalogs or from the numerous computer on-line shopping sites instead of going out and physically shopping. First do mental shopping and know what you want to buy for everyone, then go out and buy the presents. Don't spend hours on your feet looking for them. If you are in the malls or stores, take frequent rest breaks and actually sit down for at least five to ten minutes for every

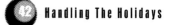

hour of shopping. Carefully organize your time so that you do not find yourself spending several hours on your feet before your realize so much time has passed.

Be careful about carrying packages through the store as these assorted boxes of different weights quickly multiply and become a burden to your muscles, making it difficult to follow proper fibronomics. Take advantage of shopping carts to haul your merchandise around. Ask the stores if you can leave your newly purchased items behind the counter while you finish your shopping, then gather up all the packages in one final sweep. Get two oversized shopping bags and distribute packages evenly between the bags, carrying one in each arm to balance the weight on your body.

Watch out for the mall parking where the only available parking spot is practically in a different city. It is a good idea to have a non-fibromyalgia person drop you off at the mall's main entrance so you can avoid the long walking. Shop during low volume times at the stores (early morning) so you can park closer and spend less time waiting in line. Remember where you park. Instead of wrapping all your gifts, take advantage of the free gift-wrapping at the stores or use decorative gift bags or boxes that require no wrapping. I bribe my daughter to do my gift wrapping. If I wrap my own gifts, I definitely leave my perfectionist tendencies in the other room!

3. **Baking:** When baking or cooking, make sure that you practice your fibronomics. Instead of baking cookies, try buying them or paying someone else to bake. By the time you figure the time and cost, particularly the intangible costs of increased pain/flare-up, you would be amazed that buying your cookies will be cost-effective.

Make sure your kitchen work area is ergonomically efficient; that is, you are not putting yourself into prolonged unnatural positions to accomplish a task. Store the pans where they can be reached easily. Have someone else get the heavy pots and pans down from the high shelves or bring them up from the basement.

One of my patients "recycles" cookies. She puts cookies others have given her on a nice plate and takes them somewhere else! You can freeze your extra cookies to use over the next few months when you have company.

4. **Decorating:** Spread out your decorations over a two-week period instead of trying to cram it into one day. Use ladders to put your body and arms closer to your decorations. Be creative to maintain fibronomics: place decorations at lower levels instead of up high; use decorations that wrap instead of those that need to be hung, clipped or nailed. Hire your neighbor's kid to put up your outside lights while you supervise. Have someone carry up your holiday boxes from the basement. Get a smaller tree; it's a lot less work but still gives the Christmas spirit. It's exciting to put up decorations; but remember they will have to come back down in January, so plan ahead.

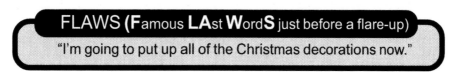

FLAWS (**F**amous **LA**st **W**ord**S** just before a flare-up)

"I'm going to put up all of the Christmas decorations now."

5. **Job:** Be particularly attentive to your job's fibronomics. If possible, schedule vacation time, or at least schedule a long weekend. Try to protect your weekends as much as possible so that you do not find yourself working six or seven days a week. If you can, bring some of your work duties home to a less stressful environment.

6. **Parties:** Prioritize the parties that you must attend. Do not commit yourself to any party you don't feel you need to attend. If you go to parties, avoid prolonged standing and take frequent sitting breaks. If you are unable to sit in a chair, make sure that you take frequent bathroom breaks and sit on the commode for a few minutes, even if you don't have to go! It's okay to leave the party early (or go to the party fashionably late). For your own parties, try to do pot-luck instead of assuming all the responsibility. If you are able, hire a caterer to handle your party.

7. **Dressing:** Dress warmly, making sure that the neck and hands are covered. If it is icy, make sure you have one free hand at all times to hold on to something. Wear good traction shoes or boots. Try to soak up any sunlight, as it can be invigorating. Plan a vacation to a hot, dry area!

8. **Family:** Pay special attention to family stresses and family needs. Keep communication open. Schedule a private night out with your spouse for just the two of you. Take family time-outs where everyone takes a break from their hectic schedules, catches up, and relaxes.

9. **Depression:** Watch for depression. See your doctor or counselor if it develops. Antidepressant medications may be necessary. Attend support group meetings, and discuss with others problems and strategies for handling the holidays.

10. **Procrastination:** To avoid procrastination, buy a monthly planner calendar and write your necessary events, highlighting those areas, and committing only to those dates. Get together with a group of your fibromyalgia friends and plan a shopping outing as a group in July. Make a list of things that you absolutely must do and eliminate those things that are not really necessary.

11. **Finances:** Set financial limits on what you will spend during the holidays. Participate in your bank's Christmas Saver's Club to save throughout the year. Don't be tempted by such offers as "90 days, same as cash," since, if you can't afford it now, you can't afford it in 90 days. Plan how much you will spend for each gift. Be careful with your credit cards. Force yourself to add to your savings account in the month of December, rather than depleting it.

12. **Eating:** Instead of eating large amounts of everything, eat less and have more frequent, smaller meals. Promise yourself that you will not gain any weight over the holiday season. Don't neglect your exercise program since you need to burn off calories. If you are increasing your carbohydrate consumption, make sure you eat adequate protein as well to minimize the chance of hypoglycemia and carbo craving. So if you are eating sugar cookies, eat some cottage cheese also. Heck, try dipping your sugar cookies in cottage cheese!

Don't forget to enjoy the holidays! Just because you have fibromyalgia does not automatically mean you will be miserable. You can take some active steps in preparing for the holidays and assuring that you have as much control of your fibromyalgia as possible during this difficult time.

▶ If You Want To Know More

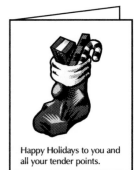

Happy Holidays to you and all your tender points.

Pellegrino MJ. *Inside fibromyalgia*. Columbus OH: Anadem Publishing, 2001.

Becoming A Fibromyalgia Victor

Personal Snapshot—Hearing

by Mark J. Pellegrino, M.D.

Let's *"ear"* it

Have you noticed the multitude of expressions with the word "ear" in them? Do you really know the true (literal?) meanings?

Play it by ear is a familiar one that means improvise as the situation develops. It is not part of the directions on a Q-tip box.

Being up to one's ear can mean deep involvement and serious trouble, especially if one happens to be in quicksand. *Out on your ear* also means trouble, and is not necessarily indicating a deep sleep in the lateral recumbent position.

If you are *on one's ear*, that person is definitely irritated with you, most likely because he doesn't like you standing on his ear. Perhaps when this expression was first invented, it was common practice to indicate disapproval of one's remarks by standing on the person's ear. Probably the left ear meant mild disgust, but the right ear, you see, that meant big trouble; *up to one's ear (while on one's ear?)*.

If you say an *earful*, you are spreading gossip, and you will find that everyone will be *all ears*, or eager to listen to your every word.

When you *lend an ear* to someone, you are listening intently. This does not refer to loaning your hearing aid to a friend (which we all know we shouldn't do anyway, right?)

Good news for me? Well then that's *music to my ears*.

continued on next page...

Personal Snapshot—Hearing

continued from previous page...

Did you ever *turn a deaf ear* or ignore someone? Did your comments ever *fall on deaf ears*, or get completely ignored? I do not use these particular expressions (except in an editorial!) because of the not-so-subliminal association between hearing impairment and ignorance. That's another editorial though! Perhaps we should get more specific and sophisticated and denote *turn a corn ear* to those who refuse to listen to the importance of vegetable nutrients, and *fall on deaf cauliflower ears* when being ignored by a hearing impaired ex-boxer?

Although these expressions are the more common ones, I've found a few that may not be as well known. For example, *"ear" today and gone tomorrow* means "I can hear today with my hearing aids, but tomorrow they are being sent for repairs and I don't have any functioning loaners to use in the meantime.

"Ear" goes is an unheralded expression that indicates inability to fully understand all the spoken words due to hearing impairment.

If you *score a bull's "ear"*, you correctly "guess" what is being said by speech-reading and getting lucky!

And my favorite, *take my ear*, or try to understand what it's like to have a hearing impairment because it can be difficult at times, but it does not prevent me from living a normal life.

Thanks for *lending me your ears*. I hope this didn't *go in one ear and out the other!*

Everyone has a unique story about trying to deal with a chronic condition. I have listened to thousands of patient stories and my ongoing hope is that the end of the story will always be better than the beginning of the story. I want each person to be able to cross the finish line, break the tape, and feel victorious. My own story doesn't start with fibromyalgia, but with hearing impairment.

I have a hearing impairment, specifically nerve deafness caused by damage from an antibiotic, streptomycin. I lost most of my hearing at a young age, but fortunately I was born with normal hearing and was able to develop language skills before I lost most of my hearing. Also, I have enough residual hearing that allows me to benefit from hearing aids. I have worn hearing aids since I was 14 years-old (about ten years ago . . . I think!).

I also have fibromyalgia.

I accept "both" conditions, but I first learned to deal with my hearing impairment. Ultimately, coping with my hearing impairment prepared me to deal with fibromyalgia when "it" came around in my late twenties (just a few years ago . . . I think!).

Hearing impairment and fibromyalgia are very similar in many ways. Both conditions cause chronic impairment. They both have been called "invisible conditions" because we look normal. Both conditions have controversial origins which have lead to present day confusions and uninformed perceptions.

Fibromyalgia was first described as an inflammation of fibrous tissue (which is not the case). For a while fibromyalgia was considered a "psychogenic" disorder. (Today we better understand its physical abnormalities.) Many doctors still do not accept fibromyalgia as a "real" condition (and they are wrong).

A hearing impairment has had a negative stigma attached to it which dates back to 355 B.C. when the great Greek philosopher Aristotle was translated to have said, "Those who are born deaf all become senseless and incapable of reason." What Aristotle actually said was, "Those who are deaf from birth cannot learn speech even though they may have a voice." Unfortunately, the Greek words meaning "deaf" and "speechless" also meant "dumb" and "stupid" in certain instances. It was these negative meanings that were translated by writers of that time. Because Aristotle was considered a genius, his writings were accepted without question for hundreds of years, even though they were sometimes incorrectly translated.

Today, those with fibromyalgia and hearing impairment strive to overcome negative stereotyping and to enlighten those who are uninformed. Education remains the key weapon in attacking these obstacles. Effective coping strategies and successful lifestyle changes are needed to deal with these conditions that can be treated even if they cannot be cured yet. My hearing impairment has contributed to my "profile" in many ways, so I have included it here.

Sometime during my third year of life, I rapidly lost 85% of my hearing. As far as memories go, things seemed to have gone fairly normally for me up to that point. I do not remember anything that specifically registered in my mind to the effect that, "Gee, Mark, you used to hear well, and now you can hardly hear anything."

My pediatrician did not understand what had happened either. I was a healthy baby who would get periodic earaches, sore throats, and sniffles. For these I would get injections of a pediatric medicine that included the combination of penicillin and streptomycin. It seemed that many kids got injections of this combination medicine in the early 1960's, as it was commonly prescribed by some pediatricians.

It would not be until years later, as a third year medical student, that I finally learned that the true cause of my hearing impairment: these seemingly innocuous injections that contained streptomycin. It turns out that I have a hereditary susceptibility to hearing loss caused by streptomycin. Nestled in my body's DNA structure is a defective gene that prevents normal metabolism of streptomycin into harmless by-products. Because of this hereditary defective gene, streptomycin cannot be degraded properly, and the by-products accumulated specifically in their favorite place, the inner ear fluid.

The by-products interfered with the formation of key inner ear proteins vital to my hearing, and thus caused hearing loss. Because it usually takes 3 to six months for the damage to result, it is difficult for one to make an association of a delayed hearing loss to a specific event that occurred six months earlier. After all, who is going to think about something that happened six months ago when your mother brings you to the doctor because you can no longer hear the tea kettle whistle, and you are not saying your "S" sound correctly anymore?

One of my earlier childhood memories was my first haircut. That was the first time I noticed my ears. Up to that point I had long honey-colored locks that covered my ears. I did not want to get a haircut (not a single hair cut) let alone having my head completely shaved except for a little tassel in the front, the Princeton. (Representing what, their graduation hats?)

I had to be bribed with a banana to sit still. I was probably the only kid in the United States who would endure such torture by being offered a banana. I would have done anything for a banana.

("May I cut your arm off, Mark?" "Of course not, don't be silly." "I'll give you a banana." "Well, okay.") A hair-covered banana, or more appropriately in my case, banana-flavored hair, did the trick, and my head was shaven, and lo and behold, my ears were acutely exposed!

Symbolically, my first haircut made me focus on my ears. I didn't like my ears at first and it wasn't too long after that I began to realize that I had a problem hearing, certainly because of my abnormal ears.

The normal human ear can distinguish some 400,000 different sounds; hearing is a marvelous physiologic accomplishment. The inner ear organ, the organ of Corti, is a beautiful microscopic harp, composed of tens of thousands of strings called hair cells which transmit hearing signals to the brain.

If you happen to have most of your hair cells wiped out due to streptomycin damage, it is as if thousands of the harp strings have been cut, particularly the ones forming the high pitch sounds.

Of course I didn't know any of this at the time. Heck, I was still working on my number two potty training! Years later when I got my first hearing aid, I always wanted to "cover my ears" to hide this abnormality. It would not be until I was an adult when I could comfortably "show my ears" again.

In my early childhood I was able to piece together clues that I was not hearing as well as the other kids. I couldn't hear the bells on the ice cream truck when it was a few blocks away, so I always got a late start in running to greet the ice cream truck, and I had to wait my turn in line. (Undoubtedly this caused severe psychological scars!)

My speech was affected by my hearing impairment. Normal voicing is related to normal hearing and if one does not hear sounds normally, then it is difficult for one to speak normally. My speech has a characteristic nasal distortion, as if a person has a bad cold. In my case it was more like a combination of Alf and Rocky Balboa. As a child, though, it must have sounded more like a muzzled Donald Duck.

Other kids noticed my different speech, and being the incredibly honest and blunt kids they were, they would always ask, "Why do you talk funny?" And then, being an incredibly insightful kid, I figured something was wrong with my speech because my ears were not working right. For reasons beyond my control, something was wrong with me and I could not hear like everyone else could.

I had various hearing checks and evaluations and saw specialists. I worked with a speech therapist. I was a kid who had something wrong with him and I indeed felt abnormal. The real world was a constant reminder that I was abnormal. Grownups always offered honest observations about my "behavior." Usually these comments were directed to my parents.

"I have asked your son several times how old he is, and he hasn't answered me." Translation: "You son is a snobby little brat who is ignoring me."

Another favorite: "Oh, is he sick, he sounds all stuffed up." Translation: "Why does your son talk funny?" Once in awhile I would be asked questions directly. A typical scenario would be:

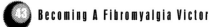

Any older lady: "Why, you cute little boy, what might your name be?"

Me: "Mark."

(Smile, confused look): "What did you say?"

Me: "Mark."

(Puzzled expression, with facial contortions): "Mud?"

Me: "No! Mark."

"Mike?"

(Heart palpitations, facial flushing): "It's Mark!"

(Total befuddlement): "You're going to have to speak more clearly."

At times like that I wished my parents would have named me "Bob."

My inability to hear well caused me a lot of stress. It made me feel abnormal and fostered a negative self-image and lack of confidence. My unwanted hearing impairment was making me feel inferior, abnormal and stupid, so I devised a beautifully simple plan to deal with my hearing loss: I would simply pretend that everything was okay. I became friends with "Mr. Denial" to deal with my ongoing stress.

Fortunately for me I was able to excel in areas other than hearing well! I was a good athlete and a good student, capabilities that helped me feel more like a normal person as I tried to forget my hearing impairment.

However, I had daily reminders that I could not hear well, whether it be missed conversation, or someone asking me why I talked funny.

To minimize the effect of my hearing loss, I developed valuable communication skills, which I would sharpen over the years. These skills were listening and speech reading.

To listen is to pay attention to sound and to be alert to catching an expected sound. Everyone listens and hears sounds: a student listens to a lecturer and listens for the bell; the doctor listens to a heartbeat; a musician listens to the rhythm. But how does one listen if he does not hear well?

Ironic as it may seem, the best listeners in the world are those who have a hearing impairment. In order to understand what is being said, the hearing impaired individual must quickly learn to make that extra effort to listen carefully, to maximize the meaning of what is being heard.

Through necessity I had to invent good listening skills. I used my vision and my remaining hearing to best understand words, expressions, and gestures everywhere in the world.

Eighty percent of communication is non-verbal, and I had to learn to read the clues. I paid close attention to facial expression, to eyes, to lips, to voice tones that hinted at underlying meanings. I learned to be patient. If at first I didn't catch all the meaning, rather than completely lose concentration and thereby lose the further communication, I would continue concentrating and wait until familiar words (with meaning!) finally arrived to my brain.

I learned that 80% percent of conversation actually consists of connecting, helping, and qualifying words that assisted the other 20% that actually carried meaning. My goal became simple. Match the 33% of conversation I actually heard to the 20% that had actual meaning! (I was good at rationalizing back then.)

I became good at relaying non-verbal clues from me back to the speaker, such as smiling, nodding, looking puzzled. The speaker would get feedback from me whether I was following completely or not and could re-direct a conversation more effectively based on the feedback I provided.

Another listening skill I developed was to continuously repeat in my mind what was being said. Like assembling pieces of a jigsaw puzzle, I was trying to comprehend the complete picture, even if there were some pieces missing. I learned to anticipate "delayed realization," when I finally would understand the first sentence after using clues from the third sentence and backtracking in my mind.

The other communication skill I learned was speech reading, also known as lip reading. This ties in with listening, but focuses more on the art of observing and recognizing sounds as they are produced by characteristic and predictable mouth movements. Even if I was unable to hear all the sounds, I could still understand by "seeing" the sounds.

Fortunately I was able to acquire this skill naturally, and it became my best friend in communication. The lip, chin, tongue, teeth, cheeks, and eyes all interact to provide characteristic speech reading clues that I learned to automatically decipher.

There are some drawbacks to speech reading. Many sounds have a similar "look." For example, P, B and M look exactly alike, but obviously sound different. Inevitably many words exist that look alike on the lips when spoken and can lead to confusion.

Words such as "chews," "shoes" and "juice" all sound different, but look exactly alike. My common sense usually allowed me to figure out the correct choice and temporize my confusion. Once I swore a teacher asked me to chew an orange shoe, and I was ready to oblige (she was a teacher after all) when I saw a carton of orange juice being passed to me and realize she had said, "choose orange juice."

There are other situations where speech reading becomes impossible, and I quickly learned who was not "speech readable." Anyone who had an overhanging mustache, mouth full of food or chewing gum, cigarette, cigar or pipe hanging from the mouth, or a microphone obstructing the mouth were all situations where physical barriers prevented speech reading. Persons with foreign accents were also very difficult to speech read because my speech reading and understanding skills were based on a familiar English frame of reference.

My speech reading skills would sometimes give me an advantage over my normal hearing counterparts. I can "hear" slang words uttered by angry athletes and coaches during televised sporting events, even though the sounds are not picked up by the TV microphone. (I have yet to figure out how to speech read ventriloquist dummies!) At best, speech reading alone allows half the words to be understood. However, speech reading has become a valuable coping strategy for dealing with my hearing impairment.

Hearing aids were recommended when I was young to improve my residual hearing. However, I resisted any attempt to wear hearing aids. How could I continue to hide my hearing loss and look normal if I wore obvious hearing aids? I was doing fairly well with my communication skills; why did I need to put a spotlight on myself that would make me appear even more different to my peers?

In retrospect, getting hearing aids was the single most important event that improved my overall effective communication. At first I viewed hearing aids as punishment. To me they were highly visible radio antennas sticking out of my ears with a sign on them that said "abnormal kid below." When I was 14 years old, I ultimately allowed myself to be fitted with bilateral in-the-ear hearing aids. And yes, I hated them and would continue to hate them for seven years. Sure they helped me, but I would prefer that nobody knew I had them.

I let my hair grow long over my ears to hide my hearing aids. I vividly remember cringing every time the wind would blow my hair for fear that someone would see my hearing aids.

Years later I would come to realize that it didn't matter whether I wore hearing aids or not, and whether anybody saw them or not, because I was still the person who I was and I'm not such a bad guy after all!

Getting a hearing aid was one of the traumatic experiences I had when I was 14. The other traumatic experience (literally) that happened when I was 14 was that I fell and broke my shoulder. This introduced me to the world of medicine and from that point on I knew that I wanted to be a physician.

Now I had a goal in life and one that seemed so natural for me. I wondered if my severe hearing impairment would matter, but deep down I felt that because of my hearing impairment I would be able to better understand problems that people had when they saw me as a doctor. I believed in my dream and I was fortunate that in the fall of 1980, I found myself in medical school.

By the time I got to medical school, I already had some pretty good survival skills for dealing with my hearing impairment. On the first day of class, I staked out my lecture seat in the very front row nearest to the podium, just to the right. Others quickly learned that no one sits in Pellegrino's seat. Quite frankly, no one sits in the front row except Pellegrino! For some reason the front row is not a highly prized commodity in an education environment. For me, though, it was the optimal place where I could hear and speech read, and basically soak up medical information.

Special preparations were necessary to improve my understanding of lecture topics. I found that reading about the material the night before it would be presented helped increase my familiarity with the new concepts and the new words. This also lessened the dreaded "Am I in the right room? … On the right planet?" feeling during the actual talk.

It is not an easy task, speech reading words like "meningofacial angiomatosis." Actually, it is not an easy task reading words like "meningofacial angiomatosis." To be honest, I still have no idea what "meningofacial angiomatosis" is!

Luckily, modern medical teaching was dominated by use of visual aids, which are perfect tools to complement my preparation ritual, my speech reading skills, and my devoted note-taking. I managed to survive the lecture barrage.

I began my clinical years of medical school eager to interact with patients. Armed with an amplified stethoscope and a digital vibrating beeper, I quickly learned that I loved working with the patients. I perfected a routine upon entering a patient's room that included meticulously turning off all background noise-makers (TV, air conditioner, radio) to enable maximum effective communication with patients who I discovered often had hearing impairments themselves.

During hospital rounds I mastered the art of walking in front of the talking physician with my head turned to focus on speech reading. I routinely walked into moving and stationary objects in the hallway, but the damage was minimal!

And of course, I told people I had a hearing impairment, reminding them to slow down and face me so that I could speech read. Numerous patients asked me where I was from because of my "accent."

I even survived my surgical rotation, which included a great deal of operating room time. Speech reading undulating shadows on surgical masks was a technique I could not master. Not surprisingly, I was not interested in a career as a surgeon.

One of the highlights of medical school, and perhaps my biggest confidence booster, occurred during a cardiology rotation. My amplified stethoscope had been a lifesaver for me up to that point; I could crank up the volume and bring the heart-lungs sounds into my ears at a comfortable level.

One day our cardiology instructor challenged my team, which included a cardiology fellow, a second year resident, and me. We each listened to the patient and the patient's heart rhythm, and told the instructor what we heard. I was last, and my description was the only one of the three that exactly matched what the cardiology instructor heard. I think I knew then I could be a "normal" physician.

Another highlight of my medical school years was the introduction to a specialty called physical medicine and rehabilitation. This specialty deals with patients who have a disability of some sort, with the focus on optimizing quality of life by improving function. After being introduced to this specialty, I knew that I wanted to be a physiatrist (a specialist in physical medicine and rehabilitation).

Having lived with a hearing impairment nearly all my life, I felt able to understand patients when they become disabled in some way. Just as I try to live my life to the fullest despite my hearing impairment, I wanted to help others live their lives to the fullest. I was fortunate to be accepted into The Ohio State University Physical Medicine and Rehabilitation Program, one of the best in the world.

My hearing impairment has shaped who I am. I've had my whole life to first deny, then accept my hearing impairment; educate myself and others; develop coping strategies, communication skills, and the ability to use adaptive equipment; and most importantly, doing the best with what I did have to try to overcome any difficulties the hearing impairment caused. I realize that I am a normal person who just happens to have a hearing impairment.

I spent a long time trying to constantly detach my hearing impairment from the rest of me, but I could never get away from the reality of the situation: I have a hearing impairment.

I eventually realized that my biggest problem was not to get others to accept me, but to get me to accept myself, hearing impairment and all. There is nothing wrong with having a hearing impairment, and no one is to blame for it, either. It is my responsibility to deal with my difficulties, not to avoid them.

I didn't change overnight; adjusting to an impairment is a slow ongoing process. It's like climbing a ladder, where improvement comes a rung at a time. I hope I can keep moving up the ladder as I continue to deal with my hearing loss and the challenges that it brings.

My fibromyalgia came second. Even though I can look back and realize I had childhood symptoms related to fibromyalgia, my persistent fibromyalgia pain did not develop until long after I had been dealing with my hearing impairment. My hearing impairment laid the groundwork for coping with any other chronic disorder that would come along.

And, along came fibromyalgia! Since my coping roads were already laid and being traveled by hearing impairment, I basically said, "Okay, here I go again." I was able to steer my fibromyalgia car down the roads already built. Sure, I had to add a few new speeds, fill in some potholes, and build a bridge here and there, but I found it easier to make the transition coping-wise, the second time around. I continue to deal with my fibromyalgia and hearing impairment on a daily basis and await cures for both of them!

Fibromyalgia can be a scary condition. It is not life-threatening, but the pain it causes can lead to severe problems with everyday functioning. One can be overwhelmed with the difficulties of dealing with fibromyalgia, from understanding and living with the diagnosis each day, to wondering what will happen tomorrow and the next year. Physicians try to help fibromyalgia patients by prescribing medicines, therapies, and anything that we think may work. We have an unlimited array of treatments we can try, but I believe the most important thing we can prescribe for fibromyalgia patients is hope. Hope: to cherish a desire with the expectation of fulfillment.

Hope means something different to each of us. Each person's interpretation of hope is shaped by that individual's experiences, backgrounds, and influences. Like our fibromyalgia, hope is unique for each individual.

Everyone has "basic" experiences and influences such as growing up, puberty, school, family, and heritage. Many share common experiences and backgrounds that impart a general flavor to a "hope recipe," but each adds secret ingredients that ultimately give hope its unique individual flavor.

My three secret ingredients to my hope recipe which provide me with unique influences and experiences are: (1) hearing impairment; (2) fibromyalgia; (3) rehabilitation specialty. Each gives me a different perspective on the meaning of hope and has defined for me my expectation to be fulfilled.

My hearing impairment has taught me that *understanding* is hope. I literally strive to understand what is being said because I can't hear well. When someone speaks to me, I hope I can understand what was said so I can effectively communicate. My association of hope with understanding began at a young age when I first lost most of my hearing.

When I listen to songs on the radio, I can hear music and voices, but I cannot quite understand the words. If I could only turn the "clarity notch" up just a bit more so that I could understand the words and symbolically understand the music of life. Each day I hope to understand the words to the songs.

My fibromyalgia has taught me that *knowledge* is hope. Unknown pains can trigger the worst fears. Knowing about fibromyalgia, knowing that it is not life-threatening, deforming, or paralyzing, starts the education process. With education and knowledge comes opportunity to improve the pain, to gain successful experiences, and to accept the fibromyalgia.

My emphasis has been on educating people about their fibromyalgia. The diagnosis of fibromyalgia is the start of the education; finding successful treatments is continuing the education process. Knowing as much as possible about fibromyalgia and educating others on fibromyalgia allows me to have hope. If we understand more, we fear less, do better and have hope. Someday I hope all of our combined knowledge will lead to a cure for fibromyalgia.

My rehabilitation specialty has taught me that *ability* is hope. Disabilities, or focusing on what we can't do, are the opposite of hope. Focusing on our abilities is hopeful, for it motivates us to do what we can. It also lets us anticipate that we can do even more, that we have the ability to improve.

Ability as hope can help erase the negative stereotypical comments, "There's nothing to do for your fibromyalgia," "You just have to learn to live with your pain," "You can't do this anymore," or "You'll probably get worse." Use your abilities to achieve positive rewarding goals.

I have taken my hope "ingredients" and realized my individual hope definition or hope philosophy: learn and understand everything you can about your fibromyalgia. Apply this knowledge to improve your quality of life and expect even better knowledge, abilities and understanding.

I have already talked about being a fibromyalgia survivor. This symbolically means that despite fibromyalgia, we continue to live our lives as best we can, having learned successful "survival" strategies. We must connect with fibromyalgia on a very personal level, as it is an inherent part of our very being. As we strive to improve our knowledge, abilities and understanding of this condition, we may find that we become successful; that we do more than just "survive" our fibromyalgia. We have earned a better quality of life and deserve to call ourselves victorious in the battle against the "enemy."

I am not alone, and you are not alone. We do not have to bear the burden alone. Whatever our backgrounds, whatever our differences, we all share the same painful problem. Because we live each day facing the same challenges and the same obstacles, we have developed a unique understanding of each other, despite never having met one another! We are an invisible army connected by our desire to conquer fibromyalgia. When people with fibromyalgia first meet each other, there is almost a magical ability to immediately open the doors that lead to our most innermost sensitivities, fears, and hopes. On the outside we may be perfect strangers, but given the opportunity to look inside and help each other, we may find that we are indeed perfect friends and comrades.

Fibromyalgia has caused a lot of changes in our lives. Living with fibromyalgia has given us very personal experiences. We need to remind each other that we are not alone, that we understand the pain, that we can do better even if we hurt, that the sun can shine brighter tomorrow, and that there is hope for a better tomorrow.

We need to have hope that we will soon be Fibromyalgia Victors and take a victory lap together!

▶ If You Want To Know More

1. Pellegrino MJ. *Inside fibromyalgia*. Columbus OH: Anadem Publishing, 2001.

2. Pellegrino MJ. *A sunnier tomorrow*. Columbus OH: Anadem Publishing, 1998.

Note: Chapter titles are in bold